# Acute Management of the Burned Patient

## J. A. J. Martyn, M.D.

Associate Professor of Anaesthesiology,
Harvard Medical School, and
Massachusetts General Hospital;
Associate Director of Anesthesia,
Shriners Burns Institute,
Boston, Massachusetts

1990

## W. B. SAUNDERS COMPANY

Harcourt Brace Jovanovich, Inc.

*Philadelphia, London, Toronto, Montreal, Sydney, Tokyo*

**W. B. SAUNDERS COMPANY**
Harcourt Brace Jovanovich, Inc.

The Curtis Center
Independence Square West
Philadelphia, PA 19106

**Library of Congress Cataloging-in-Publication Data**

Acute management of the burned patient /
[edited by] J. A. Jeevendra Martyn.

p.    cm.

1. Burns and scalds—Treatment.    2. Critical care
medicine.    I. Martyn, J. A. Jeevendra.
[DNLM: 1. Burns—therapy.    WO 704 A189]

RD96.4.A28 1990

617.1'106—dc20

DNLM/DLC                                        89–70051
                                                    CIP

ISBN 0–7216–2774–9

*Sponsoring Editor:*   Richard Zorab

*Manuscript Editor:*   Donna Walker

*Production Manager:*   Frank Polizzano

Acute Management of the Burned Patient                ISBN   0–7216–2774–9

Printed in the United States of America.

Last digit is the print number:     9    8    7    6    5    4    3    2    1

This book is thankfully dedicated
to my parents
Lily Beatrice Martyn and the late Joseph Frederick Martyn

# Contributors

NAOKI AIKAWA, M.D., D.M.Sc., F.A.C.S.
Associate Professor, Department of Emergency Medicine, School of Medicine, Keio University; Director, Emergency Medical Services, Keio University Hospital, Tokyo, Japan
*Complications of Burn Injury*


STACEY J. BELL, M.S., R.D.
Nutrition Support Dietitian, New England Deaconess Hospital, Boston, Massachusetts
*Nutritional Support of the Burn Patient*


GEORGE L. BLACKBURN, M.D., Ph.D.
Associate Professor of Surgery, Harvard Medical School; Chief, Nutrition Metabolism Laboratory, New England Deaconess Hospital, Boston, Massachusetts
*Nutritional Support of the Burn Patient*


SUSAN E. BRIGGS, M.D.
Assistant Professor of Surgery, Harvard Medical School; Assistant Surgeon, Massachusetts General Hospital; Assistant Chief of Staff, Shriners Burns Institute; Director, Surgical Consult Service, Spaulding Rehabilitation Hospital, Boston, Massachusetts
*First Aid, Transportation, and Immediate Acute Care of Thermal Injuries; Rationale for Acute Surgical Approach*


SUE S. CAHNERS, M.S.W.
Director of Social Service, Shriners Hospital for Crippled Children, Burns Institute, Boston Unit, Boston, Massachusetts
*The Social Worker and the Family: A Long-Term Relationship in Burn Care*


ROBERT H. DEMLING, M.D.
Professor of Surgery, Harvard Medical School; Director, Longwood Area Trauma/Burn Center at Brigham and Womens, Beth Israel, and Boston Children's Hospitals, Boston, Massachusetts
*Pathophysiological Changes After Cutaneous Burns and Approach to Initial Resuscitation; Management of the Major Burn in the Intensive Care Unit*

v

GARY C. du MOULIN, Ph.D., M.P.H.
Assistant Professor of Anaesthesia, Harvard Medical School; Director, Anaesthesia/
Respiratory Therapy, Equipment Assessment Unit, Beth Israel Hospital, Boston, Massa-
chusetts
*Minimizing the Potential for Infection in the Hospitalized Burned Patient: Architectural,
Engineering, and Environmental Considerations*

AMY E. FLYNN, R.P.T.
Director of Rehabilitation, Shriners Hospital for Crippled Children, Burns Institute,
Boston Unit, Boston, Massachusetts
*Rehabilitation of the Burn Patient*

N. GOUDSOUZIAN, M.D.
Associate Professor of Anaesthesia, Harvard Medical School; Director, Pediatric Anaes-
thesia, Massachusetts General Hospital, Boston, Massachusetts
*Management of Upper Airway Following Burns*

JOHN A. GRISWOLD, M.D.
Assistant Professor of Surgery, Department of Surgery, University of Mississippi Medical
Center; Attending Surgeon, University Medical Center, Jackson, Mississippi
*Toxic Epidermal Necrolysis*

LAURIE L. GUNTER, O.T.R.
Staff Occupational Therapist, Shriners Hospital for Crippled Children, Burns Institute,
Boston Unit, Boston, Massachusetts
*Rehabilitation of the Burn Patient*

CHARLES A. HALES, M.D.
Associate Professor of Medicine, Harvard Medical School; Associate Director, Pulmonary
Unit, Massachusetts General Hospital, Boston, Massachusetts
*Pulmonary Disorders in the Burn Patient*

JOHN T. HERRIN, M.B.B.S., F.R.A.C.P.
Associate Clinical Professor of Pediatrics, Harvard Medical School; Chief, Pediatric
Nephrology and Pediatrician, Massachusetts General Hospital, Chief, Pediatrics, Shriners
Hospital for Crippled Children, Burns Institute, Boston Unit, Boston, Massachusetts
*Renal Function in Burns*

PATRICIA P. KARTIGANER, M.S.W.
Deputy Director, Social Service, Shriners Hospital for Crippled Children, Burns Institute,
Boston Unit, Boston, Massachusetts
*The Social Worker and the Family: A Long-Term Relationship in Burn Care*

JEEVENDRA MARTYN, M.D.
Associate Professor of Anaesthesiology, Harvard Medical School and Massachusetts General Hospital; Associate Director of Anesthesia, Shriners Burn Institute, Boston Unit; Director, Clinical Pharmacology, Department of Anesthesia, Massachusetts General Hospital, Boston, Massachusetts

MARJORIE McETTRICK-MALONEY, R.N., B.S.N., M.P.A./H.
Clinical and Discharge Coordinator, Shriners Hospital for Crippled Children, Burns Institute, Boston Unit, Boston, Massachusetts
*Intensive Care Nursing of the Burn Patient*

JOSEPH A. MOLNAR, M.D., Ph.D.
Instructor of Surgery, Division of Plastic Surgery, Medical College of Virginia Hospitals, Richmond, Virginia
*Toxic Epidermal Necrolysis*

PATRICIA F. OSGOOD, Ph.D.
Assistant Professor, Harvard Medical School; Assistant Pharmacologist (Anaesthesia), Massachusetts General Hospital Staff Scientist, Shriners Hospital for Crippled Children, Burns Institute, Boston Unit, Boston, Massachusetts
*Management of Pain*

EDWARD G. PAVLIN, M.D.
Associate Professor, Department of Anaesthesiology, University of Washington Medical School; Associate Professor and Attending Anesthesiologist, Harborview Medical Center, Seattle, Washington
*Perioperative Fluid Requirements in the Thermally Injured Patient*

JOHN P. REMENSNYDER, M.D.
Associate Professor of Surgery, Harvard Medical School; Chief of Staff, Shriners Hospital for Crippled Children, Burns Institute, Boston Unit, Boston, Massachusetts
*Acute Electrical Injuries*

MARISSA SELIGMAN, Pharm. D.
Manager, Scientific Publications, Miles Inc., Pharmaceutical Division, West Haven, Connecticut
*Burn Wound Infections*

YOTARO SHINOZAWA, M.D.
Instructor in Surgery and Deputy Chief Surgeon, Department of Surgery, School of Medicine, Keio University, Tokyo, Japan
*Complications of Burn Injury*

FREDERICK J. STODDARD, M.D.
Assistant Professor of Psychiatry, Harvard Medical School; Chief of Psychiatry, Shriners Hospital for Crippled Children, Burns Institute, Boston Unit; Associate Psychiatrist, Massachusetts General Hospital, Boston, Massachusetts
*Psychiatric Management of the Burned Patient*


JONATHAN STRONGIN, M.D., Ph.D.
Clinical Instructor, Harvard Medical School; Clinical and Research Fellow, Massachusetts General Hospital, Boston, Massachusetts
*Pulmonary Disorders in the Burn Patient*


S. K. SZYFELBEIN, M.D.
Associate Professor, Harvard Medical School; Anesthetist, Massachusetts General Hospital; Director of Anesthesia, Shriners Hospital for Crippled Children, Burns Institute, Boston Unit, Boston, Massachusetts
*Management of Upper Airway Following Burns; Management of Pain*

# Foreword

Acute care physicians constantly deal with severely ill patients, sometimes unexpectedly, sometimes on a scheduled basis. Burned victims fit this category well, presenting urgent, unexpected problems to the anesthesiologist and the surgeon as well as all members of the care-giving team. Additionally, burned individuals react paradoxically to conventional anesthetic medications and agents, a field pioneered by Dr. Martyn, who has edited this volume. As early surgical excision, and coverage of major thermal burns becomes established therapy, acute care physicians must become familiar with the vagaries, difficulties, and pitfalls of the care of those unfortunate enough to have been burned. Dr. Martyn perceived the need—hence, this book. Authored by a coherent group of physicians with broad burn-care experience, the information contained in the following chapters is designed to provide a basis for the thorough understanding necessary to ensure safe conduct of extensively burned patients through the combined anesthesia/surgical experience.

JOHN P. REMENSNYDER, M.D.
*Shriners Burns Institute*
*Boston Unit*

# Preface

During the last several years tremendous advances have been made in the care of the acutely burned patient, a direct product of clinical and basic research. This information and the rationale for these new approaches have been published in many different journals and publications. The W.B. Saunders Company has given me an opportunity as editor, to invite some of the foremost scientists/clinicians in the field to summarize these advances. The result you see in this volume. These authors, experts in their field, have succeeded in providing state-of-the-science as well as state-of-the-art approaches to acute burn care. I am most grateful to them for their contributions to this publication.

The aim of this book is to disseminate this new information to medical and paramedical personnel involved in the care of these burned patients. I myself have tremendously enjoyed the reading and have learned much from these contributions. I hope that this publication will be widely accepted, will stimulate further research, and most importantly will help improve the care and alleviate the suffering of burned patients.

I would like to express once again my appreciation and thanks to my wife Raji and my sons Rajeeve, Sanjeeve, and Tréjeeve, who were so kind in encouraging all my academic endeavours and accepting my frequent absence to finish the different tasks.

JEEVENDRA MARTYN, M.D.

# Contents

## 1
First Aid, Transportation, and Immediate Acute Care of
Thermal Injuries .......................................................... 1
  *Susan E. Briggs*

## 2
Pathophysiological Changes After Cutaneous Burns and
Approach to Initial Resuscitation ....................................... 12
  *Robert H. Demling*

## 3
Pulmonary Disorders in the Burn Patient ............................. 25
  *Jonathan Strongin and Charles A. Hales*

## 4
Management of Upper Airway Following Burns ...................... 46
  *N. Goudsouzian and S. K. Szyfelbein*

## 5
Acute Electrical Injuries .................................................. 66
  *John P. Remensnyder*

## 6
Management of the Major Burn in the Intensive Care Unit ......... 87
  *Robert H. Demling*

## 7
Intensive Care Nursing of the Burn Patient ........................... 97
  *Marjorie McEttrick-Maloney*

# 8
Rationale for Acute Surgical Approach ............................. 118
*Susan E. Briggs*

# 9
Toxic Epidermal Necrolysis .......................................... 128
*John A. Griswold and Joseph A. Molnar*

# 10
Nutritional Support of the Burn Patient ............................. 138
*Stacey J. Bell and George L. Blackburn*

# 11
Complications of Burn Injury ......................................... 159
*Yotaro Shinozawa and Naoki Aikawa*

# 12
Clinical Pharmacology and Therapeutics in Burns ............... 180
*Jeevendra Martyn*

# 13
Management of Pain .................................................. 201
*Patricia F. Osgood and S. K. Szyfelbein*

# 14
Anesthetic Management of the Burned Patient ................... 217
*Jeevendra Martyn and S. K. Szyfelbein*

# 15
Perioperative Fluid Requirements in the Thermally
Injured Patient ........................................................ 231
*Edward G. Pavlin*

# 16
Renal Function in Burns .............................................. 239
*John T. Herrin*

# 17
Psychiatric Management of the Burned Patient ................... 256
> *Frederick J. Stoddard*

# 18
Minimizing the Potential for Infection in the Hospitalized
Burned Patient: Architectural, Engineering, and Environmental
Considerations ......................................................... 273
> *Gary C. duMoulin*

# 19
Burn Wound Infections .................................................. 288
> *Marissa Seligman and Jeevendra Martyn*

# 20
The Social Worker and the Family: A Long-Term Relationship
in Burn Care ........................................................... 306
> *Sue S. Cahners and Patricia P. Kartiganer*

# 21
Rehabilitation of the Burn Patient ..................................... 320
> *Amy E. Flynn and Laurie L. Gunter*

Index ................................................................. 333

1

# First Aid, Transportation, and Immediate Acute Care of Thermal Injuries

SUSAN E. BRIGGS

Burns are a major cause of traumatic injury in all ages of the population. Burns may be caused by a variety of scalding agents, chemicals, electricity, and radiation. Extreme cold can also produce an injury similar to a burn. Regardless of the etiology of the burn, certain initial practices remain the same for all patients. The same general principles of resuscitation apply to burns as to other forms of traumatic injury. Cardiopulmonary stability must be the initial priority. Definitive care of the burn wound is a secondary priority.

The first priority in the care of the burn at the scene of the accident is to stop the burning process. It is important to remember that clothing, especially smoldering clothing or clothing soaked with chemicals, can be the source of continued burning of the patient's skin unless the clothes are promptly removed (Fig. 1–1). In flame burns, the extent of injury is proportional to the intensity and size of the flame burn and the duration of exposure. Extinguishing the source of the flame burn promptly is the obvious first priority of treatment. Methods of accomplishing this goal are rolling of the patient on the ground, application of a blanket or coat, use of cool water or other extinguishing liquids, and the use of gelatinous impregnated blankets. The gel penetrates hot and burning clothing and stops the burning process by transfer of heat from the skin to the blanket.[1–3] Scald burns are usually self-limiting injuries. The degree of injury is proportional to the age of the patient, anatomical location of the burn, and temperature of the scalding agent. Viscous liquids such as grease and spaghetti sauce often need to be removed mechanically in order to stop the burning process. In very young and old patients with thin skin, scald burns often produce a deep thermal injury. In general, scald burns in individuals under two years of age will have a significant proportion of third-degree burn.

Patients sustaining chemical burns should have clothing removed as quickly as possible to stop the continued injury due to absorbed chemical agents. Copious irrigation of the affected area with water, not neutralization of the offending agent, is the key to the emergency treatment of chemical burns. Following copious irrigation of the affected area with water, utilizing any type of irrigating system available at the scene of the accident, the burn should be covered with clean dry sheets. In chemical burns, the concentration of the agent and the duration of exposure are the key factors in determining the extent of thermal

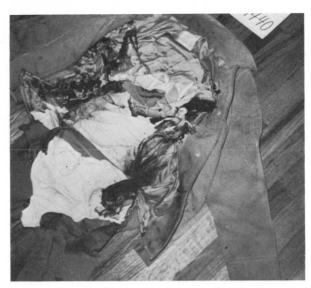

**FIGURE 1–1.** Smoldering fabric left on burned individual during transport to hospital.

injury. Therefore, if the patient is hemodynamically stable, copious irrigation at the scene rather than the emergency room of the hospital is the initial key priority.

Electrical injuries require special consideration at the scene of the accident. In electrical injuries it is important to stop the burning process by removing the patient from the source of electrical current. Caution must be utilized so that the rescue team does not become part of the electrical circuit while attempting to free a person still in contact with a live wire. The victim must not be touched by the rescuers until the current source is either deactivated or pushed away from the patient by means of nonconducting materials such as wood.[1–5]

It is important to remember that four types of injuries may occur in electrical accidents. Deep conductive electrical injuries involve extensive muscular injury, the extent of which may not be obvious at the scene. They may also involve remote areas of the body such as the central nervous system and the thoracic and abdominal cavities. The presence of entrance and exit wounds should make one suspicious of deep conductive injury (Fig. 1–2). Arc injuries produce limited, deep areas of coagulation damage, especially in flexion areas such as the axilla and groin. Surface thermal burns occur as a result of the flash ignition of clothing and must be treated as such with prompt stoppage of the burning process. Patients with electrical injuries often present with extensive total body surface area (TBSA) thermal burns. Associated injuries are quite common in patients with electrical burns, especially those who are thrown from the electrical source or fall from a high point. The patient must be evaluated for associated traumatic injury, especially cervical spine injury, long bone fractures, and intrathoracic or intra-abdominal injuries.[1, 2, 5]

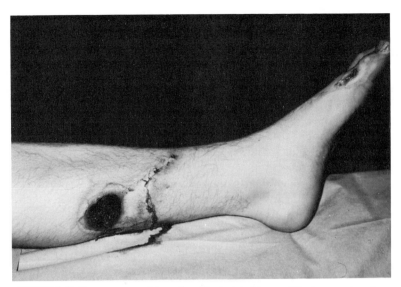

**FIGURE 1–2.** Entrance wound in male with electrical burn of the lower extremity.

Numerous cardiac abnormalities are common with electrical injuries, such as asystole and ventricular fibrillation. Therefore, once the patient is removed from the source of electrical contact, cardiopulmonary resuscitation must be promptly initiated if indicated. If the patient is asystolic, rapid institution of cardiopulmonary resuscitation when a pulse cannot be palpated is mandatory. Ventricular fibrillation is not uncommon and the use of the chest thump may be valuable in reversing this dysrhythmia at the scene.

Various factors influence the degree of tissue damage in electrical burns, including the type and voltage of the circuit, resistance, pathway of transmission within the body, duration, and contact.

Cooling of the thermal burn continues to be a controversial subject. Early cooling of small burns can be accomplished by application of cool water (20°C) or gelatinous impregnated dressings to transfer heat from the wound into the dressing. Such dressings can be stored in areas where water is not readily available (e.g., planes). The dangers of hypothermia must be considered when cooling large burns, especially in the pediatric population. Ice packs or ice water must be used judiciously and only with small burns, as they may cause a cold injury more serious than the thermal burn, or significant hypothermia with associated cardiac dysrhythmias may occur. In general, cool solutions may reduce the pain of partial-thickness injuries with intact nerve endings but should be instituted with caution in burns greater than 20 per cent TBSA or if the air temperature is below 50°F.[1–3]

At the scene of the accident the patient should be wrapped in clean, dry dressings. Sterile dressings are not necessary, as the main goal of the dressings is to minimize contamination at the scene of the accident and to diminish the pain from exposure to the air, especially in partial-thickness burns. Application of topical agents should be avoided until the wound has been adequately debrided and evaluated as to further treatment. Oral fluids should not be given, as the patient may develop an ileus with burns greater than 15 per cent TBSA.

The final priority at the scene is to establish whether the patient should be treated on an outpatient basis or referred to an appropriate facility for further evaluation or treatment. All patients with burns greater than 15 per cent TBSA, electrical burns, inhalation burns, and burns with a high risk of cosmetic or functional deformities, such as on face, hands, and joint surfaces, should be referred to a hospital facility. A brief history of the burn may prove extremely valuable in triaging the patient. Explosive burns or burns associated with motor vehicle accidents or falls should alert the physician to the possibility of associated internal injuries. A history of a fire in a closed space, e.g., a bedroom or a car with the windows up, should raise suspicion of inhalation injury. Patients with chemical and electrical burns should be sent to an appropriate facility, as damage is usually deeper than can be visualized.

## CLASSIFICATION OF BURNS

Proper triage and treatment of thermal injuries require a knowledge of the pathophysiology of burn injury. A first-degree burn involves only the epidermis and is characterized by cutaneous erythema and mild pain. Tissue damage is minimal, and protective functions of the skin, located in the dermis, remain intact. The chief symptom, pain, usually resolves in 48 to 72 hours. In 5 to 10 days the damaged epithelium peels off, leaving no residual scarring. The most common causes of first-degree burns are overexposure to sunlight and brief scalding by hot liquids.

A second-degree burn involves injury to the entire epidermis and variable portions of the dermal layer. Vesicle (blister) formation is characteristic of second-degree burns. A superficial second-degree burn is extremely painful because large numbers of remaining viable nerve endings are exposed. Superficial second-degree burns heal in 7 to 14 days owing to regeneration of epithelium by the epithelial cells that line the hair follicles, sweat glands, and other skin appendages deep in the dermis. A mid-level to deep second-degree burn heals spontaneously, but re-epithelialization is extremely slow. Pain is present but to a lesser degree than in more superficial burns because fewer intact nerve endings remain. Fluid losses and metabolic effects of deep dermal burns are essentially the same as those of third-degree burns.

A full-thickness or third-degree burn involves destruction of the entire epidermis and dermis, leaving no residual epidermal cells to repopulate. The wound will not epithelialize and can heal only by wound contraction or skin grafting. The lack of painful sensation in a third-degree burn is due to heat destruction of nerve endings.

## MAJOR BURNS

All patients with burns greater than 10 to 15 per cent TBSA require fluid resuscitation and referral to a hospital. The initial priorities in the management of a major thermal injury are (1) establishment of an adequate airway and assessment of inhalation injury; (2) calculation of burn size and institution of fluid resuscitation; and (3) determination of the need for escharotomy or fasciotomy.

## AIRWAY MANAGEMENT AND ASSESSMENT OF INHALATION INJURY

The first priority at the scene of the injury is the establishment of an adequate airway. Oxygen should be administered by face mask or endotracheal tube. Indications for intubation are the presence of massive facial swelling or inhalation injury (Fig. 1–3). Pulmonary damage due to smoke inhalation and carbon monoxide intoxication is the leading cause of early death in burns and is probably a more important determinant of survival at present than the actual size of the burn. Understanding of the distinct pathophysiology of the different types of inhalation injury has enabled the physician to better assess and treat such injuries.

The hallmarks of smoke inhalation injury are hypoxia and hypercapnia. There are two distinct mechanisms of pulmonary injury following inhalation: (1) smoke toxicity and (2) carbon monoxide intoxication. Smoke toxicity is further divided into direct thermal injury and smoke poisoning. Direct thermal injury involves the inhalation of superheated, incomplete products of combustion such as soot and particulate matter, which causes direct mucosal damage to the tracheobronchial tree. Smoke poisoning results from the thermodegradation of both natural and man-made materials. The end result of the thermodegradation is the production of noxious gases such as hydrogen cyanide.[1, 4] The effects of carbon monoxide intoxication are due to the tissue hypoxia, and no pathological changes are seen in the tracheobronchial tree. Carbon monoxide has a greater affinity for the hemoglobin-binding sites. Increased carboxyhemoglobin levels are useful in evaluating the extent of carbon monoxide intoxication if the patient has not received oxygen during transport to the hospital. The half-life of carbon monoxide on the hemoglobin molecule is one-half hour if 100 per cent oxygen is breathed. Therefore, many patients with significant carbon monoxide intoxication have normal carboxyhemoglobin levels if they have been treated with oxygen on the way to the hospital.

Clinical signs that should alert the physician to the presence of inhalation

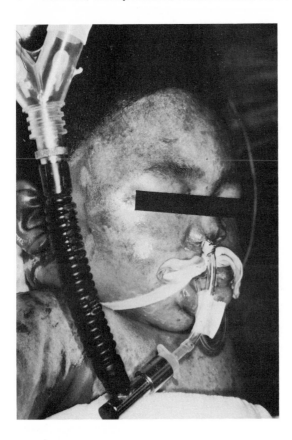

**FIGURE 1–3.** Significant facial swelling 2 hours post burn in patient with 70 per cent TBSA thermal burn and superficial second-degree burns of the face.

injury include (1) upper body, especially facial, burns; (2) singeing of the eybrows and nasal hair; (3) soot in the oropharynx; (4) history of impaired mentation and/or confinement in a burning environment ("closed space injury"); (5) carbonaceous sputum.

Survival from inhalation injury is dependent on the extent of pulmonary parenchymal damage. The physician's role is to prevent additional complications that further compromise the patient's pulmonary reserves. Prevention of aspiration, pulmonary edema, pneumonia, and hypoxia secondary to inadequate ventilation, mechanical ventilation, and aggressive use of bronchoscopy (flexible and rigid) to clear pulmonary secretions if needed are important adjuncts in the treatment of inhalation injuries.

## CALCULATION OF BURN SIZE AND INITIATION OF FLUID RESUSCITATION

Calculation of the fluid requirement for resuscitation in the burned individual is based on the extent of second- and third-degree burns only. First-degree burns do not involve the loss of body fluids. In children, the relative body surface area of the head and neck is much larger than in adults, and the body surface area associated with the lower extremities is much less. The "rule of nines" is a useful and practical guide for determining the extent of the burn. The adult body configuration is such that anatomical regions represent 9 per cent of a multiple of the TBSA. The following chart indicates the "rule of nines" in adults and the adjustment of per cent of body surface in children according to age.

### Rule of Nines—Adults

| Anatomical Area | Per Cent of Body Surface |
| --- | --- |
| Head | 9% |
| Anterior trunk | 18% |
| Posterior trunk | 18% |
| Right leg | 18% |
| Left leg | 18% |
| Right arm | 9% |
| Left arm | 9% |
| Perineum | 1% |

### Per Cent of Body Surface According to Age

| | Newborn | 3 Years | 6 Years | 12+ Years |
| --- | --- | --- | --- | --- |
| Head | 18% | 15% | 12% | 6% |
| Trunk | 40% | 40% | 40% | 38% |
| Arms | 16% | 16% | 16% | 19% |
| Legs | 26% | 29% | 32% | 36% |

Fluid resuscitation should be initiated with the administration of isotonic electrolyte solution such as lactated Ringer's solution. The rate of fluid administration in children should be approximately 400 to 500 ml per square meter of body surface or a sufficient quantity of fluid to maintain urine output at 1 ml per kilogram of body weight per hour in infants and children. In older children, the standardized burn formulas, such as the modified Parkland Formula listed below, may be utilized. The major problem with weight-related formulas is that surface area and weight relationships are not constant in the growing child.

### Fluid Resuscitation

| Fluid | Amount | Rate | Renal Response |
| --- | --- | --- | --- |
| First 24 hours: lactated Ringer's solution | 4 ml/kg body wt/% second- and third-degree burns | ½ first 8 hr; ½ second 16 hr (¼ second 8 hr; ¼ third 8 hr) | 1 mg/kg/hr (child) 50–70 ml/hr (adults) |

Immediately following the thermal injury, there is a rapid loss of volume from the vascular space and concomitant expansion of the interstitial space. The loss of fluid from the vascular space is rapid and maximal at 6 to 12 hours. This physiological response is the basis of the administration of one-half the calculated 24-hour fluid requirement the first 8 hours following thermal injury, one-fourth the second 8 hours, and one-fourth the third 8 hours. After 24 hours post injury, fluid requirements decrease to a constant that remains as long as the burn wound is open. Continued controversy exists over the role of colloid replacement in acute thermal injury. Colloid is valuable, however, as an adjunct to fluid replacement in hypovolemic patients who do not respond adequately to crystalloid replacement, but it need not be utilized routinely in any burn patient.

## DETERMINATION OF NEED FOR ESCHAROTOMY AND/OR FASCIOTOMY

Full-thickness burns of the thorax and extremities, including digits, result in significant loss of tissue elasticity with subsequent constriction of underlying structures. The most reliable method for measuring distal pulses in the burned extremity is with a Dopper ultrasonic flow meter. Escharotomies are linear incisions extending through the full depth of the burned skin which allow separation of constricting eschar. Escharotomies should be performed in the emergency room in all full-thickness circumferential burns of trunk and extremities, including the digits, regardless of the pulse status. Failure to relieve a constricting eschar of the thorax may result in life-threatening respiratory depression (Fig. 1–4). Failure to relieve a constricting eschar in the extremities may result in limb loss or permanent damage to underlying neurovascular structures. If escharotomy does not restore adequate circulation in the extremities, the possibility of compartment syndrome and need for fasciotomy should be considered (Fig. 1–5).

## SECONDARY PRIORITIES

### Antibiotics

Prophylactic antibiotics have no proven role in burn patients and are not utilized routinely. All burns are potentially contaminated soft-tissue wounds. Tetanus toxoid (0.5 ml) should therefore be given to all burn victims. Prior immunization status is important information to obtain. Unimmunized individuals should receive 250 units of human tetanus immunoglobulin as well as tetanus toxoid, and provisions should be made for additional tetanus boosters following discharge.[5]

### Gastric Decompression

Most patients with burns greater than 20 per cent develop a reflex paralytic ileus during the first 24 hours following thermal injury and require nasogastric tube decompression for varying periods of time.

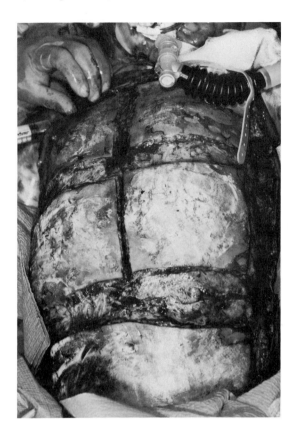

**FIGURE 1–4.** Chest escharotomies in a patient with full-thickness burns of thorax.

## Minor Burns

First-degree burns are generally treated on an outpatient basis except for extensive first-degree burns, which require inpatient hospitalization for control of pain. Superficial second-degree burns less than 15 per cent TBSA can generally be treated on an outpatient basis with the exception of the very young or old, immunosuppressed patients, or patients with associated injuries. The same basic principles of resuscitation apply to minor burns as to major burns but are less frequently utilized.

The following represent guidelines for outpatient management of minor burns:

1. At the scene of the accident cooling of small burns may be utilized to diminish the pain of partial-thickness burns. Ice water or ice packs should be avoided to stop the burning process. Smoldering clothing and chemicals should be removed from the skin as promptly as possible. Copious irrigation of the affected parts should be utilized in viscous scald burns and chemical burns.

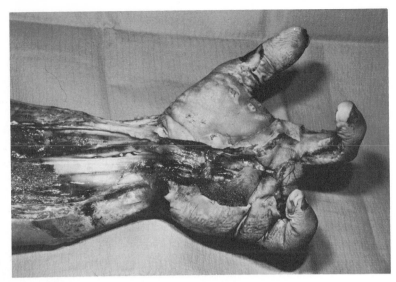

**FIGURE 1–5.** Fasciotomy of the upper extremity in a patient with electrical burn of the arm.

 2. Wrap the burn in clean cloth until appropriate treatment is available either at home or in the emergency ward.

 3. Guidelines for tetanus prophylaxis are the same as for a major burn. A tetanus toxoid booster is recommended for any patient who has not received one for 5 years or cannot recall the date of the last immunization. Patients who have not been previously immunized should receive 250 units of tetanus immunoglobulin and the first of a series of active immunizations with tetanus toxoid.

 4. No antibiotics should be utilized prophylactically.

 5. Adequate debridement is more important than the choice of topical agents in minor burns. The burn should be washed gently with mild soap and water prior to application of any topical agent. Removal of tar and asphalt can be accomplished with products such as Medrisol (a citrus and petroleum distillate with hydrochlorothiazide structure). Mineral or petroleum ointments may be also used to remove tar. It is often helpful to shave hair in areas adjacent to burns in order to promote better dressing application.

 6. Blisters may be left intact and the underlying wound allowed to heal if the fluid environment is small. Large blisters in areas where it is unlikely they will remain intact are better debrided early so as to obtain the maximal effect of any topical or burn dressing. A major cause of delayed burn wound infection is undebrided blisters.

 7. Burn dressings should be done twice a day after the washing with soap and water. Numerous agents may be utilized depending on patient compliance (Bacitracin, Xeroform, Silvadene). In general, partial-thickness burns are better covered with a dressing or an ointment to relieve pain.

8. Follow-up should be performed daily until the extent of thermal injury is apparent. Small chemical burns may often take a week to ten days to reveal the extent of thermal injury.

9. Direct exposure to the sun in the areas of the burn should be avoided during the healing process.

10. Pruritus is a common complaint following thermal injury, and Benadryl may be useful.

11. The use of synthetic skin substitutes in the treatment of small partial-thickness burns in outpatients is encouraging. These diminish pain and promote healing. In particular, Biobrane has been used effectively in the treatment of small partial-thickness burns.

## SUMMARY

All burns are surgical wounds, and basic principles of adequate debridement apply. Major burns should be considered traumatic injuries and the same priorities of resuscitation utilized in each case. Minor burns may be treated in a variety of effective manners provided that the wound is kept clean and observed for evidence of extensive injury not identified on initial examination.

## REFERENCES

1. Artz CP, Moncrief JA: The Treatment of Burns. Philadelphia, WB Saunders Company, 1969.
2. Boswick JA Jr (ed): The Art and Science of Burn Care. Rockville, MD, Aspen Publications, 1987.
3. Heimbach DM, Engrav LH: Surgical Management of the Burn Wound. New York, Raven Press, 1984.
4. Kemble JVH, Lamb BE: Practical Burn Management. London, England, Hodder and Stoughton, 1987.
5. Richardson JD, Polk HC Jr, Flint LM: Trauma: Clinical Care and Physiology. Chicago, Year Book Medical Publishers, 1987.
6. Dineen JJ, Moncure AC, Gross PL: MGH Textbook of Emergency Medicine. 2nd ed. Baltimore, Williams & Wilkins, 1983.

# 2

## Pathophysiological Changes after Cutaneous Burns and Approach to Initial Resuscitation

ROBERT H. DEMLING

### Anatomy and Function of the Skin

The skin is the largest organ of the body, ranging from 0.025 square meters ($m^2$) in the newborn to 1.0 $m^2$ in the adult. It consists of two layers—epidermis and dermis, or corium (Fig. 2–1). The outermost cells of the epidermis are dead cornified cells that act as a tough protective barrier against the environment. The second, thicker layer, the corium (0.60 to 1.2 mm), is composed chiefly of fibrous connective tissue. The dermis contains the blood vessels and nerves to the skin and epithelial appendages of specialized function. Since the nerve endings that mediate pain are found only in the dermis, partial-thickness injuries are extremely painful, whereas full-thickness injuries are often anesthetic. The dermis is a barrier that prevents loss of body fluids by evaporation and loss of excess body heat. Sweat glands help maintain body temperature by controlling the amount of heat loss by evaporation. Both the continued loss of water through burned skin and the loss of heat play a major role in the pathophysiological changes seen post burn. The skin is also our primary protective barrier against invasive infection, preventing penetration of microorganisms into the subdermal tissues. Burn wound infection is a major cause of mortality and morbidity. Another protection the skin provides is adaptation to changes in the physical environment initiated by the sensory nerve endings in the dermis which detect sensations of touch, pressure, pain, cold, and heat. The degree of impairment in the above protective characteristics of normal skin is dependent on the depth of burn injury and extent of injury, i.e., the size of the burn relative to that of total body skin surface area (TBSA).

### Depth of Burn Injury

Traditionally, burn depth has been classified in degrees of injury. A *first-degree* burn involves only the thinner outer epidermis layer and is characterized by erythema and mild discomfort. Tissue damage is minimal, and protective functions of the skin are intact. Pain, the chief symptom, usually resolves in 48 to 72 hours, and healing takes place uneventfully. The pain is believed to be in large part due to local vasodilator prostaglandin production. In 5 to 10 days the

12

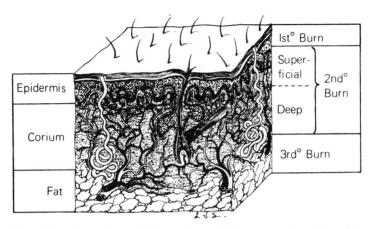

**FIGURE 2–1.** Scheme of normal skin histology and the categorization of burn injury.

damaged epithelium peels off, usually leaving no residual scarring. The common causes of first-degree burns are overexposure to sunlight and brief scalding by hot liquids.

*Second-degree* burns are defined as those in which the entire epidermis and variable portions of the dermis layer are heat destroyed. A *superficial* second-degree burn is classified as the heat destruction of the upper third of the dermis. The microvessels perfusing this area are injured and permeability is increased, resulting in the leakage of large amounts of plasma into the interstitium. This fluid in turn lifts off the thin heat-destroyed epidermis, leading to blister formation. The blisters continue to increase in size in the post-burn period as cell and protein breakdown occurs, increasing the content of osmotically active particles in the blister fluid, which subsequently attract additional water. A superficial second-degree burn is extremely painful, as the large number of sensory nerve organelles present below the epidermis are exposed. Despite loss of the entire basal layer of the epidermis, a burn of this depth will heal in 7 to 14 days owing to repopulation by the epithelial cells that line the hair follicles, sweat glands, and other skin appendages anchored deep in the dermis. Minimal scarring is expected to occur, as the wound inflammation that stimulates excessive collagen deposition is short-lived owing to the rapid wound closure.

A mid- to *deep dermal* second-degree burn extends well into the dermal layer, and fewer viable epidermal cells remain. Therefore, re-epithelialization is extremely slow, sometimes requiring months. Blister formation does not characteristically occur with a burn this deep, as the dead tissue layer is sufficiently thick and adherent to underlying dermal collagen that it cannot be readily lifted off the surface. The exception is the very young or very old patient who already has a very thin dermis. The residual dermis is usually red in appearance with some evidence of plasma leakage from remaining intact blood vessels. Remaining blood supply is marginal, and progression of the burn to a deeper injury can occur. Pain is present but to a lesser degree than that in the more superficial burns, as most of the nerve endings have been heat destroyed. Fluid losses and the metabolic effects of deep dermal burns are basically the same as those seen with third-degree burns. Dense scarring often occurs if the wound is allowed to heal primarily instead of by skin grafting. The subsequent function of the very thin healed skin is poor, and the epidermis readily shears off from the underlying dermis with only minimal trauma.

A full-thickness, or *third-degree*, burn is defined as destruction of the entire epidermis and dermis, leaving no residual epidermal cells to repopulate. This wound therefore does not re-epithelialize, and whatever area of the wound is not closed by wound contraction will require skin grafting. The dermal blood vessels are heat-coagulated, thereby leaving the tissue avascular. The characteristic appearance of the burn tissue is a waxy white color and a dry surface. If the burn extends into the fat or has had prolonged contact with a flame source, a leathery brown or black appearance can be seen, characterizing charred tissue. A short exposure to a very high temperature, such as direct contact with a flame, is the usual cause of a third-degree burn. However, prolonged contact with only a moderate temperature, e.g., 130°F water for 1 to 2 minutes, can result in a third-degree burn. This type of prolonged contact, as seen in an immersion scald burn, also leads to hemolysis of red cells as well as release of myoglobin from underlying muscle. Full-thickness burns usually result in occlusion of the wound blood flow. The lack of any painful sensation found with a full-thickness burn is due to heat destruction of all the nerve endings.

A *zone of ischemia* is usually present below the dead tissue and above the deeper living tissue in the early post-burn period. This zone is composed of cells that have been heat-injured but are not destroyed. The vasculature to this area is also compromised, with some vessels thrombosed and others patent but with endothelial cell damage. This marginally viable tissue can be readily converted to nonviable tissue (eschar) by a further insult such as hypoxia, a further decrease in blood flow, or infection. Prevention of wound conversion from viable tissue to eschar is of major importance in the resuscitation period and a topic of considerable recent research interest.[1]

## Severity of Injury

The size or surface area of the body involved, the depth of injury, the location of injury, the patient's age, and the presence of associated injuries determine morbidity and mortality.[2] Age and presence of associated injury appear now to be the most significant parameters dictating survival, as new aggressive approaches to the burn wound have decreased the role of the wound itself in burn morbidity and mortality.[2] A burn not complicated by smoke inhalation in a young person 10 to 30 years old has the best survival prognosis. Superimposed smoke inhalation injury markedly increases mortality rate.

A simple determination of the burn surface area can be obtained using the "rule of nines," considering each arm to be 9 per cent, each leg 18 per cent, anterior trunk 18 per cent, posterior trunk 18 per cent, and head 9 per cent of TBSA. In small children, the determination needs to be modified, as their head size approaches 18 per cent of TBSA. Age becomes a major factor in survival with children under 2 and adults over 60 years of age. An uncomplicated 50 per cent TBSA burn in the toddler population has a mortality rate in excess of 50 per cent. The higher death rate in small children results from a number of factors. First, the TBSA relative to body weight is much greater than in adults, resulting in a comparably greater physiological impact on the child. Second, an incompletely developed immune system, e.g., in the infant, decreases resistance to infection. Third, immature kidneys and liver have less ability to remove the high solute load from injured tissue and to rapidly produce new protein and maximally utilize exogenous nutrients. A 50 per cent TBSA burn in the elderly has a mortality rate approaching 100 per cent. Inability of the elderly to tolerate stress, due to pre-existing cardiac or pulmonary disease or other chronic diseases such as diabetes and general immune incompetence, increases mortality.

## ACUTE CARDIOPULMONARY CHANGES

### Fluid Shifts and Hemodynamic Instability

Adequate initial volume resuscitation is clearly critical to the survival of a major body burn. Hypovolemia can rapidly lead to conversion of a viable but ischemic deep dermal burn to a nonviable full-thickness burn, further increasing mortality. Today, with improving knowledge of the massive fluid shifts and vascular changes that occur, mortality related to burn-induced volume loss has decreased considerably.

The problem of hypovolemia, when aggressively corrected, can be replaced by a generalized burn edema formation, a problem clearly less lethal than shock, but one that can result in serious morbidity. Massive tissue edema results in an increase in tissue pressure and a decrease in tissue oxygen tension, leading to a further ischemic insult to already damaged cells. Edema formation in the chest wall results in an increased chest wall stiffness. Edema in the upper airway after severe burns is well recognized, as is small airway edema after inhalation injury. Both can lead to a rapidly fatal respiratory failure if not controlled. Hypoprotein-emia characteristically occurs owing to the loss of protein from the leaky capillaries in burn tissue, which can further accentuate edema formation in nonburned tissues.[4]

Although the exact pathophysiology of the post-burn vascular changes and volume shifts remains to be determined, there are clearly three processes involved: (1) an increase in microvascular permeability localized to the burned tissue, (2) a generalized impairment in cell membrane function resulting in cell swelling, and (3) an increase in burn tissue osmotic pressure leading to further fluid accumulation.

Clinically evident cardiovascular instability arises from the microvascular and cell membrane alterations just described. There is a noticeable early reduction in plasma volume. This plasma loss has been measured by Mason et al[5] to be in excess of 4 ml per kilogram of body weight per hour in a burn exceeding 30 per cent TBSA. There is no functional semipermeable membrane in burn tissue to allow for maintenance of a colloid osmotic gradient generated by protein. Therefore, functional plasma volume within burn tissue can be restored only with expansion of the extracellular space as well. During this period, some extracellular sodium and water are also being depleted by a shift into the cells. There is a further sodium loss into the burn eschar as described above. The quantity of sodium lost from the extracellular space during the 24-hour period after the burn has been measured by Baxter[3] to be 0.4 to 0.5 mEq per kilogram of body weight per per cent of body burn. The rate of loss of plasma volume is the greatest during the first 4 to 6 hours, decreasing substantially by 18 to 24 hours if adequate perfusion has been maintained.

Edema in nonburned tissues occurs later in the resuscitation period, out of phase with burn edema, indicating a different mechanism of formation. Protein loss, as reflected by hypoproteinemia, is at its greatest during the first 8 hours.[4] Experimentally, plasma volume loss into the nonburned interstitium is minimized if colloid osmotic pressure and interstitial protein stores are maintained, which, of course, is not totally feasible in the initial period after a massive burn.

Cardiac output is initially depressed as a result of hypovolemia. Increased systemic and, to a lesser extent, pulmonary vascular resistance also occurs owing to release of catecholamines. A decrease in cardiac contractility from a circulating myocardial depressant factor has also been reported, but the factor has yet to be identified and its presence remains controversial.[3, 5] Positive-pressure ventilation, frequently required in the early post-burn period, may further decrease ventricular output. Cardiac output is usually restored toward normal before restoration of a normal plasma volume owing to an increased heart rate typical of the increased stress response. Central venous pressure and pulmonary artery wedge pressure usually remain low even when cardiac output and perfusion are adequate, indicating that blood volume is less than normal. This fact is important to recognize when selecting appropriate rescuscitation monitors, as an overzealous attempt at restoring blood volume over and above that necessary for adequate perfusion can markedly accentuate edema-related complications. Fluid and protein losses in burn tissue are markedly aggravated by increases in venous pressure produced by excessive fluid infusion or by the released venoconstrictor mediators. Blood volume in severe burns can remain decreased for days in view of the ongoing losses. Even with massive fluid replacement, blood hematocrit of 50 to 55 per cent is not uncommon in the early post-burn period.

## Temperature Change

With a deep burn, the barrier to the loss of water by evaporation is markedly impaired. The loss of the evaporation barrier also means loss of the barrier to *heat loss*, a fact extremely important to recognize in the resuscitation period.[6] The protective mechanism of vasoconstriction in the skin is also absent. Body heat is lost by the mechanisms of convection, conduction, and radiation, all of which are magnified after burns diminish the skin barrier. Transfer of heat to a moving system, such as air or water, is known as *convection*. If body surface temperature is higher than air temperature, heat flows from body to air until the gradient is gone. However, warm air rises and is replaced by cooler air. The faster the air moves across the skin, the greater the gradient and the greater the heat loss. Air movement by a fan, a laminar airflow unit, or an air-fluidized bed can play a major role in heat loss, depending on the size of the gradient. Heat loss can be decreased by closing the wound under dressings, thereby limiting the air movement and decreasing the air-wound temperature gradient. Owing to increased heat conductivity in water, the rate of loss of body heat in water (wet dressings or hydrotherapy) is 25 times greater than that in air.

Heat is also exchanged by direct contact with an object, e.g., bed or dressing table. This process is known as *conduction*, and heat loss is again dependent on the temperature gradient. The increased wound blood flow seen after burns accentuates conduction heat loss. *Radiation* is emission of energy from the body surface as heat. The loss is dependent on body heat production, surface blood flow, and surface area. Radiation losses are increased post burn as a result of hypermetabolism and increased blood flow. Both of these processes are not maximized until the inflammation stage. Heat lost by any or all of these mechanisms leads to hypothermia, which results in an exaggerated stress response and increased energy requirements to correct the problem.[6]

An increase in body temperature can also occur during this period. Intermittent spiking temperature, usually initiated by manipulation of the burn wound, is a frequent occurrence. This hyperthermic response is the result of a pyrogen such as interleukin-1, a 15,000 molecular weight polypeptide released from the macrophages in injured tissue which subsequently alters the hypothalamic temperature regulator via prostaglandin $E_2$ production.[8]

## Burn-Induced Pulmonary Changes

Pulmonary dysfunction is a major cause of morbidity and mortality in the burn patient. This subject will be covered in more detail in Chapters 3 and 4. A decrease in arterial oxygen tension is frequently seen on admission.[1, 7] Alterations in lung function in the early period have been characteristically attributed to an increase in lung water due to burn-induced changes in the lung microcirculation or to superimposed smoke inhalation injury.[9, 10] The presence of a body burn clearly accentuates smoke injury.[11–19] The lack of a significant increase in lung water early post burn in the absence of a smoke inhalation injury has been demonstrated in man[11–13] using the double-indicator dilution technique. The validity of the indicator dilution technique as a measure of lung water, however, has been questioned.[14] Increased lung water will, of course, occur if massive fluid overload is produced.

Some modest lung circulatory and ventilatory changes are evident in large burn injuries without inhalation injury.[7, 15] These changes include an increase in pulmonary artery pressure and a decrease in arterial oxygen tension. Ventilatory changes include an increase in closing volume and an increase in airway resistance, indicating small airways pathology. Several bronchoconstrictors and vasoactive mediators are released from burn tissue.[16, 17] These agents, which have an effect on smooth muscle constriction in the lung, include histamine, serotonin, and thromboxane $A_2$. There is also a measurable increase in the lipid peroxide content of lung parenchyma beginning several hours after injury, reflecting an oxygen radical production and secondary lung changes post burn.[19]

Chest wall edema that decreases total lung compliance is also a significant problem.[18] Deep circumferential burns to the chest wall can severely impair ventilation.

## Early Metabolic Changes

The immediate post-burn period is known as the ebb phase, as nutrient flow and $O_2$ delivery to cells is decreased, leading to a decrease in metabolic rate. A massive catecholamine release occurs immediately after burn injury, both from the adrenal medulla and from the autonomic nervous system. The catechol discharge is, in large part, responsible for the systemic vasoconstriction and increased vascular resistance.[20, 21]

Glucagon is released during the same response as well as corticosteroids, resulting in mobilization of liver glycogen to glucose and a resulting hyperglycemia. The effect of the insulin released in response is overwhelmed by these anti-insulin hormones. Burn-induced hypovolemia increases renin production by the kidney and, in turn, increases aldosterone production. The net result is a decrease in free water clearance and a concentration of urine with conservation of sodium. The only readily available energy store is liver glycogen, which is rapidly depleted during the resuscitation phase. Pain and anxiety potentiate the stress response. Loss of body heat due to the removal of the skin barrier can add yet another stimulus to the release of these stress hormones. A cold or wet environment stimulates muscle shivering, utilizing any residual glucose to restore body temperature. Anaerobic metabolism ensues if oxygen demands are further increased, leading to a metabolic acidosis.

## Hematological Response

As for hematological disorders, there is frequently evidence of hemolysis, particularly after deep third-degree burns or any prolonged exposure to a heat source, with free plasma hemoglobin and hemoglobinuria.[22] Increased red cell lipid peroxidation is evident, and fragmented cells are often seen on smear.[23]

Many of these injured red cells have a markedly shortened life span, leading to an anemia beginning during the first week. Red cell hematopoiesis is markedly impaired and remains so until the burn is closed, leading to a persistent anemia. A leukocytosis is also characteristic during this early phase. An activation of clotting and consumption within the wound of platelets, fibrinogen, and other clotting factors are seen. Frequently, a hypercoagulable state is present in the initial period in moderate burn injuries. A hypocoagulable state, reflected in a depletion of clotting factors, is seen with massive burns. A decrease in the fibrinogen half-life in these patients indicates ongoing intravascular clotting. Even massive doses of heparin have been unsuccessful in restoring fibrinogen half-life to normal. This is most likely the result of the tremendous stimulus to clotting as a result of the large area of exposed injured collagen in burn tissue.

## TREATMENT IN THE ACUTE PHASE

### Removal of Burn Source

The first objective is to stop the burning process, as the deeper the burn the greater potential for mortality and morbidity. With a flame or scald burn, the clothing can retain heat for considerable periods of time, as is evident when one sees clothes still smoldering on admission. Rapid removal of clothing is, therefore, essential. At the scene, frequently the fire is put out with water by firemen or emergency medical technicians, after which the patient should be kept warm to decrease further heat loss.

Removal of the injury source is of particular importance with chemical burns, as the chemicals remain in fabric and on the skin for long periods of time. For most chemicals, in particular most acids and alkali, flushing the injured tissue with water for considerable periods of time is necessary. For acid burns, the length of irrigation time should be 30 minutes. With alkali, improvements in the degree of injury can be seen for up to an hour of wound irrigation. Corrosive powders, of course, should be removed prior to the addition of water. Of concern is not only the skin burn but also the absorption of chemicals that can cause systemic toxicity, such as neurological dysfunction, red cell hemolysis, and liver or kidney failure, as is seen with such agents as white phosphorus. Of importance during this period is the avoidance of hypothermia, which itself will result in significant morbidity. Therefore, once the source is removed, the patient should be initially covered with clean and dry dressings or blankets.

### Initial Fluid Resuscitation

A peripheral vein catheter through nonburn tissue is the preferable route of administration of fluids. A central line need be placed only for monitoring purposes and may be removed as soon as the need for monitoring ceases. An extremely high complication rate with central catheters occurs in burn patients due to both infection and embolic episodes from the hypercoagulable state. Owing to a high rate of infection complications, an intravenous catheter should *not* be placed through burn tissue unless no other possible route exists.

In general, isotonic salt solutions that are free of glucose, in view of early glucose intolerance, are appropriate for resuscitation from burn injury if given in sufficient amounts. The oral route can be used for smaller burns, but intestinal ileus occurs after deep burns in excess of 20 per cent TBSA, limiting the early use of the gastrointestinal tract.

It is quite clear that both crystalloid and colloid solutions are effective in restoring tissue perfusion based on their successful past and continued use. However, it makes no more sense to use one fluid for all patients than it does to use one antibiotic for all infections. Each of the following solutions has particular properties that make it advantageous for specific circumstances. *Isotonic salt solutions* are cheap and readily available. *Lactated Ringer's solution,* although slightly hypotonic, is used predominantly because of a more neutral pH plus the addition of other electrolytes besides sodium and chloride. Increased edema in nonburned tissue is the major disadvantage.[24, 25] *Hypertonic salt solutions* can decrease the fluid requirements needed to maintain perfusion by extracting intracellular water.[26, 27] The *increased osmotic pressure* may also help to counteract the increased flux of water into the eschar caused by the increased osmotic pressure in burn tissue. Because this is still a crystalloid, hypoproteinemia and blood volume are not as well maintained as with colloid.[25] *Nonprotein colloids,* such as *dextran* and *hetastarch,* have the molecular size and increased oncotic pressure sufficient to maintain blood volume and cardiac output while borrowing water from the interstitial space of nonburned tissues rather than from intracellular fluid. This results in less total fluid and less nonburn edema.[28-30] No real effect is seen on burn tissue edema due to the increased permeability. Blood volume is better maintained than with crystalloid alone, owing to the marked water-retaining capacity of these solutions, particularly dextran. However, the other properties of protein, such as clotting and opsonic activity, are not provided and the volume effect rapidly dissipates once the solution is discontinued.[31, 32] *Protein solutions,* when used with crystalloids, also decrease total fluid requirements and maintain vascular stability if initiated after the marked fluid and protein shifts seen in the first 6 to 8 hours. If colloids are needed immediately, nonprotein colloid is more economical, followed later by protein.

Given these characteristics, the appropriate solution can be chosen. Most young burn patients (the exception being the very young child) with less than 50 per cent TBSA without a pulmonary burn can be resuscitated with isotonic crystalloid. Patients with burns in excess of 50 per cent TBSA may benefit from the use of hypertonic salt solutions, which will maintain extracellular volume but limit the amount of edema. A severe hyperosmolar state, however, must be avoided. Protein restoration may be necessary to improve blood volume, particularly if early excision is to be performed. This approach may also be useful for the patient with a respiratory burn, again to minimize edema. An alternative fluid for the massive burn in the young patient or major burn in the elderly is dextran or *hetastarch* and salt-containing *crystalloid*, followed at 8 to 12 hours by protein infusion and crystalloid as needed.[23] The amount of dextran or starch which can be infused without leading to potential complications is limited to several liters over a 24-hour period. This regimen is also very useful for the patient admitted in shock to more rapidly restore adequate volume and perfusion. Familiarity with the properties of the various solutions allows one to choose the regimen with desired characteristics, including economy as well as effectiveness. Inotropic agents are usually not needed except for the elderly, for patients with pre-existing cardiac dysfunction, or for the massive burn patient with myocardial depression.

The fluid requirements for the first 24 hours vary between 2 and 4 cc per kilogram of body weight per per cent body burn, depending on the type of fluid used, the age of the patient, the size of the burn, and the presence of an inhalation injury.[34] Fluids should be infused at a constant rate rather than given as fluid challenges, since the latter transiently increase pressure in excess of that required for adequate perfusion and thereby accentuate edema formation. Fluid requirements in the first 6 to 8 hours will clearly exceed those in the subsequent 18 hours as the largest fluid shifts occur early. The ideal fluid infusion rate is one that maintains adequate perfusion as reflected by a urine output of 0.5 cc per kilogram per hour, a pulse rate of around 120, no significant base deficit, and usually a venous oxygen tension not less than 35 mm Hg.[33] Rate of infusion should be very gradually decreased over the 24-hour period when possible so as to maintain adequate perfusion, giving as little volume as necessary. It is important to remember that excess fluid, i.e., above the predicted values, given early in the resuscitation cannot be compensated for by a decrease in the subsequent infusion rate, as the initial fluid is in large part already in the tissues and cannot be retrieved. Decreasing the infusion rate only produces hypoperfusion.

## Pulmonary Support

The combination of an increase in airways resistance, a decrease in chest wall compliance due to edema or to the inelastic burn tissue itself, pain-induced splinting, and narcotic-induced hypoventilation can result in a significant lung dysfunction.[18] Elevation of the head and chest 20 to 30 degrees is very helpful. Endotracheal intubation and mechanical ventilation may be very advantageous for maintaining both airway patency and oxygenation.[35] Ventilator settings must be aimed, however, at maintaining lung volume while avoiding excessive increases in mean airway pressure, which will impair cardiac output. Since the lung parenchyma is usually normal, the increased airway pressure is readily transmitted to the mediastinum.

## Wound Management

The initial objectives are to maintain both perfusion and tissue oxygen delivery at optimal levels to protect the zone of ischemia in the burn tissue. The remaining viable dermis in the partial-thickness burn wound also needs to be protected from desiccation if it is partial thickness.[37] Large blisters can be left intact to help prevent the desiccation of the underlying dermis.[38] Removal of dirt and devitalized tissue is essential. Tetanus protection is also essential as with any soft-tissue injury. Systemic antibiotics will not prevent burn tissue infection because the wound itself is devitalized or severely ischemic, and adequate antibiotic levels cannot be achieved in dead tissue by the intravenous route. The application of soluble topical antibiotics to the surface of deep burns or the use of occlusive or biological dressings on superficial burns at least temporarily controls wound bacterial growth.[37–39] The addition of topical agents such as cyclo-oxygenase inhibitors to block thromboxane $A_2$–induced vasoconstriction is currently being studied.[40]

## Management of Metabolic and Hematological Changes

Decreasing the stimuli that accentuate the early stress response is the goal of resuscitation. Adequate fluid resuscitation minimizes the hypovolemia-induced catecholamine release. Prevention of hypothermia by avoidance of cold or wet dressings in large burns and placement of the patient in a warm temperature-controlled environment is necessary.[21, 41] Adequate control of pain and anxiety further controls the catecholamine release.[36] In the intubated and ventilated patient, a narcotic infusion can be very advantageous if the patient is hemodynamically stable.[36] Hypoxia also needs to be prevented, as this evokes a very potent stress response.

As for hematological abnormalities, replacement of clotting factors appears to be the only therapy necessary; this is indicated primarily if excision of burn tissue the following day is planned. Spontaneous bleeding as a result of the decrease in clotting factors is very uncommon during this early period but may be seen in massive burns. Thrombocytopenia resulting from consumption coagulopathy needs to be treated if excision and grafting are to be performed.

## REFERENCES

1. Demling RH: Improved survival after massive burns. J Trauma 23:179–184, 1983.
2. Pruitt BA, Tumbusch W, Mason A: Mortality in 1100 consecutive burns treated at a burns unit. Ann Surg 159:396–401, 1964.
3. Baxter CR: Fluid volume and electrolyte changes in the early post-burn period. Clin Plast Surg 1:693–709, 1974.
4. Birke G, Liljedahl SO, Plantin LO: Distribution and losses of plasma protein during the early stage of severe burns. Ann NY Acad Sci 150:895–904, 1968.
5. Mason AD, Pruitt BA, Moncrief JA: Hemodynamic changes in the early post-burn period: The influence of fluid administration and vasodilator. J Trauma 11:36–46, 1971.

6. Ruch T, Patton H: Physiology and Biophysics. Philadelphia, WB Saunders Company, 1966.
7. Petroff P, Pruitt BA: Pulmonary disease in the burn patient. *In* Artz C, Moncrief W, Pruitt B (eds): Burns, A Team Approach. Philadelphia, WB Saunders Company, 1979, pp 95–160.
8. Wilmore D, Mason A, Johnson D: Effect of ambient temperature on heat production and heat loss in patients. J Appl Physiol 38:593–600, 1975.
9. Moylan JA, Alexander LG: Diagnosis and treatment of inhalation injury. World J Surg 2:185–191, 1978.
10. Nash G, Foley FD, Langlinais P: Pulmonary interstitial edema and hyaline membrane in adult burn patient. Hum Pathol 5:149–160, 1974.
11. Kramer GC, Harms BA, Gunther R, et al: The effects of hypoproteinemia on blood-to-lymph fluid transport in sheep. Circ Res 49:1173–1180, 1981.
12. Tranbaugh RF, Elings VB, Christensen J, Lewis FR: Effect of inhalation injury on lung water accumulation. J Trauma 23:597–604, 1983.
13. Tranbaugh RF, Lewis FR, Christensen J, Elings VB: Lung water changes after thermal injury: The effects of crystalloid resuscitation and sepsis. Ann Surg 192:479–488, 1980.
14. Prien T, Traber LD, Herndon DN, et al: Pulmonary edema with smoke inhalation, undetected by indicator-dilution techniques. J Appl Physiol 63:907–911, 1987.
15. Asch MJ, Feldman RJ, Walker HL: Systemic and pulmonary hemodynamic changes accompanying thermal injury. Ann Surg 178:218–221, 1973.
16. Demling RH, Wong C, Jin L, Lalonde C: Early lung dysfunction after major burns (role of edema and vasoactive mediators). J Trauma 25:959–966, 1985.
17. Demling RH: Role of prostaglandins in acute microvascular injury. Ann NY Acad Sci 384:517–534, 1982.
18. Demling RH: Respiratory injury. Pulmonary dysfunction in the burn patient. J Burn Care Rehabil 7:277–286, 1986.
19. Demling RH, Katz A, Lalonde C, et al: The immediate effect of burn wound excision on pulmonary function in sheep: The role of prostanoid, oxygen radicals and chemhetastarch. Surgery 101:44–55, 1987.
20. Wilmore DW, Long JM, Mason AD: Catecholamines: Mediator of the hypermetabolic response to thermal injury. Ann Surg 180:653–659, 1974.
21. Wilmore D, Aulick L, Mason A: Influence of the burn wound on local and systemic responses to injury. Ann Surg 156:444–459, 1977.
22. Eurenius K: Hematologic changes in burns. *In* Artz C, Moncrief J, Pruitt B (eds): Burns, A Team Approach. Philadelphia, WB Saunders Company, 1979, pp 132–148.
23. Sasaki J, Cottam G, Baxter C: Lipid peroxidation following thermal injury. J Burn Care Rehabil 4:251–255, 1983.
24. Harms BA, Kramer GC, Bodai B, et al: Effect of hypoproteinemia on pulmonary and soft tissue edema formation. Crit Care Med 9:503–508, 1981.
25. Demling RH: Burns. N Engl J Med 313:1389–1398, 1985.
26. Monafo, WW, Halverson, JD, Schectman F: The role of concentrated sodium solutions in the resuscitation of patients with severe burns. Surgery 95:129–134, 1986.
27. Monafo WW, Chunktrasakul C, Ayvazian VH: Hypertonic sodium solutions in treatment of burn shock. Am J Surg 126:778–783, 1973.
28. Lamki LO, Liljedahl SO: Plasma volume changes after infusion of various plasma expanders. Resuscitation 5:93–102, 1976.
29. Haupt M, Rackow E: Colloid osmotic pressure and fluid resuscitation with hetastarch, albumin and saline solutions. Crit Care Med 10:159–162, 1982.
30. Gelin LE, Solvell L, Zederfeldt B: The plasma volume expanding effect of low viscous dextran and Macrodex. Acta Chir Scand 122:309–318, 1981.
31. Warden GD, Stratta RJ, Saffle JR, et al: Plasma exchange therapy in patients failing to resuscitate from burn shock. J Trauma 23:945–951, 1983.
32. Schnarro RH, Cline CW, Goldfarb IW, et al: Plasma exchange for failure of resuscitation in thermal injuries. J Burn Care Rehabil 3:230–234, 1986.
33. Agarwal N, Petro J, Salisbury R: Physiologic profile monitoring in burned patients. J Trauma 23:577–583, 1983.
34. Scheulen J, Munster A: The Parkland formula in patients with burns and inhalation injury. J Trauma 22:869–871, 1982.
35. Venus B, Matsuda T, Copiozo J: Prophylactic intubation and continuous positive airway pressure in the management of inhalation injury in burn victims. Crit Care Med 9:519–523, 1981.

36. Demling RH: What are the functions of endorphin following thermal injury? J Trauma 24:S172–S176, 1984.
37. Alvarez A, Mertz P, Eaglstern W: The effect of occlusive dressings on collagen syntheses and re-epithelialization in superficial wounds. J Surg Res 35:142–148, 1983.
38. Wilson J, Moncrief J: Vapor pressure of normal and burned skin. Ann Surg 162:130–136, 1965.
39. Lamke L: Evaporative water loss from normal and burnt skin. Scand J Plast Reconstr Surg 5:17–22, 1971.
40. Robson M, Del Becraro E, Heggers J: Increased dermal perfusion after burning by decreasing thromboxane production. J Trauma 20:722–726, 1980.
41. Wilmore DW, Mason AD, Johnson DW, et al: Effect of ambient temperature on heat production and heat loss in burned patients. J Appl Physiol 38:593–597, 1975.

# 3

# Pulmonary Disorders in the Burn Patient

## JONATHAN STRONGIN* and CHARLES HALES

## RESPIRATORY COMPLICATIONS OF BURN INJURY AND SMOKE INHALATION

The lethal effects of smoke inhalation have been known for centuries. Pliny the Elder recorded that prisoners in the Second Punic War were placed in cages directly above green wood fires for execution. In more modern times several fires have helped establish the fact that smoke inhalation itself, with or without body surface burns, is a major killer. Among them were the Cleveland cellulose fire in the early 1930s and the Coconut Grove Nightclub fire in Boston in 1942, in which 75 of the 114 victims died within hours of injury, many without significant surface burns.[1, 2] With increases in survival of patients in the post-burn period from improved management of burn shock and wound sepsis, pulmonary complications have emerged as a major cause of morbidity and mortality, occurring in up to 25 per cent of hospitalized burn patients and responsible for up to 70 per cent of thermal injury deaths.[3] In a recent prospective study, 9 of 28 patients with fire-related injuries developed respiratory failure that required intubation, and 4 of the 28 died, all from pulmonary complications.[4] Since an estimated 7000 to 10,000 people per year in the United States are killed in fires and 100,000 are injured, fire-related lung injury contributes heavily to the approximately 150,000 annual cases of adult respiratory distress syndrome.

The Coconut Grove fire helped establish a recognized pattern of pulmonary injury which has subsequently been amplified and extended.[2, 5, 6] Three broad categories of lung injury after surface burns and/or smoke inhalation have emerged: (1) the acute effects that occur from 0 to 24 hours after exposure and involve direct inhalation damage with bronchospasm, airway swelling, atelectasis, and pulmonary edema, as well as tissue hypoxia; (2) adult respiratory distress syndrome (ARDS) beginning two to five days after injury; and (3) complications (primarily pulmonary emboli and pneumonia) delayed five days or more post injury. Further, the combination of smoke injury with burns of greater than 25 to 40 per cent of total body surface area (TBSA) is synergistic in producing injury to the lungs.[7] In this chapter we will describe the anatomical and pathophysio-

Supported by an NIH training grant in Pulmonary Pathophysiology (HLO 7354)* and by a grant from the NIH (HL36829) and from the Shriners Burns Institute.

logical patterns of injury as they occur temporally, review the diagnosis and management of inhalation injury, and outline the treatment of diseases of the lung related to burn trauma.

## Early Injury

In the first hours following fire exposure the lung injury is due mainly to smoke with or without associated cutaneous burns. The uppermost airway easily buffers the heat of smoke, and thus thermal injury is usually confined to the larynx and upper trachea.[8] An important exception to this is when smoke is delivered as steam.[9] In this situation, direct thermal injury can readily occur below the larynx. More commonly, the parenchymal lung damage that occurs after smoke inhalation is a result of the chemical content of smoke.[10, 11] Smoke is a composite substance of various liquid and solid particles suspended in gas. The magnitude of lung or airway injury depends on the duration of exposure as well as the chemical content of the smoke.

### Carbon Monoxide

In the first minutes to hours after a fire, carbon monoxide poisoning is the most frequent cause of death.[12, 13] Carbon monoxide (CO) has a binding affinity for hemoglobin which is 210 to 240 times greater than that of oxygen ($O_2$). The carbon monoxide thus displaces $O_2$ from hemoglobin, resulting in tissue hypoxemia. For example, the addition of only 0.1 per cent carbon monoxide to inspired air will produce at equilibrium 40 per cent oxyhemoglobin and 60 per cent carboxyhemoglobin, resulting in a significant (60 per cent) reduction in the $O_2$-carrying capacity (Fig. 3–1). Carbon monoxide also shifts the $O_2$-hemoglobin dissociation curve to the left (Fig. 3–2), further compromising the $O_2$ delivery capacity and leading to tissue hypoxemia. Therefore the $O_2$ delivery to tissues is worse with 60 per cent carboxyhemoglobin than with an anemia with a hemoglobin 40 per cent of normal, since the remaining hemoglobin in the presence of carbon monoxide is much less capable of releasing $O_2$ to the tissues. With very low concentrations of carbon monoxide in the ambient air, these changes are apparent at a cellular level, even though the partial pressure of inspired oxygen ($P_{O_2}$) is only minimally reduced (for 0.1 per cent CO, there is less than 1 mm Hg reduction in $FI_{O_2}$). Thus, the alveolar and arterial $P_{O_2}$ tensions are virtually normal, but the $O_2$ content is markedly reduced (Fig. 3–2). This is because the $P_{O_2}$ in blood reflects the gas in solution, not the $O_2$ bound to hemoglobin. Further, very high concentrations of carbon monoxide are believed to have a direct toxic effect by interfering with the cytochrome system.[14] At the scene of a fire, combustion can lower the fraction of inspired oxygen from 0.21 to 0.10, and this hypoxia can magnify the effects of carbon monoxide poisoning.[12] The resulting tissue hypoxia affects all end organs. Arrhythmias are the most common fatal occurrence.

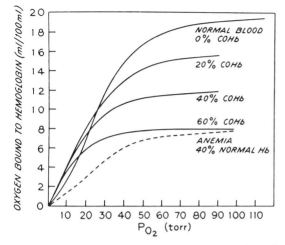

**FIGURE 3–1.** Calculated $O_2$ binding/dissociation curves of human blood containing varying amounts of COHb, expressed as $O_2$ bound to hemoglobin. Note that the reduction of oxygen bound to hemoglobin is a function of the percentage of carboxyhemoglobin and is independent of the $Po_2$ of the blood within the normal physiological range. Additionally note that the presence of carbon monoxide on the hemoglobin alters the way the remaining binding sites hold onto oxygen. In blood containing 60 per cent COHb, the remaining hemoglobin holds on more tightly to oxygen at any given $Po_2$, as can be seen by comparing the 60 per cent COHb curve (40 per cent residual hemoglobin) to the 40 per cent normal Hb curve. This is expanded in Figure 3–2. (From Comroe JH Jr: Physiology of Respiration. 2nd ed. Copyright 1974 Year Book Medical Publishers, Inc., Chicago. Used by permission (redrawn from Roughton FJW, Darby RC: Am J Physiol 141:17, 1944).)

## Toxins in Smoke

Besides carbon monoxide, the most frequently encountered toxic constituents of smoke are hydrogen chloride (HCl), hydrogen cyanide (HCn), nitrogen dioxide ($NO_2$), carbon dioxide ($CO_2$), acrolein, benzine, and suspended particulates.[15, 16] The exact concentration of each is a function of the material being burned and the temperature of the fire. In a study of structural fires in Boston, acrolein and carbon monoxide were found to occur most often in life-threatening concentrations. Less hazardous concentrations of HCl, HCn, and $NO_2$ were

**FIGURE 3–2.** Oxygen-hemoglobin dissociation curve. Note the "left shift" of the carboxyhemoglobin curve. This in effect means that, as arterial blood arrives at the tissues where the mean $Po_2$ is around 40 torr, each molecule of carboxyhemoglobin releases less $O_2$ to the tissues than normal hemoglobin. For example, at a $Po_2$ of 40 torr, normal hemoglobin releases 25 per cent of its oxygen, but carboxyhemoglobin releases less than 10 per cent. (Data from Comroe JH Jr.: Physiology of Respiration. 2nd ed. Copyright 1974 Year Book Medical Publishers, Inc., Chicago.)

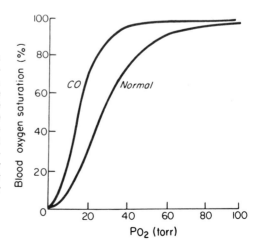

found, although synergistic effects of these substances were not addressed.[17] Data from other types of fires are scant, but smoke produced from the burning of modern substances such as plastic and electrical equipment probably has increased concentrations of acrolein and other organic aldehydes. Table 3–1 lists common toxic products of combustion.

The acute effects of these chemicals and particulates on the airway are irritation and bronchoconstriction.[10] Airway obstruction may be further enhanced by the resulting tracheal bronchitis and edema. Impairment of mucociliary clearance has also been demonstrated.[18] This along with mucosal sloughing may further exacerbate the acute effects of airway constriction.

Upper airway obstruction is a serious complication of inhalation injury, and its occurrence is increased by head and neck injury and burns. Particularly treacherous is glottic edema. The outward expansion of the glottis is limited by cartilaginous rings. Thus any swelling that occurs is displaced inward. When the airway is narrowed below 8 mm, there is a precipitous fall in achievable peak flow rates (Fig. 3–3).[19] A further small increase in local swelling and edema may change a patient from a stable, relatively asymptomatic state at an airway diameter of 7 or 8 mm to one of critical obstruction. Soot in the pharynx and nares, stridor over the upper airway, or any type of facial burn should prompt special evaluation of the upper airway either with flow-volume loops, lateral overpenetrated neck films of the air column, or direct visualization. The evidence of upper airway burns may influence the decision to admit an asymptomatic patient to the hospital.

The components of smoke may dissolve in the airways and produce local irritation.[20] Highly soluble compounds such as ammonia, sulfur dioxide, chlorine, and hydrogen chloride most often predominate in the upper airways, whereas less soluble substances such as aldehydes, phosphorus, and oxides of nitrogen make their way to the lower airways.[15, 16] Some of these substances have specific toxic effects besides local irritation. Cyanide, for example, inhibits cellular oxidation.[10] The soluble toxins can produce airway sloughing, which can occlude both large (central) and small (peripheral) airways. This can lead to hypoxemia, atelectasis, and increased right-to-left shunting. At this stage the atelectasis may not be radiographically apparent. In addition to the mechanical effects of

## TABLE 3–1. Common Toxic Products of Combustion

| Substance | Toxic Products |
|---|---|
| Polyvinyl chloride | Hydrogen chloride, phosgene, chlorine |
| Wood, cotton, paper | Acrolein, acetaldehyde, formaldehyde, acetic acid, formic acid |
| Petroleum products | Acrolein, acetic acid, formic acid |
| Nitrocellulose film | Oxides of nitrogen, acetic acid, formic acid |
| Nitrogen-containing compounds (polyurethane) | Isocyanate, hydrogen cyanide |
| Polyfluorocarbons (Teflon) | Octafluoroisobutylene |
| Melamine resins | Ammonia, hydrogen cyanide |

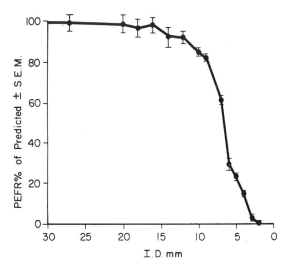

**FIGURE 3–3.** Mean peak expiratory flow rate (PEFR) in five normal volunteers as a function of progressive reduction in the inner diameter (I.D.) of an external airway. Note the precipitous decline in flow rates as the airway is reduced below 8 mm. (Adapted with permission from Al-Bazzaz F, Grillo H, Kazemi H: Response to exercise in upper airway obstruction. Am Rev Respir Dis 111:631, 1975.)

absorption atelectasis from the occlusion of distal airways, alveolar collapse may also occur from the inactivation of surfactant, a direct effect of smoke.[21, 22] The less soluble toxins may reach more peripherally in the airways and produce pulmonary edema.

### Experimental Data on Smoke-Induced Pulmonary Edema

Data from our laboratory suggest that, when inhaled as part of a synthetic smoke, HCl and acrolein are injurious to airways and that acrolein also causes pulmonary edema. By using synthetic smoke we are able to control the chemical composition and size of particulate matter so that we can examine the influence of one toxin at a time in smoke rather than the multiple toxins present in real smoke. When hydrogen chloride smoke with HCl concentration of 200 to 2500 ppm, impregnated on carbon particles of 4.3 ± 2 microns, was given to anesthetized dogs, there were unremarkable hemodynamic and extravascular lung water changes for up to 24 hours of observation. Postmortem examination after sacrifice showed an even distribution of carbon particles down to the alveolar level. HCl damage to the mucosa of the trachea and carina, as well as to the intralobar bronchi, was present. Additionally, there was some suggestion of alveolar wall thickening. Blood-corrected wet/dry lung weight ratios as a measurement of pulmonary edema were normal, however. We conclude from these studies that aerosolized HCl and carbon can cause airway damage but do not produce pulmonary edema. This is at variance with lung injury models, in which HCl instilled directly as a bolus into the lung causes extensive damage.[23] The difference is likely due to the diffuse presentation of the HCl when it is a smoke, to binding of the HCl to the carbon soot from which it is only slowly released, and to the fact that HCl as a vapor is very soluble and probably does not reach the alveoli.

When the aldehyde acrolein is given in a similar manner as a smoke, the following pattern of injury results. At lower doses (less than 25 ppm) there were no remarkable changes up to 18 hours. With concentrations between 225 and 300 ppm, there was an initial small rise in pulmonary artery pressures for 10 minutes, followed by a return to baseline. Cardiac output and pulmonary capillary wedge pressure remained stable. Extravascular lung water (EVLW) began to rise at a slow constant rate over the next three hours. This rise in EVLW peaked at two and one-half to three times baseline, at which point tracheal fluid was evident. In our model, alveolar/plasma protein concentrations were 0.8, suggesting that acrolein smoke does produce a permeability protein edema. Histologically the acrolein smoke–injured lung showed severe airway mucosal damage with epithelial desquamation, intraluminal mucus and exudate, and submucosal edema with a mild neutrophilic infiltration. Airway injury was a constant feature and showed a damage gradient most severe proximally, with minimal involvement of the distal respiratory bronchioles and alveolar ducts at low doses of acrolein (100 ppm). With high doses of acrolein (100 to 300 ppm) a distinctive localizing pattern of morphological injury was noted. This pattern was zonal and centered on small bronchi, bronchioles, and the juxtaposed alveoli that abutted the adventitia of these bronchi and bronchioles. The latter disclosed transmural injury characterized by mucosal sloughing, prominent interstitial edema, marked dilatation, and congestion of the bronchial plexus and venules. Frequent hemorrhage and extravascular fibrin deposits were found within the peribronchial sheath. Juxtaposed alveolae showed deposits of fibrin, high protein intra-alveolar fluid, slight infiltration of neutrophils, and occasional hemorrhage. Alveolar ducts and their contiguous sacs appeared uninvolved.[24]

The bronchial circulation may play an important role in this model of injury in edema formation, since the bronchial vessels supplying the terminal bronchioles are noticeably engorged.[25] Monastral Blue B,[26] a tracer that targets vessels with endothelial gaps, leaks from bronchial vessels of acrolein smoke–exposed dogs but not from normals and not from pulmonary vessels, suggesting the bronchial arteries may be the important site of acrolein injury.

To further elucidate the role of the bronchial circulation in edema formation in inhalation injury, we have ligated the bronchial arteries before smoke exposure. In some animals there was no detectable increase in extravascular lung water after acrolein smoke. In other dogs edema did occur, but in general this edema was more delayed in onset than usual after acrolein smoke exposure. The histology in these latter dogs still showed the peribronchial focal edema. We are thus uncertain at present whether our bronchial artery ligations were incomplete or collateral retrograde flow from the pulmonary circulation played a part in the edema formation. When the acrolein is delivered unilaterally, the resultant pattern of injury is unilateral; the contralateral lung shows no sign of injury. The model of acrolein injury supports the hypothesis that edema formation seen in smoke inhalation may be a local phenomenon and that the bronchial circulation (venules) may be the major site of fluid leakage. Final conclusive proof of the importance of the bronchial circulation to pulmonary edema after acrolein smoke exposure is the occurrence of the edema in an exposed lung even though the pulmonary artery to that lung had been occluded.

The effects of inhalation injury with smoke obtained from burning cotton in a sheep model have been analyzed in a series of experiments at the Shriners Burns Institute at Galveston, Texas.[27, 28] These experiments also show similar results with a 10-fold increase in bronchial blood flow and a threefold elevation in protein-rich lymph flow. Cardiac index and pulmonary artery and left atrial pressures were unchanged. With smoke inhalation, volume increases were noted in the vascular and extravascular compartments of the lung with a substantial increase in lung lymph neutrophil counts, which were greater in magnitude and duration than systemic increase when compared to sham controls. Furthermore, antiprotease activity, seen as a measure of the animal's capacity to minimize neutrophil-mediated injury, was depressed and lung lymph concentrations of 6-keto $PGF_1$ were elevated, although no systemic changes were detected. 6-Keto $PGF_1$ is the stable metabolite of prostacycline, which is a vasodilator that has been shown to decrease pulmonary microvascular permeability in sheep. While this may not be sufficient to explain the edema formation, it does provide evidence that the arachidonic acid pathway was activated and that the alternate complement pathway may play a role, findings that have been suggested by the in vitro stimulation of the arachidonic acid cascade and activation of pulmonary macrophages by acrolein.[29]

The finding of increased interstitial neutrophils is important and may indicate that the neutrophil plays some role, perhaps late in the pathogenesis of lung injury from inhalation alone, and in a similar manner to that which it plays when scald burn injury occurs. Further work needs to be done to corroborate these findings, especially histopathological demonstrations. The acute exposure to acrolein smoke, however, does not seem to need polymorphonuclear cells, at least in any noticeable number, to cause injury.

## Acute Injury

Lung injury can develop in fire victims from smoke inhalation alone.[11] However, unlike the delayed diffuse pattern of lung injury seen in patients with cutaneous burns, in patients with smoke inhalation the pattern of injury may be localized about the airways, suggesting that direct toxic effects of inhaled chemicals and particulates may be responsible. Additionally, the lung injury that occurs from smoke inhalation alone usually appears within 24 hours, whereas when skin burns are involved, it appears 24 to 72 hours later. The importance of polymorphonuclear leukocytes to the lung injury after inhalation burns may be minor, since the lungs have only minimal white cell agglutination and margination within vessels. A leukocyte infiltration does occur but is limited to airways and is not seen in vessels around alveoli, as in other forms of acute lung injury.[61]

## Delayed Injury

Typically within one to five days after fire injury (but in some cases almost immediately or delayed up to a week) a pattern of injury can develop which is described as "delayed," differentiated from the acute effects of early airway obstruction. The underlying feature of this pattern of injury is a noncardiogenic pulmonary edema characterized by progressive hypoxemia, normal cardiac function with normal left atrial and pulmonary capillary wedge pressures, and the radiographic appearance of bilateral interstitial infiltrates. The constellation of these clinical findings has suggested that the delayed form of inhalation injury is a form of the adult respiratory distress syndrome (ARDS). It is believed that the underlying pathophysiological defect is hypoproteinemia and increased vascular permeability, but whether this is a pulmonary vascular process, a result of disruption of the bronchiolar circulation, or a combination of these is not resolved. Head, in a study using albumin tagged with indocynine green given intravenously, found bronchoscopic washings positive for the dye in patients following smoke inhalation. This led him to conclude that the primary defect was an increased vascular permeability to protein.[30] The exact mechanism by which this leakage occurs is not completely understood, but recent studies have suggested that there is a spectrum of pathogenic responses that produce the syndrome of pulmonary capillary damage and increased extravascular lung water.

The delayed pattern of pulmonary injury related to fire and smoke inhalation occurs in two situations: (1) body surface burns without smoke inhalation, (2) a combination of smoke inhalation and surface burns. Smoke inhalation alone usually causes the acute injury profile of bronchospasm, atelectasis, and pulmonary edema. The mechanism underlying the leakage may differ in surface burn–induced lung injury from that seen with smoke inhalation.

Scald burns involving 25 to 30 per cent TBSA can produce the ARDS-like syndrome even in the absence of smoke inhalation.[10, 31–35] However, when smoke inhalation occurs in conjunction with scald burns, the incidence of pulmonary damage and vascular leakage is increased and is seen to occur with decreased extents of body surface burns, thus suggesting that smoke inhalation and surface burns can act synergistically.[7]

In the lung, injury occurring secondary to body scald burns probably occurs through a common pathway of injury involving hypoproteinemia and complement activation (probably C5a or its metabolites) with subsequent leukocyte aggregation and deposition in the lung vasculature, where the activated leukocytes disgorge their products (including proteolytic enzymes and free radicals of oxygen). These, along with activation of the arachidonic acid cascade, produce changes in pulmonary vasoreactivity and permeability, resulting in ARDS.[36–46]

The precipitating events that involve this final common pathway of pulmonary injury in burn patients are probably multifactorial. Plasma hypoproteinemia in major surface burns, at least in sheep, seems to predispose to an increase in transudation of fluid into the lung and lung lymph, perhaps providing a boggy lung unable to deal well with other injury. Disseminated intravascular coagulation (DIC) mediated by oxygen radical formation released from activated neutrophils and/or infection from gram-negative bacteria (a frequent complication of surface burns) may be important clinically.[42, 43, 47, 48] Work from our own laboratory with endotoxin in a dog model has shown in vivo evidence of hydroxyl radical release after administration of endotoxin; this hydroxyl radical release is associated with the appearance of cyclo-oxygenase products that mediate changes in pulmonary vasomotor tone.[49, 50] We believe that these eicosanoids can act as chemoattractants for leukocytes and induce pulmonary vasospasm and permeability edema. These eicosanoids are also released in burn injury and may play a role in lung injury too, but data in this regard are still preliminary.[51]

In animals, scald burns have also been shown to produce activation of the alternate complement pathway, resulting in enhanced circulatory leukocyte aggregation with pulmonary sequestration of the leukocytes in a lung that becomes hemorrhagic and edematous.[40] Depletion of complement by administration of cobra venom factor largely prevents this injury.[41]

In sheep, scald burns of 25 to 40 per cent TBSA produce a low-protein pulmonary edema, suggesting that pulmonary venospasm may be responsible for the edema formation. When these events are followed beyond 48 hours, it appears that this low-protein edema is a transient phenomenon and does not lead to ARDS.[52] When larger burns of 50 to 75 per cent are produced, an increased amount of lymph flow without an increase in measured lung water, as well as a fall in $PaO_2$, transient pulmonary hypertension, and a significant reduction in compliance, has been reported to occur.[46] This may be related to measured increases in plasma thromboxane, since animals treated with ibuprofen both pre- and post-burn exhibited less dysfunction. When nonlethal doses of endotoxin are given in conjunction with the scald burn, however, there is a marked increase in pulmonary morbidity and mortality.[53] In this instance, the pattern of injury resembles that of the neutrophil-mediated acute lung injury seen in a number of circumstances. Thus, cutaneous burns may fit the white cell mode of acute lung injury, but cutaneous burns alone, unless very extensive, probably are not enough of a stimulant to produce lung injury unless another white cell stimulant such as a mild endotoxemia also occurs. This may well be the case in humans as well. Pulmonary edema can follow acutely after smoke inhalation,[5] but after body surface burns alone it is uncommon unless accompanied by sepsis.[35]

In humans, however, postmortem examination of lungs of patients dying of surface scald injury shows the usual picture of ARDS with hyaline membranes, proliferating type II pneumocytes, and edema but may not be notable for leukocyte infiltration.[54-56] This may be related to the remote stage after injury at which the autopsied lungs have been examined, or it may suggest that the white cell is not as important in human burn ARDS as animal models suggest. Of note are recent case reports of non–burn-related ARDS occurring in granulocytopenic patients[57–59] as well as an animal model of ARDS in neutropenic sheep.[60] This suggests that in patients with cutaneous burns, ARDS may be the culmination of several pathways of response to injury, only one of which is via the activated polymorphonuclear leukocyte.

## Late Complications

With improvements in the recognition and management of inhalation injury, as well as improvements in burn management technique, more patients are surviving the acute and delayed phases of lung injury. This has led to an increase in the occurrence of late-phase pulmonary injury, which is characterized by atelectasis, pneumonia, and pulmonary embolism.

During the late phase the most frequent pulmonary complication is pneumonia, which occurs in 1 to 15 per cent of cases.[8, 62] Several factors are believed to be related to the late occurrence of pneumonia. Foremost is a depression of cellular immunity which has been demonstrated in the sera of burn patients exposed to mitogen stimulation assays.[63] It is now known that this is secondary to an increase in the number of suppressor lymphocytes, which affect humoral immunity as well.[64–66] In part, this is probably a nonspecific phenomenon that is seen in altered physiological states related to stress such as malnutrition, surgery, childbirth, anesthesia, chronic disease, and bereavement.[67] Increased sensitivity to $PGE_2$ may play a role, as shown in some preliminary data, and is particularly appealing since, in vitro at least, these changes can be reversed by prostaglandin inhibitors such as indomethacin. However, there is some evidence to suggest that an immunosuppressive factor is found in the sera of burn patients which may be responsible for these changes.[68, 69]

The change in immune function clearly correlates with the degree of body surface area affected by burns.[63, 68] Whether this finding is due to a "stress"-related factor or is specific to the pathophysiology of burns needs further elucidation. In one retrospective study of 1018 consecutive admissions to the Galveston Shriners Burns Institute, mortality was correlated with a rising percentage of TBSA involved.[70] However, more striking increases were observed if inhalation injury was also a factor (Table 3–2). Inhalation injury was also noted to increase with age, and the authors of this study postulated that younger individuals were more likely to be outside when injured and less likely to ingest alcohol and drugs, which they believe predispose individuals to inhalation injury.

Acrolein has also been demonstrated to exert a direct immunosuppressive effect in mice by decreasing antibacterial defenses at low concentrations.[71] It may also predispose to an increased incidence of postviral or secondary bacterial pneumonia. This suggests that there are local direct toxic effects of smoke inhalation in host defenses as well as generalized systemic factors.

Other factors may also be responsible in the development of pneumonia.

**TABLE 3–2.** Incidence and Mortality of Inhalation Injury as Related to TBSA Burn

| | | | Mortality | |
|---|---|---|---|---|
| Per Cent TBSA Burn | No. of Patients | With Inhalation Injury | *Without Inhalation Injury* | *With Inhalation Injury* |
| 0–20 | 627 | 2% | 1% | 36% |
| 21–40 | 200 | 11% | 2% | 38% |
| 41–60 | 102 | 20% | 18% | 50% |
| 61–80 | 56 | 32% | 24% | 67% |
| 81–100 | 33 | 55% | 47% | 83% |

Incidence and mortality as related to per cent TBSA are shown. Both incidence and mortality increase with increasing size of burn.

Hematogenous spread of organisms from infected wounds, decreased mucociliary clearance in the setting of stress and intubation, and the effects of aspiration and poor pulmonary toilet have also been implicated. Generally, the causative organisms of pneumonia in burn patients reflect the occurrence of infection at the wound site.[72, 73] With improved methods of wound care, however, there has been a reduction in hematogenously spread infection relative to airborne pneumonias. Nevertheless, causative organisms generally reflect the microbiology of the wound.

Pulmonary emboli are also important causes of late mortality in burn patients, occurring in 5 to 30 per cent of patients.[74] It is generally believed that their origin is attributable to immobilization from prolonged bedrest. Other possible etiologies are hypercoagulable states associated with burn trauma and shown by thrombocytosis and increased levels of Factors V and VII.[75] An increased incidence of central venous thrombosis from central line insertion occurs, supporting the concept of a hypercoagulable state. It is also possible that smoke-induced abnormalities in the pulmonary circulation and microthrombi may predispose to endothelial injury and pulmonary thrombosis.

Atelectasis is also common during this stage. It may occur as a consequence of immobilization, poor pulmonary toilet, and poor inspiration. The latter may occur from chest wall restriction, which occurs occasionally as circumferential wounds heal and scar.[4] Additionally, elevated concentrations of C-reactive protein found in the lavage fluid of ARDS patients may interfere with surfactant function and thus lead to the development of atelectasis.[76]

## Patient Assessment and Management

### Clinical Examination

The initial evaluation of patients who have substantial burns and/or inhalation injury, or are thought to have sustained such, should be directed toward identifying patients with serious injury and those at risk for developing delayed sequelae. Both groups of patients should be hospitalized.[10]

As in other types of injury, the history is of primary importance. Whether or not the fire occurred within a closed space is a key factor in patients suspected of having inhalation injury. Closed fires and the consequent lack of ventilation increase the chance of inhalation injury.[70] Additionally, the source of combustion is important, i.e., whether it is a structural fire or occurs from the combustion of petroleum products, chemicals, or plastics. These latter factors increase the risk of later injury. Similarly, inebriation and unconsciousness increase the risk of smoke inhalation. As mentioned earlier, the risk also increases with age. None of these factors, however, commonly predicts which patients are at risk for delayed complications. Factors (established by examination of the patient on presentation) which suggest pulmonary injury are the presence of cutaneous body burns including facial burns and singed eyes, soot in the oropharynx, hoarseness, rales, wheezing, and visible airway edema.[77] Cyanosis may or may not be present. Carbonaceous sputum is also particularly suggestive of airway injury, although, as in the case of facial burns, its presence does not predict the extent of airway injury. As is always the case, general principles of emergency medical care should be followed, beginning with an assessment of airway patency.

Besides airway patency, in the initial period carbon monoxide poisoning is of particular concern.[12] Signs of carbon monoxide poisoning are often not grossly obvious. Careful neurological evaluation, including formal mental status testing, may be necessary to uncover subtle signs. There is a loose correlation between the degree of carbon monoxide poisoning as measured by the percentage of carboxyhemoglobin and neurological findings. At mild levels of poisoning (CO levels between 10 and 20 per cent), headache, confusion, and nausea are the most common presenting signs. At moderate levels of exposure (between 20 and 40 per cent CO), irritability, dizziness, fatigue, dimming of vision, and impaired judgment may become apparent. Severe levels of exposure (40 to 60 per cent CO) are characterized by hallucinations, ataxia, convulsions, or coma. Tachypnea may be present at this level. Higher levels are generally believed to be fatal, since the resultant $O_2$ transfer at the tissue level is very severely disrupted. Even if tissue hypoxemia is severe, tachypnea may not be present until acidosis occurs. This is because the carotid body, the sensor for atrial $Po_2$, with its very high rate of perfusion, is affected by $Pao_2$ rather than $O_2$ content, and the $Pao_2$ of the carbon monoxide–intoxicated patient is usually normal. Only when tissue hypoxemia is so severe that lactic acidosis occurs does an increase in minute ventilation occur in response to the acidosis. The classic cherry red color associated with carbon monoxide poisoning is rarely seen except in the capillary or blood collection tube. Most often the affected patients appear gray.

### Laboratory Tests

If possible, carboxyhemoglobin levels should be measured, since many cases of carbon monoxide poisoning go undetected initially.[13] Routine blood gases should also be obtained to search for other reversible causes of hypoxemia. They can also point out a metabolic acidosis, a strong clue to the presence of carboxyhemoglobinemia.

Oxygen content or saturation should be measured by a technique that corrects for carboxyhemoglobin. Unfortunately, most standard laboratory spectrophotometers cannot distinguish between oxy- and carboxyhemoglobin, and they may not give reliable values. In the presence of carboxyhemoglobin, oxygen saturations calculated from the $PaO_2$ alone are inaccurate and misleading.

Initial chest radiographs are mandatory. Although they may at first be normal even in patients with pulmonary injury, they should be obtained to rule out the occasionally treatable abnormality. Furthermore, they serve as baseline films for later comparison. Early films may reveal subtle signs of interstitial edema such as perivascular fuzziness and peribronchial cuffing, which are often manifest during the first 24 hours.[78]

A recent review suggests that a widened vascular pedicle documented on serial chest films predicts which patients will develop pulmonary edema.[79] Pulmonary function tests are helpful in assessing the presence of airway obstruction but can be reasonably done only on nonintubated patients. If possible, a flow-volume loop should be obtained. This is a graph of respiratory flow rates plotted against lung volumes obtained from a forced vital capacity maneuver. It is a sensitive, noninvasive way of assessing for both upper and lower airway obstruction. If flow-volume measures are not available, a peak expiratory flow rate (PEFR) and forced expiratory volume in one second ($FEV_1$), both measured with a single handheld inexpensive piece of equipment, should be obtained. Although without the visual pattern suggestive of airway obstruction seen on the flow-volume loop, PEFR (in L/sec) depressed out of proportion to the $FEV_1$ (0.6 PEFR < $FEV_1$) is also suggestive of upper airway obstruction.

In patients with inhalation or facial burn injury, the respiratory tract airway should be visualized by laryngeal mirror, laryngoscopy, or bronchoscopy for evidence of injury. If an endoscopist is not immediately available, initial evaluation should be completed with a flashlight and mirror. In patients without an obvious need for intubation, but in whom there is a high suspicion of substantial inhalation injuries such as seen with facial burns, singed eyes, or carbonaceous sputum, bronchoscopy should be considered. Endoscopy is also a direct means of assessing airway patency.

Xenon-133 lung scanning may be undertaken to diagnose inhalation injury.[80] Inhalation injury is suggested by a delayed clearance of $^{133}$Xe and inequality in its pattern of clearance. Pre-existing lung disease, however, may yield false-positive results. Although patient co-operation is not necessary to perform this study, patients for whom the scan might be considered are often too ill to justify moving them to the radiology suite.

In a sense bronchoscopy and $^{133}$Xe scanning may be considered complementary procedures. Bronchoscopy identifies large airway injury, and $^{133}$Xe scanning reveals smaller airway injury. $^{133}$Xe scanning will not detect upper airway injury until almost complete obstruction has occurred, whereas bronchoscopy gives no direct indication of distal airway damage. The presence of positive or negative signs at bronchoscopy does not necessarily reflect changes at the small airway or alveolar level.

## Treatment

There are few hard and fast rules of management in patients known or suspected to have pulmonary damage in the setting of burn or inhalation injury. Two principles, however, are paramount. First, an adequate airway must be maintained or established if not already present. Second, 100 per cent oxygen should be supplied at the earliest possible moment. If the patient is comatose, then intubation to deliver a high concentration of $O_2$ should be done, as face mask $O_2$ usually has an $FIO_2$ of only about 0.6. Initial treatment with 100 per cent inspired oxygen reflects the fact that the half-life of carboxyhemoglobin is approximately five hours at an $FIO_2$ of 0.21, which is room air. Breathing oxygen with an $FIO_2$ of 1.0 will significantly decrease this half-life to less than one hour, thus restoring adequate tissue oxygenation at the earliest possible moment. Hyperbaric chambers capable of delivering 100 per cent oxygen at three atmospheres of pressure will aid in the treatment of carbon monoxide poisoning by further shortening the half-life of carboxyhemoglobin to 25 minutes. The overall utility of this modality has not been assessed in a prospective manner.[81]

One hundred per cent oxygen therapy should be continued for at least two hours or until carboxyhemoglobin and $O_2$ saturation levels are known.[12] In certain patients with chronic obstructive pulmonary disease and a history of carbon dioxide retention, the high $FIO_2$ may decrease, since these patients are dependent upon hypoxic drive to maintain adequate ventilation. If a history of $CO_2$ retention is known, then these patients should be intubated prophylactically.

Intubation as a matter of routine should also be considered in all comatose patients as well as those who have an altered sensorium or depressed gag reflex. Further, patients who may exhibit evidence of mild obstruction by either the flow-volume loops or clinical assessment should be monitored closely, since mild airway obstruction can become very severe in a matter of minutes. If upper airway narrowing proceeds from a moderately narrowed 7-mm passage, which may be asymptomatic, to a 4-mm airway, there will be a precipitous fall in achievable peak flow rates (Fig. 3–3).[19] This can lead to acute respiratory failure, even in alert patients. Clinical signs that may herald severe upper airway obstruction are increasing tachypnea, dyspnea, and hoarseness. In these patients, intubation should be undertaken electively.

In burn patients and patients with inhalation injury, airway patency is best assured by either orotracheal or nasotracheal intubation rather than tracheostomy, even if a long-term artificial airway is anticipated. The reasons for this are higher rates of infection and complications such as tracheal stenosis and tracheomalacia in patients with tracheostomies.[82] In one recent prospective study, permanent upper airway sequelae such as tracheal stenosis were related to an increased duration of tube placement and high cuff pressure. High-volume, low-pressure endotracheal tube cuffs are recommended.[83]

Once airway patency is established, further treatment depends on the severity of injury. For patients who have had only mild injury by laboratory and clinical assessment, humidification and usual pulmonary toilet may suffice. For patients with moderate injury, e.g., bronchospasm, frequent suctioning and bronchodilators should be included in the regimen. Bronchoscopy should be considered to assess the patient for signs of more serious inhalation damage and airway obstruction. Patients with mild and moderate obstruction who were intubated prophylactically may not require mechanical ventilation or an increased $FIO_2$ if carboxyhemoglobin levels are known to be nontoxic. In patients who are intubated, some prophylactic end-expiratory pressure may be necessary, since bypassing the glottis by intubation converts alveolar pressure to atmospheric, perhaps facilitating edema formation.[84] Some experimental data in dogs suggest that continuous positive airway pressure (CPAP) may improve pulmonary function and gas exchange, but the data are not conclusive.[85]

In patients with severe lung injury such as seen with facial burn or evidence of high carboxyhemoglobin levels, intubation and mechanical ventilation with positive end-expiratory pressure (PEEP) may be necessary. PEEP may help to decrease atelectasis and lower right-to-left shunt, thus decreasing requirements for high $FIO_2$ beyond the initial period.

The role of Swan-Ganz catheterization in burn patients is controversial. Some authorities favor placement of the catheter to monitor fluid status and optimize management. However, these patients are at risk for complications of catheter placement such as endocarditis,[86] line sepsis, and perhaps pulmonary emboli. Pulmonary artery catheterization should thus be reserved for specific indications. Often the catheter can be quickly removed after confirming that the pulmonary capillary wedge pressure is not elevated.

Those patients who are severely ill require serial arterial blood gas determinations. An arterial line should therefore be inserted at the outset, even if this requires traversing a burned area. In this case, inserting the catheter will become more difficult with time, while blood gas determinations will remain essential.

The technology for extravascular lung water (EVLW) measured by double indicator technique is operational, and EVLW determinations may become a measurement that can readily be performed in the Intensive Care Unit.[48, 87, 89] Whether this will have an impact on management and survival is unknown. For the present, these techniques are investigational.

Patients not admitted to the hospital should be advised that symptoms may develop up to two days after the fire. They should be instructed to return to the hospital at the first sign of distress, since mild airway obstruction can change quickly to very severe obstruction.

Current practice indicates that fluid resuscitation should be given to maintain adequate end-organ perfusion and urine output. The ideal fluid for resuscitation remains controversial, although there is increasing evidence for the beneficial effects of early use of colloid.[88] Other studies, however, indicate that the use of crystalloid does not necessarily lead to an increase in extravascular lung water; rather, an increase in EVLW might be a function of the severity of inhalation injury. Related to this is the observation that the presence of inhalation injury in burn patients increases fluid and sodium requirements by 30 to 40 per cent.[90] A recent study comparing high-dose fluid volume resuscitation in sheep with inhalation injury against normal-volume replacement in sheep with inhalation injury and in sham controls demonstrated that at 12 hours following inhalation injury the animals who received high-dose fluid resuscitation were not different from the sham controls with respect to lung lymph flow, lymph/plasma protein ratios, and cardiac output.[91] However, the animals who received inhalation injury and maintenance fluid replacement had a significantly higher lung lymph flow, L/P protein ratio, and lower cardiac output, as well as an increased mortality, suggesting that a low cardiac output may play a role in the development of noncardiogenic pulmonary edema seen after inhalation injury. The authors postulate that polymorphonuclear leukocytes may play a role in the development of vascular permeability, since an increased cardiac output results in increased shear rates in the pulmonary vasculature, which would tend to favor decreased margination of neutrophils in the vascular bed. With a depressed cardiac output, as in hypovolemia, there would be an increased margination of polymorphonuclear leukocytes which would serve as a focus for initiation of vascular injury as described earlier.

The use of steroids in burn or inhalation injury remains controversial. Moylan, in an N.I.H. consensus conference, concluded that their use should be avoided, since the rate of mortality in a group of 17 patients who received high-dose methylprednisolone for 48 hours was four times that of controls.[92] A prospective study of 225 patients with inhalation injury sustained in hotel fires in Nevada failed to document any beneficial effects from steroid therapy.[93] In an in vitro study in rats who received surface burns, steroids were shown to decrease white cell agglutination in the mesenteric microvasculature but had no effect on edema formation in organs as measured by wet/dry weight ratios.[94] Recently, Beeley et al observed increased survival after steroid treatment in rabbits given acrolein to produce inhalation injury.[95] Interestingly, however, there was no histopathological correlation with steroid treatment; the controls and steroid-treated groups had similar evidence of pulmonary damage. The reasons for this increase in survival are not clear, and further investigation is required.

Prophylactic antibiotics should not be given.[72] Rather, frequent sputum Gram's stains should be monitored and treatment begun based on the appearance of organisms and polymorphonuclear leukocytes in the sputum. Broad coverage and "shotgun" therapy should be avoided, since the occurrence of pneumonia and related respiratory pathogens replicates the environment of the patient (the microbiology of the ICU) and the organisms cultured from the wounds.

Bronchodilators may be useful in treating airway obstruction if present, although no studies address this issue specifically in victims of fires and inhalation injury. If wheezing is present on the physical examination or airway obstruction is documented by the flow-volume loop, we recommend treatment with inhaled beta-agonists delivered via a nebulizer as the first line of treatment. Albuterol, 0.5 ml/2.5 cc normal saline, or metaproterenol (Alupent), 0.3 cc/2.5 cc normal saline every 4 to 6 hours, should suffice if there is no co-existent coronary disease. If coronary artery disease is present, reduced doses may be utilized. The additional use of methylxanthines provides some minimal therapeutic efficacy, especially in cases of more severe bronchospasm. Intravenous administration of aminophylline, 0.4 to 0.9 ml/hr, is preferred over oral theophylline, since a steady-state concentration is attained sooner. An initial loading dose of 5 mg/kg body weight is necessary. Additionally, serum levels of theophylline may be readily monitored to attain a therapeutic nontoxic serum level (10 to 20 mg/dl).

For patients in whom no contraindication exists, minidose heparin (5000 units subcutaneously every 12 hours) should be given in an effort to reduce the risk of venous thrombosis and resultant pulmonary emboli in patients who undergo prolonged bedrest.

## Prognosis for Survivors of Fire-Related Lung Injury

The long-term prognosis is generally good, although few data specifically address this issue. Pulmonary function tests in the days following inhalation injury show both mild obstructive and restrictive defects.[4] The latter may be due to atelectasis and elevated diaphragms (especially with ileus) as well as to circumferential scars that constrict and decrease thoracic ribcage expansion. For those patients with restricting scars, distant in time from the original burn, surgical release of the scar results in return of normal pulmonary function. With resolution of noncardiogenic pulmonary edema associated with burns and inhalation injury, the prognosis for return of lung function is similarly optimistic. Again, however, follow-up data are limited.

## SUMMARY

The pulmonary complications of burns and inhalation injury can be divided into three distinct syndromes on the basis of clinical features and temporal pattern of occurrence. Early, carbon monoxide poisoning, airway obstruction, and pulmonary edema are the major concerns. The adult respiratory distress syndrome (ARDS) is usually clinically evident between 24 and 48 hours, although it can occur later. Inhalation injury and burn injury are synergistic, and their combined effects can increase morbidity and mortality. Late complications, at days to weeks, include pneumonia, atelectasis, and pulmonary emboli. Attention should be directed by history, evidence of obvious injury, and laboratory determinations of carboxyhemoglobin, arterial blood gases, and spirometry.

Treatment should initially focus on establishing and maintaining a patent airway and ensuring adequate ventilation and oxygenation as well as general principles of medical practice. Prophylactic antibiotics and steroids are not recommended.

## REFERENCES

1. Barnes BA: Mortality of burns at MGH 1939–1954. Ann Surg 145(2):210–222, 1957.
2. Cope O, Rhinebach FW: The problems of burn shock complicated by pulmonary damage. Ann Surg 117:915, 1943.
3. Teixidor HS, Novick G, Rubin E: Pulmonary complications in burn patients. J Can Assoc Radiol 34:264–270, 1983.
4. Whitener DR, Whitener LM, Robertson KJ, et al: Pulmonary function measurement in patients with thermal injury and smoke inhalation. Am Rev Respir Dis 122:731–739, 1980.
5. Achauer BM, Allyn PA, Furnas DW, Bartlett RH: Pulmonary complications of burns: The major threat to the burn patient. Ann Surg 177:311–319, 1973.
6. Zawaki BE, Jung RC, Joyce J, Rincon E: Smoke, burns, and the natural history of inhalation injury in fire victims. Ann Surg 185:100–110, 1977.
7. Bartlett RH: Types of respiratory injury. J Trauma 19:918, 1979.
8. Pruitt BA, DiVincenti FC, Mason AD Jr, et al: The occurrence and significance of pneumonia and other pulmonary complications in burned patients: Comparison of conventional and topical treatments. J Trauma 10:519–531, 1970.
9. Moritz AR: The effects of inhaled heat on the air passages of the lung: An experimental investigation. Am J Pathol 21:311–317, 1945.
10. Crapo RO: Smoke inhalation injuries. JAMA 246:1694–1695, 1981.
11. Trunkey DD: Inhalation injury. Surg Clin North Am 58:1133–1140, 1978.
12. Fein A, Leff A, Hopewell PC: Pathophysiology and management of the complications resulting from fire and the inhaled products of combustion. Crit Care Med 8:94–98, 1980.
13. Zikria BA, Budd DG, Flock F: What is clinical smoke poisoning? Ann Surg 81:151–156, 1975.
14. Chance B, Erecinska M, Wagner M: Mitochondrial response to carbon monoxide poison. Ann NY Acad Sci 174:193, 1970.
15. Dyer RF, Esch VH: Polyvinyl chloride toxicity in fire fighters: Hydrogen chloride toxicity in fire fighters. JAMA 235:393–397, 1976.
16. Morikawa T: Acrolein, formaldehyde and volatile fatty acids from smoldering combustion. J Combust Toxicol 3:135–150, 1976.
17. Treitman RD, Burgess WA, Gold A: Air contaminants encountered by fire fighters. Am Indust Hygiene Assoc J 41:796–802, 1980.
18. Warner A: Clinical aspects of mucociliary clearance. Am Rev Respir Dis 116:73, 1977.
19. Al-Bazzaz F, Grillo H, Kazemi H: Response to exercise in upper airway obstruction. Am Rev Respir Dis 111:631, 1975.
20. Zikria BA, Ferrer JM, Fluch HF: The chemical factors contributing to pulmonary damage in "smoke poisoning." Surgery 71:704–709, 1972.
21. Nieman GF, Clark WR, Stennis DW, Weff WR: The effect of smoke inhalation on pulmonary surfactant. Ann Surg 191:171–181, 1980.
22. Zhi-Yuan L, Ngao L, Pei-Feng C, et al: Pulmonary surfactant activity after severe steam inhalation injury in rabbits. Burns 12:330–336, 1986.
23. Wynne JW: Aspiration pneumonitis: Correlation of experimental models with clinical disease. Clin Chest Med 3:25–34, 1982.
24. Hales CA, Barkin PW, Jung W, et al: Synthetic smoke with acrolein but not HCl produces pulmonary edema. J Appl Physiol 64:(3):1121–133, 1988.
25. Pietra GG, Szidor JP, Carpenter HA, Fishman AP: Bronchial venular leakage during endotoxin shock. Am J Pathol 77:387–406, 1974.
26. Joris I, DeGirolami U, Wortham K, Majno G: Vascular labeling with monastral blue B. Stain Technol 57:177–183, 1982.
27. Herndon DN, Traber DL, Niehaus GD, et al: The pathophysiology of smoke inhalation in a sheep model. J Trauma 24:1044–1051, 1984.

28. Traber DL, Herndon DN, Stein MD, et al: The pulmonary lesion of smoke inhalation in an ovine model. Circ Shock 18:311–323, 1986.
29. Grundfest CC, Chang J, Newcombe D: Acrolein: A potent modulator of lung macrophage arachidonic acid metabolism. Biochem Biophys Acta 713:149–159, 1982.
30. Head JM: Inhalation injury in burns. Am J Surg 139:508–512, 1980.
31. Hatherill JR, Till GO, Bruner LH, Ward PA: Thermal injury, intravascular hemolysis, and toxic oxygen products. J Clin Invest 78:629–638, 1986.
32. Heideman M: The effect of thermal injury on hemodynamic, respiratory and hematologic variables in relation to complement activation. J Trauma 19:239–247, 1979.
33. Morgan A, Knight D, O'Connor N: Lung water changes after thermal burn. Ann Surg 187:288–293, 1978.
34. Stone HH, Martin JD: Pulmonary injury associated with thermal burns. Surg Gynecol Obstet 129:1242–1246, 1969.
35. Tranbaugh RF, Lewis F, Christensen JM, Elings VB: Lung water changes after thermal injury. Ann Surg 192:479–490, 1980.
36. Brigham KL, Meyrick B: Interactions of granulocytes with the lungs. Circ Res 54:623–635, 1984.
37. Brigham KL, Owen PJ: Increased sheep lung vascular permeability caused by histamine. Circ Res 37:647–657, 1975.
38. Demling RH: Burns. N Engl J Med 313:1389–1398, 1985.
39. Demling RH: Role of prostaglandins in acute pulmonary microvascular injury. Ann NY Acad Sci Vol 384: 517–534, 1982.
40. Gelfand J, Donelan M, Hawiger A, Burke J: Alternative complement pathway activation increases mortality in a model of burn injury in mice. J Clin Invest 70:1170–1176, 1982.
41. Gelfand J, Donelan M, Burke J: Preferential activation and depletion of the alternative complement pathway by burn injury. Ann Surg 198:58–62, 1983.
42. Sacks T, Moldow C, Craddock P, et al: Oxygen radicals mediate endothelial cell damage by complement-stimulated granulocytes: An in vitro model of immune vascular damage. J Clin Invest 61:1161–1167, 1978.
43. Staub NC, Schultz EL, Albertine KH: Leukocytes and pulmonary vascular injury. Ann NY Acad Sci 384:332–342, 1982.
44. Till GO, Beauchamp C, Menapalc D, et al: Oxygen radical dependent lung damage following thermal injury of rat skin. J Trauma 23:269–277, 1983.
45. Till GO, Johnson K, Kunkel R, Ward P: Intravascular activation of complement and acute lung injury: Depending on neutrophils and toxioxygen metabolites. J Clin Invest 69:1126–1135, 1982.
46. Demling RH, Wong C, Jin EJ, et al: Early lung dysfunction after major burns: Role of edema and vasoactive mediators. J Trauma 25:959–966, 1985.
47. Hechtman HB, Valeri CR, Shepro D: Role of humoral mediators in adult respiratory distress syndrome. Chest 86:623–627, 1984.
48. Tranbaugh RF, Elings VB, Christensen JM, Lewis FR: Effect of inhalation injury on lung water accumulation. J Trauma 23:597–604, 1983.
49. Hales CA, Sonne L, Peterson M, et al: Role of thromboxane and prostacyclin in pulmonary vasomotor changes after endotoxin in dogs. J Clin Invest 68:497–505, 1981.
50. Statton GW, Snider MT, Hales CA, Watkins WD: Low dose endotoxin in vivo results in hydroxyl radical formation and stimulation of prostaglandin release. Am Rev Respir Dis 123:199, 1981.
51. Perkowski SZ, Havill AM, Flynn JT, Gee MH: Role of intrapulmonary release of eicosanoids and superoxide anion as mediators of pulmonary dysfunction and endothelial injury in sheep with intermittent complement activation. Circ Res 53:574–583, 1983.
52. Demling RH, Well JA, Bolzer FO: Effect of thermal injury on the pulmonary microcirculation. Surgery 83:746–751, 1978.
53. Nerlich M, Flynn J, Demling RH: Effect of thermal injury on endotoxin-induced lung injury. Surgery 93:171–181, 1980.
54. Foley FD, Moncrief JA, Mason AD: Pathology of the lung in fatally burned patients. Ann Surg 167:251–264, 1968.
55. Nash G, Foley FD, Langlinais PC: Pulmonary interstitial edema and hyaline membranes in adult burn patients. Human Pathol 5:149–160, 1974.
56. Socher FM, Mallory GK: Lung lesions in patients dying of burns. Arch Pathol 75:303–308, 1963.
57. Laufe MD, Simon RH, Flint A, Keller JB: ARDS in neutropenic patients. Am J Med 80:1022–1026, 1986.

58. Ognibene FP, Martin SE, Parker MM, et al: ARDS in patients with severe neutropenia. N Engl J Med 315:547–551, 1986.
59. Rinaldo JE, Sorovetz H: Deterioration of oxygenation and abnormal lung microvascular permeability during resolution of leukopenia in patients with diffuse lung injury. Am Rev Respir Dis 131:579–583, 1985.
60. Dyer EL, Snapper JR: Role of circulating granulocytes in sheep lung injury produced by phorbol myristate acetate. J Appl Physiol 60(2):576–589, 1986.
61. Rowland RR, Yamayuchi KT, Santibanel AS, et al: Smoke inhalation model for lung permeability studies. J Trauma 26(2):153, 1986.
62. Pruitt BA, Flemma RJ, DiVincenti FC, et al: Pulmonary complications in burn patients. J Thorac Cardiovasc Surg 59:7–20, 1970.
63. Munster AM, Eurenius K, Katz RM, et al: Cell-mediated immunity after thermal injury. Ann Surg 177:139–143, 1973.
64. Miller CL, Baker CC: Changes in lymphocyte activity after thermal injury. J Clin Invest 63:202–210, 1979.
65. Munster AM: Immunologic response of trauma and burns. Am J Med 76(3A):142–145, 1984.
66. Wood JJ, O'Mahoney JB, Rodrick ML, et al: Abnormalities of antibody production after thermal injury. Arch Surg 121:108–115, 1986.
67. Goodwin JS, Bromberg S, Staszak C, et al: Effect of physical stress on sensitivity of lymphocytes to inhibition by prostaglandin $E_2$. J Immunol 127:518–522, 1981.
68. Constantian WB: Association of sepsis with an immunosuppressive polypeptide in the serum of burn patients. Ann Surg 188:209–215, 1978.
69. Wolfe J, Saporoschitz A, Young A, et al: Suppressive serum, suppressor lymphocytes and death from burns. Ann Surg 193:513–520, 1981.
70. Thompson PB, Herndon DN, Traber DL, Abston S: Effect on mortality of inhalation injury. J Trauma 26:163–165, 1986.
71. Astry CL, Jakab GJ: The effects of acrolein exposure on pulmonary antibacterial defenses. Toxicol Appl Pharmacol 67:49–54, 1982.
72. Pruitt BA, McManus AT: Opportunistic infection in severely burned patients. Am J Med 76(3A):146–154, 1984.
73. Shirani KZ, McManus AT, Vaughan GM, et al: Effects of environment on infection in burn patients. Arch Surg 121:31–36, 1986.
74. Coleman JB, Chang FC: Pulmonary embolism: An unrecognized event in severely burned patients. Am J Surg 130:697–699, 1975.
75. Curreli PW, Kate AJ, Gotin LN, Pruitt BA: Coagulation abnormalities in the thermally injured patient. Curr Top Surg Res 2:401, 1970.
76. Li JJ, Hales CA, Sanders L, et al: C-reactive protein elevations in ARDS interfere with surfactant function. Clin Res 32(2):468A, 1985.
77. Wroblewski DA, Bower GC: The significance of facial burns in acute smoke inhalation. Crit Care Med 7:335–338, 1979.
78. Teixidor HS, Rubin E, Novick GS, Alonso DR: Smoke inhalation: Radiographic manifestations. Radiology 149:383–387, 1983.
79. Haponik EF, Adelman M, Munster AM, Bleecker ER: Increased vascular pedicle width preceding burn-related pulmonary edema. Chest 90:649–655, 1986.
80. Moylan JA, Wilmore DW, Mouton DE, Pruitt BA: Early diagnosis of inhalation injury using [133]Xenon lung scan. Ann Surg 176:477–484, 1972.
81. Hart GB, Strauss WB, Lennon PA, Whitcraft DD: Treatment of smoke inhalation by hyperbaric oxygen. J Emerg Med 3:211–215, 1985.
82. Eckhauser FE, Billote J, Burke JF, Quinby WC: Tracheostomy complicating massive burn injury: A plea for conservation. Am J Surg 126:418–423, 1974.
83. Lund T, Goodwin CW, McManus WF, et al: Upper airway sequelae in burn patients requiring endotracheal intubation or tracheostomy. Ann Surg 201(3):374–382, 1985.
84. Mathay M, Venus B, Rao TLK, Matsuda T: Non-cardiac pulmonary edema precipitated by tracheal intubation in patients with inhalation injuries. Crit Care Med 11:804–806, 1983.
85. Davies LK, Poulton TJ, Modell JH: Continuous positive airway pressure is beneficial in treatment of smoke inhalation. Crit Care Med 11:726–729, 1983.
86. Ehrie M, Morgan AP, Moore FD, O'Connor NE: Endocarditis with the indwelling balloon tipped pulmonary artery catheter in burn patients. J Trauma 18:664–666, 1978.

87. Lewis FR, Elings VB, Sturm JA: Bedside measurement of lung water. J Surg Res 27:250–261, 1979.
88. Trautman ED: Assessment and implications of pulmonary edema. *In* Gravenstein JS, Newbower RS, Ream AK, Smith N (eds): Integrated Approaches to Monitoring. Boston, Butterworths, 1983, pp 79–97.
89. Peitzman AB, Shires III GT, Corbett WA, et al: Measurement of lung water in inhalation injury. Surgery 90:305–312, 1981.
90. Navar PD, Saffle JR, Warden GD: Effect of inhalation injury on fluid resuscitation requirements after thermal injury. Am J Surg 150:716–720, 1985.
91. Herndon DN, Traber DL, Traber LD: The effect of resuscitation on inhalation injury. Surgery 100:248–251, 1986.
92. NIH Consensus Conference. J Trauma 19(11):855–936, 1979.
93. Robinson NB, Hudson LD, Klein M, et al: Steroid therapy following isolated smoke inhalation injury. J Trauma 22:876–879, 1982.
94. Ferguson M, Eriksson E, Robson MC: Effect of methylprednisolone on edema formation after lung injury. Burns 5:293–298, 1978.
95. Beeley JM, Crow J, Jones JG, et al: Mortality and lung histopathology after inhalation lung injury: The effect of corticosteroids. Am Rev Respir Dis 133:191–196, 1986.
96. Mellins R: Respiratory complications of smoke inhalation in victims of fires. J Pediatr 87:1–7, 1975.

# 4

# Management of Upper Airway Following Burns

N. GOUDSOUZIAN and S. K. SZYFELBEIN

One of the major causes of morbidity and mortality from thermal accidents is injury to the airways.[1, 2] Such injuries are estimated to cause 4000 to 8000 deaths in the United States alone. In a busy burn center, about one third of the patients admitted with acute burns have this associated complication.[3, 4] The mortality attributable to an inhalation burn injury restricted to the respiratory tract is quite low (in the range of 5 to 10 per cent) but doubles or even quadruples when combined with a large cutaneous injury.[5-7]

## PATHOPHYSIOLOGY

The clinical picture of injury to the upper airway is frequently complex; a victim might inhale a variety of toxic gases, be severely burned externally, have associated injuries or fractures, or aspirate stomach contents. All will have an important bearing on prognosis and course of treatment. The toxic agents and the mechanism by which these cause damage to the upper airway have been described in Chapter 3 on "Pulmonary Disorders in the Burn Patient."

The pathological changes seen in the respiratory tract after a thermal inhalation injury vary according to the type and extent of the injury. They do, however, follow a certain pattern.[8, 9] The initial serious effect of smoke inhalation is asphyxia. The fire consumes the oxygen present in its immediate area and replaces it with such products of combustion as $CO_2$, CO, and smoke. The resultant decreased inspired oxygen concentration causes the victim to hyperventilate.

The acute response of the body to a thermal injury is edema. This edema occurs usually in and around the area of direct heat injury, but in extensive burns (more than 30 per cent of total body surface area [TBSA]) it extends away from the site of injury and includes the respiratory tract. When there is superimposed inhalation injury, marked edema and congestion of the bronchi result, causing luminal narrowing and severe airway obstruction. Bronchospasm can also occur from direct chemical irritation of the mucosa or by a reflex mechanism.[1, 5] In severe forms of injury, tracheobronchial mucosal sloughing and necrosis take place, with the possibility of airway obstruction within a few hours.[11]

The edema of the lower respiratory tract and alveoli results in decreased pulmonary compliance and increased work of breathing. The fluid formation in the lungs leads to an increased alveolar-arterial gradient. In conjunction with upper airway swelling, the pulmonary pathology leads to greater hypoxia and a further deterioration of cardiopulmonary status, which may culminate in pulmonary edema and result in acute respiratory distress syndrome.[9, 12]

The victim of a burn injury may also initially suffer from the effects of carbon monoxide (CO) inhalation.[13] Because the burn victim may be swollen or covered with soot, the cherry red appearance of CO poisoning may not be discernible. Any evaluation of the victim should take this into account. At this early stage, the possibility of cyanide poisoning should also be considered.[14]

Cutaneous burns of the face and neck may adversely affect the airway, even within a few hours. This is frequently seen with scald burns. Burns of the neck and upper chest impede the lymphatic flow of the pharyngeal structures, producing edema and precipitating respiratory obstruction.[15] In addition, edema of the face and neck limits the victim's ability to move and open his mouth and may thus interfere with the clinical management of the airway.

Edema of the upper airways is of more concern in children than in adults because of the smaller dimension of their airways. Since resistance to flow is inversely proportional to the fourth power of the radius of the tube, decreasing the radius by half will increase resistance to flow 16 times. In an infant with a tracheal diameter of 4 mm, 1 mm of edema of the mucous membrane will increase the resistance to flow 16 times and decrease the cross-sectional area by 75 per cent; a similar 1 mm of edema in an adult will increase resistance only three times and decrease the cross-sectional area by 44 per cent.[16]

A deep circumferential burn of the thorax and/or abdomen restricts chest wall motion and thus precipitates respiratory failure. In addition, the development of firm, noncompliant, and constricting eschar in the presence of underlying edema markedly limits respiratory movements. This condition is usually aggravated by the presence of ileus, which further impairs the movement of the diaphragm. Escharotomy, which is axial incision of the nonyielding eschar deep to the fascial layer, releases this tightness and allows the patient to breathe more freely (Fig. 4–1).[17] Full-thickness escharotomy should extend along the length of the eschar. This procedure does not require anesthesia and can be performed at the bedside; adequate incision is evidenced by the separation of the overlying eschar and appearance of subcutaneous tissue, called "gapping."[18–20]

## CLINICAL ASSESSMENT

As soon as the patient arrives in the emergency area, all important information should be gathered. If the patient is unable to communicate, the rescue team and, if possible, the family should be questioned. It is imperative to know the location and the type of fire, the presence and extent of associated injury,

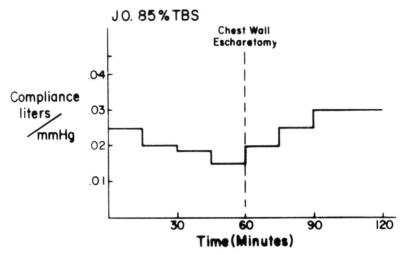

**FIGURE 4–1.** Compliance changes in a patient with circumferential burns of the chest. Because of the eschar and edema, compliance decreases with time; when an escharotomy is performed, compliance improves.

level of consciousness, and evidence of aspiration. It is also important to ascertain past medical history.

The classic signs of respiratory burns are singed nasal hairs, sooty sputum, soot in the pharynx, and burns of the face or the inside of the mouth.[5, 11, 21] None of the signs by itself is conclusive, but the presence of more than one sign strongly indicates inhalation injury. Facial burns are seen in only two thirds of inhalation injuries. Half of the patients produce carbonaceous sputum. Hoarseness is present less than 25 per cent of the time, while singed nasal hairs are an even less accurate indicator.[22, 23] Other important associated clinical findings are wheezing, dyspnea, cough, tachypnea, rales, and rhonchi.[11, 24] Complaint of chest pain or chest "tightness" usually indicates a severe inhalation injury.[21, 25]

Arterial oxygen tensions tend to be lower in the presence of inhalation injury.[12] By the time the patient arrives at the hospital, his initial hypoxia has usually been minimized by the administration of oxygen during transport. Arterial blood gases can thus be within normal limits. These patients can, however, decompensate rapidly. Changes in blood gases generally precede change seen on the chest radiograph.

Spirometry, if available, can help in identifying airway injuries in cooperative patients. Diminution of expiratory flow rates and lung volumes commonly occurs[26, 27]; hence the flow volume curves detect abnormal inspiratory and expiratory patterns with diminution of peak and expiratory flow rates as well as patterns of extrathoracic obstruction.[15]

In some centers, fiberoptic bronchoscopy is extensively used in the diagnosis of inhalation burn injury.[28, 31] The criteria for diagnosis of respiratory burn include mucosal erythema, edema, ulceration, hemorrhagic necrosis, and carbonaceous sputum. However, erythema or edema may be absent in a hypotensive patient; conversely, the presence of edema is not pathognomonic of airway burns. In mild cases, the lumen is not compromised by the edema of the upper airways. With a more serious injury, swelling is severe enough that the vocal cords are not visible because of the prolapse of the false vocal cords into the lumen of the larynx.[12] Once the false cords bulge together in the midline, the obstruction is complete.

In experienced hands, fiberoptic bronchoscopy carries a minimal risk. Its use to determine the extent and severity of the burn injury allows imminent upper airway obstruction to be detected so that endotracheal intubation can be justified and carried out.[30, 31] It is also helpful in removing debris and inspissated secretions. The value of fiberoptic bronchoscopy depends, of course, on the experience of the person performing it. It should be stressed that patients can be treated adequately without diagnostic bronchoscopy and that the lack of small fiberoptic bronchoscopes limits its use in small children.

## MANAGEMENT OF THE AIRWAYS FOLLOWING A BURN INJURY

Patients with severe inhalation burn injury require steadfast attention. The physician must evaluate rapidly the respiratory status of the patient, ascertain the extent of burn injury, and thoroughly evaluate the patient, remembering that the presence of burn does not preclude other injuries. A mild injury in the absence of physical signs of obstruction should require only careful periodic evaluation of the airway and administration of humidified oxygen. The administration of racemic epinephrine may also help. In a severe case of airway injury, the burn victim will have a rapidly increasing airflow resistance from edema and spasm of the bronchi. If respirations are failing and stridor, severe dyspnea, and tightness of the chest are present, the airway should be secured early by an endotracheal tube and supported ventilation should follow. Under these dire circumstances, or whenever there is doubt about the severity of the injury, the airway should be protected at once (Fig. 4–2). Patients with extensive injury to the face and neck should also be treated in this manner. Experience has demonstrated that prophylactic intubation eliminates fatal complications of upper airway obstruction in the first 72 hours of the post-burn period.[21]

## ENDOTRACHEAL INTUBATION

Guidelines for endotracheal intubation are broad. Difficulty should be expected because the airway structures may be swollen and covered with soot. A patient's condition may worsen very quickly, and repeated instrumentation will aggravate swelling and cause bleeding from damaged mucosa. It is of critical

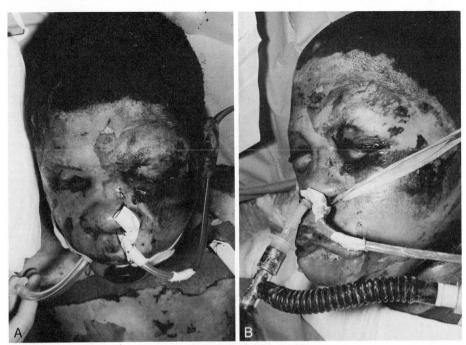

**FIGURE 4–2.** Swelling of face following a head and neck burn. *A*, Patient on admission to hospital with an orotracheal tube. Shortly after admission to hospital the orotracheal tube was changed to a nasotracheal tube. *B*, Face and neck 8 hours after burn. Note the marked swelling of the area, including intraoral structures; endotracheal intubation is virtually impossible at this stage. Thus early intubation is mandatory.

importance, then, that endotracheal intubation be carried out by an experienced practitioner as deftly and efficiently as possible.

The requisite equipment for safely managing endotracheal intubation under these circumstances is the following:

1. Face masks: Masks of various sizes need to be available. Most helpful are the transparent kind with a soft inflatable cushion (Fig. 4–3). These masks fit more easily to the contour of a swollen face.

2. Laryngoscopes of various sizes and types: The curved (McIntosh) type is probably the blade of choice for most clinicians. Although this blade is generally less traumatic, it does not always provide adequate exposure. If this is the case, a straight (Miller) blade should be employed. The straight blade is particularly helpful when the mouth cannot be fully opened due to edema and contracture. This blade can also be used to good effect in infants and small children because of the high position of the larynx and further, in infants, to lift the epiglottis if it interferes with one's view. The choice of laryngoscope is ultimately a matter of personal preference, depending upon the experience of the individual.

3. Endotracheal tubes: Several tubes should be available. A large-bore tube

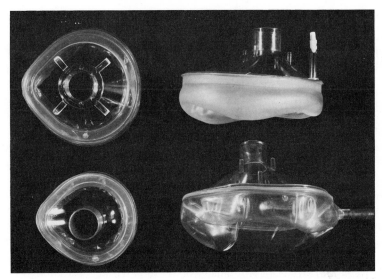

**FIGURE 4–3.** Face masks with inflatable cushions. These are useful in patients with facial burns and/or scars, since they more easily fit the varying contours of the face.

may help in the aspiration of tracheobronchial secretions, but a smaller tube might be better employed to avoid unnecessary trauma. We tend to use cuffed endotracheal tubes even in children because of the frequent need for high positive end-expiratory pressures. When the patient does not need high positive pressures, the cuff should be deflated. Cuffed tubes also provide a guard against the tendency to inflate the stomach. The exception to the use of cuffed endotracheal tubes is in small children less than two years of age.

4. Oral and nasal airways.

5. A system to provide manual positive-pressure ventilation with a high concentration of oxygen. Ideally, this is best provided by an anesthetic machine or a Mapelson T-piece. Ambu bags, however, are generally discouraged, since it is difficult to achieve the high positive pressures with them.

6. Suction catheters.

7. Nasogastric tubes.

8. Magill forceps.

9. Stylet: When orotracheal intubation is attempted in the burn victim, an introducer inside the endotracheal tube is always helpful, since the swelling may diminish the area of manipulation inside the mouth. A fixed curve on the stylet helps direct the endotracheal tube toward the larynx. Care should be taken that the tip of the stylet is not protruding beyond the proximal end of the tube. If edema is not severe and cords are easily visualized, then nasal intubation is preferable. Application of topical cocaine (4 per cent) is a useful adjunct for prevention of nasal bleeding.

10. Drugs: Atropine or other antisialagogues are strongly recommended, since manipulations of the airway will increase secretions.

Thiopental or a short-acting intravenous anesthetic agent. Muscle relaxants, succinylcholine, atracurium, or vecuronium.

## Guidelines for Intubation

CARDIOVASCULAR STABILIZATION. The importance of hydration (see Chapter 2 on fluid resuscitation) in the burned patient cannot be overstressed. Accessible intravenous lines and adequate monitoring are needed. The management of the patient is much easier and safer if the cardiovascular status is stable.

MANAGEMENT OF HYPOXIA. Prior to instrumentation of the airway, adequate oxygenation of the patient is mandatory. The oxygen saturation monitor is the most helpful. It will noninvasively provide beat-to-beat information on the saturation of the arterial blood. In the emergency situation, it is important to remember that agitation is a frequent sign of hypoxia.

ANALGESIA AND SEDATION. Any analgesic or sedative agent should be titrated intravenously with a continual assessment of the patient's ventilation. It is usually started when the patient is breathing a high concentration of oxygen. In our experience, incremental doses of morphine, 0.1 mg/kg up to a dose of 0.5 mg/kg, will provide adequate sedation and analgesia. If needed, incremental doses of diazepam (0.1 mg/kg) or midazolam (0.05 mg/kg) can be added.

VENTILATION. In the early stage of management, the adequacy of respiration and the posssibility of administering positive-pressure ventilation need to be evaluated. If gentle positive-pressure ventilation can be maintained, one can safely administer anesthesia and a muscle relaxant.

ANESTHESIA. As the adequacy of respiration is ascertained, secretions from the upper airways are suctioned. During this maneuver, the reflexes and the responses of the patient can be evaluated. If the patient swallows, coughs, or moves, an inhalation anesthetic can be initiated. It is futile to attempt intubation in a moving or coughing patient. Alternatively, incremental doses of thiopental (2 mg/kg) are administered until the patient is anesthetized and his corneal reflexes ablated. It is advisable to give an antisialagogue (atropine 0.01 mg/kg or glycopyrrolate 0.005 mg/kg) if secretions are excessive; these agents will also ablate vagal reflexes.

MUSCULAR RELAXATION. If positive-pressure ventilation can be maintained, a muscle relaxant can then be administered. Our practice is to give a relatively large dose of atracurium (1 to 1.5 mg/kg) or vecuronium (0.15 to 0.2 mg/kg).[32–35a] Alternatively, pancuronium (0.15 to 0.2 mg/kg) can be used to good effect but with the expectation of a longer duration of action. If a nondepolarizing drug is unavailable, succinylcholine in the early stages of treatment (24 hours) is not contraindicated, although not recommended[32]; a dose of 2 mg/kg should suffice.

A burned patient, like any trauma victim, may have a full stomach at the time of injury; hence, the possibility of regurgitation and aspiration is ever present. Cricoid pressure may prevent regurgitation. Laryngospasm, however, would be disastrous, for if not treated immediately it causes both the hypoxia and the edema to worsen. It is therefore preferable to administer a muscle relaxant, both to ensure an immobile patient and, more importantly, to avoid laryngospasm.

**LARYNGOSCOPY.** The actual practice of laryngoscopy and intubation in the injured patient does not differ significantly from that in the electively intubated patient. It needs to be done gently but firmly, with concern for both the patient's needs and the demands of the situation. First, the head must be braced (with, for example, a firm blanket) in the best position possible. Laryngoscopy is performed with care, the presence of edema sometimes requiring a more constant force than usual. If the larynx cannot be visualized, gentle pressure on the anterior larynx is helpful. An assistant contributes by holding the larynx externally in the best position that can be managed. Unless the structures are clearly defined, the route should be orotracheal with a relatively narrow tube with a stylet.

**SECURING THE ENDOTRACHEAL TUBE.** The importance of securing the tube cannot be overemphasized; establishing an airway and then losing it a few hours later when the edema is at its peak jeopardizes the life of the patient. The usual forms of adhesive tape are not effective in the burned patient because they do not adhere adequately even to nonburned skin. Usually, a soft string ribbon (Harrington or umbilical tape) is used. It is tied at the back of the head (not the neck) and gauze padding should be added to avoid constriction of soft tissues (Fig. 4–4). Its tightness must be frequently checked, since swelling may cause the ribbon to cut into the tissues. The position of the endotracheal tube should be confirmed with a radiograph.

**NASOGASTRIC SUCTION.** Patients with extensive burns usually have ileus and distention of the abdomen. This condition may easily jeopardize cardiorespiratory status. Therefore, when the airway is secured, a nasogastric tube needs to be inserted if it is not already in place. Administration of antacids is also made possible by the presence of a nasogastric tube.

**RESPIRATORY THERAPY.** With the airway safely secured, the patient is managed as any patient with respiratory failure. Special needs, however, may require a more intensive approach. It is necessary, for example, to liquefy and remove secretions and debris. In the burned patient, sloughing casts of tissue are also to be expected. These must be removed immediately or they will cause obstruction and atelectasis. Aggressive chest physiotherapy is imperative.[36] In patients with alveolar injury, pulmonary edema can develop within 5 minutes of endotracheal intubation.[37] This is noncardiac in origin, resulting instead from a disruption of the alveolocapillary membrane integrity. Following intubation, expiratory retard by the glottis, which maintains end-expiratory pressures, is lost, resulting in pulmonary edema. Continuous positive airway pressure (CPAP) or positive end-expiratory pressure (PEEP) can reverse this condition.

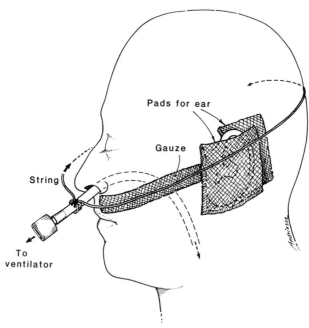

**FIGURE 4–4.** A practical way of securing the airway in burn patients. Sticky tape is not useful because of the wet surfaces. A soft ribbon is used to hold the tube and is tied around the head with gauze padding. Note also the ventral direction of the tube to avoid pressure on the nose.

## Oral Versus Nasal Endotracheal Intubation

In general, it is easier to perform endotracheal intubation through the mouth than through the nose, the main reason being that the axis of insertion of the tube is practically the same as the axis of laryngoscopy. With edema of the upper airway and larynx, attempts to pass the endotracheal tube through the nose tend to kink the endotracheal tube. Furthermore, the extent of manipulation of the tube is limited by the space and structure of the nostril. Nasal intubation can also cause bleeding. Comparatively, the mouth provides a larger area for manipulation of the tube. If, however, nasotracheal intubation can be managed, it offers several advantages. It is much better tolerated by the patient, the tube is easier to secure, and the patient cannot chew on it. If the tube must remain for longer periods of time, the laryngeal complications are less frequent than with orotracheal tubes,[38] since nasal tubes are more stable and less affected by the patient's head movements. Ulcerations of the corniculate tubercles, the arytenoid cartilages, the epiglottis, and the posterior tracheal wall, as well as paraglottic edema and the incomplete closing of the larynx seen after removal of the endotracheal tube, are most likely due to movement of the tube.

If edema has already developed, it is advisable to perform an orotracheal intubation first and then do a nasotracheal one electively. In the presence of severe swelling, or following a difficult orotracheal intubation, one should probably wait two to three days or until the edema subsides before making any change. When an orotracheal tube has been placed, it is important to keep the patient adequately sedated with or without neuromuscular blockade to prevent clamping the tube with the teeth. An oral airway can prevent the clamping, but its use for prolonged periods can cause pharyngeal ulceration.

If tracheal intubation has proved difficult previously and the endotracheal tube needs to be changed, a nasogastric tube might be usefully employed to effect a change. A relatively long small-bore, well-lubricated nasogastric tube is inserted through the tracheal tube already in place in the airway. Oxygen from a different source is connected to the nasogastric tube. Laryngoscopy is performed and the opening of the larynx is visualized as much as possible. A nasal or oral tracheal tube may then be introduced and placed in the pharynx. The endotracheal tube in the trachea is then removed, while the nasogastric tube remains in the trachea. The new endotracheal tube is now slid into the trachea next to the narrow nasogastric tube. Once the position of the new tracheal tube is confirmed, the nasogastric tube is removed. This technique provides a measure of safety: If the new tracheal tube does not pass, then the original orotracheal tube may be slid over the nasogastric tube into the trachea while oxygenation is maintained. An advantage of this maneuver is that one can more easily identify laryngeal structures with a guiding catheter in place.

## Difficult Intubation

The keys to successful intubation are familiarity with the necessary equipment and the proper preparation of the patient. In most cases, these suffice to ensure a successful procedure. Occasionally, edema is so severe that direct endotracheal intubation becomes impossible to perform and one must resort to other methods. Choosing the appropriate method should be a deliberate decision based on the pros and cons of a given situation. The ventilatory status of the patient must be closely followed throughout.

At present, the most accessible technique is fiberoptic endotracheal intubation.[30] Here, a tracheal tube is slid over the fiberoptic laryngoscope or bronchoscope. If the nasal route is used, the latter is inserted through a cocainized nostril to enter the pharynx or larynx. Once in the larynx, the nasotracheal tube may be put in place by using the fiberoptic scope as a guide.

Another useful technique involves a retrograde translaryngeal guide wire that can be inserted through the trachea or the cricothyroid membrane. The needle of a central venous catheter is inserted through the cricothyroid membrane or between the tracheal rings. The catheter is then threaded cranially and by direct laryngoscopy picked up and brought up through the mouth or, preferably, through the nose. Alternatively, a metallic J wire (Swan-Ganz introducer) can be used.[39, 40] Once the guide wire is fished out through the nostril, the endotracheal tube is threaded over it while tension is applied on the distal end of the wire. When the endotracheal tube reaches the site of perforation at the trachea, the guide wire is removed and the endotracheal tube positioned in the appropriate location. If the endotracheal tube has a side hole, the wire can be threaded over (outside in), allowing another 1 cm of space in which to direct the endotracheal tube inside the trachea.[41, 42] The guide wire can also be used to direct the fiberoptic laryngoscope in the trachea.[43] These techniques require time and skill; during manipulations, all efforts should be made to maintain the oxygenation of the patient.

Emergency cricothyroidotomy or tracheostomy is usually used as a last resort. Cricothyroidotomy seems to be more popular, since the cricothyroid membrane is more easily identifiable and becomes more prominent when the head is extended. A 12- to 14-gauge cannula can be temporarily inserted through the cricothyroid membrane and oxygen insufflated through it. The oxygen insufflation can be facilitated by attaching the barrel of a 3-ml syringe to the cannula and an 8-mm endotracheal tube adapter to the barrel of the syringe.[42] Recently, some self-contained tools have been described (Nu-Trake, Mini-trach II, Pedi-Trake) and marketed for this purpose, but it remains to be seen if they will find a place in the emergency management of critically burned patients.

In our experience, the impending need for performing tracheotomy or cricothyroidotomy has arisen several times. In each case, however, a trained laryngoscopist has been able to insert an endotracheal tube after first positioning the patient and optimizing his condition. This should not imply that emergency surgical procedures are never really indicated. It is always possible that the condition of the patient will deteriorate suddenly and that intubation will become impossible. Under these fearful circumstances, emergency procedures should be performed whatever the risks. At the very least, transtracheal insufflation may be carried out until the airway is secured. It is important to mention that blind nasotracheal intubation is unacceptable in these emergency situations. Blind attempts are also more likely to cause more damage to the mucosa and induce bleeding.

## COMPLICATIONS OF PROLONGED INTUBATION

Complications considered to be of minor consequence in patients without thermal injury can have disastrous effects in a patient with burns.

Some of the complications of prolonged nasotracheal intubation are as follows:

### EROSION OF THE NASAL ARCHES OR THE SEPTUM

This type of complication can be avoided by using smaller-sized tubes made of softer materials.[44] Sloughing of the nasal bridge can be prevented by positioning the nasotracheal tube in a caudad direction toward the mouth, rather than curving it cranially and pointing it toward the forehead (Fig. 4–4). As a further precautionary measure, whenever possible, it is advisable to alternate the naris used for intubation.

### SINUSITIS

Sinusitis can be the cause of unexplained fever in patients with a nasotracheal intubation.[45] The tube itself and the presence of edema can cause blockade of the nasal sinuses, with subsequent retention of their secretions leading to the formation of sinus-space abscesses.

### BLOCKING OF THE AUDITORY TUBE

Since the auditory (eustachian) tubes open into the nasal cavity, their blockage can lead to middle ear infection.

### EROSION OF PHARYNGEAL AND LARYNGEAL STRUCTURES

These complications seem somehow unavoidable in a patient with severe respiratory burns. It is incumbent upon the clinician, therefore, to use proper equipment such as soft tubes with soft cuffs, to pay meticulous attention to details, and to work to avoid infection. Special anatomically shaped tubes that conform better to the shape of the airways may be advantageous in diminishing ulcerations, especially in the cricoid region.[46] As indicated previously, oral airways also can cause erosions.

### TRACHEOESOPHAGEAL FISTULA

This is a dreadful complication, the most probable cause of which is high inflation pressure in the cuff of the endotracheal tube. Hence, soft pressure cuffs offer a great advantage. In certain situations, however, the intensivist finds himself in a vicious circle of damage and attempts at repair. Because of the burn, sloughing of tracheal cartilages occurs, with consequent dilatation of the trachea; higher and higher inflation pressures are thus needed to achieve an adequate seal. Ideally, the cuff should be deflated and ventilation achieved with a leak around the tube. The pulmonary status of the patient, however, may require high inflation pressures. A contributing factor in the development of tracheo-esophageal fistula is the presence of a nasogastric tube; the soft swollen tissues compressed between this and an endotracheal tube are susceptible to necrosis and sloughing. The use of small soft (Silastic) nasogastric tubes may help to avoid this complication.

Once the condition is established, it becomes extremely difficult to treat. A gastrostomy, if possible through unburned skin, will preclude the need for a nasogastric tube. If the fistula is high, a tracheotomy may be indicated. Alternatively, high-frequency ventilation can be used. The complete repair of this complication is deferred until all the wounds are healed.

### EROSION OF VASCULAR STRUCTURES

This is a rare and potentially lethal complication of prolonged endotracheal intubation. It can occur in burned tracheotomized patients with sepsis. Erosion of the tracheal wall by the endotracheal tube perforates the innominate artery, leading to massive bleeding. For treatment, the left lung is ventilated with left endobronchial intubation, while an emergency ligation of the innominate artery is performed. Usually, however, the patient succumbs from hypoxia and hemorrhagic shock.

## PROLONGED NASOTRACHEAL INTUBATION OR TRACHEOTOMY

Even as recently as 10 to 15 years ago, tracheotomy was performed whenever the need for endotracheal intubation was expected to persist for more than two days. The assumption was that it was easier to care for a patient with tracheotomy; suctioning was easy and the trauma to the pharynx and larynx was avoided.[47] The availability of less irritating endotracheal tube materials and improved tube/cuff designs have since allowed progressively longer periods of translaryngeal intubation. Nowadays three weeks or even months is not considered an unusually long period of intubation.[48]

Each route carries its own complications. Follow-up studies on nonburned patients with prolonged intubation have shown a high incidence of tracheal stenosis after tracheotomy[49]; it is actually three times higher than in patients treated with endotracheal intubation alone. The injuries reported from endotracheal intubation are due mostly to high cuff pressures,[50] whereas the stenosis following tracheotomies is mostly cicatricial, with the stenosis occurring at the site of stoma. Cuff pressure injuries are also seen with tracheotomies.[51] In general, the use of high-volume, low-pressure cuffs with low tracheal loading forces decreases but does not abolish the incidence of cuff-related injuries.[51–54] In small children, uncuffed tubes with larger internal diameters can be usefully employed beyond the nondistensible cricoid cartilage, the result being less airway resistance.[16] In the severely burned child, however, cuffed tubes are more frequently used because of the need for higher airway pressures.

Glottic stenosis can follow endotracheal intubation even after an interval as short as 24 hours; in almost all situations it occurs if tracheotomy is performed immediately after the removal of the endotracheal tube.[55] The endotracheal tube seems to induce ulceration of the vocal cords, while the subsequent tracheotomy diverts airflow, allowing the cords to lie in apposition and heal together.

In burn patients, complications are much more frequent and severe with tracheotomy than with translaryngeal intubation.[56–58] Several factors contribute to this. Tracheotomy performed rapidly in emergency situations is likely to be complicated. Tracheotomy is ideally performed in a controlled situation with the patient adequately anesthetized and positioned. When performed through burned skin and/or a damaged tracheal wall, the incision may easily become contaminated and necrosis may develop. Paratracheal extension of the infection may occur.[58] Bronchial and alveolar sepsis is also very prevalent, particularly if the procedure is performed through the burn eschar.[58] Because of these deleterious and possibly fatal complications, tracheotomy is avoided as much as possible in burned patients. It is preferable to maintain translaryngeal intubation as long as possible. If tracheotomy has to be performed, it should be delayed until burns at and near the site have healed. If laryngotracheal stenosis develops, the patient can be treated by prolonged stenting with T-shaped silicone tubes or by tracheoplasty.[59, 60]

## EXTUBATION

The optimum time for decannulation of the endotracheal tube in a burned patient is a matter of clinical judgment. Several criteria should be taken into account before proceeding to extubation.

1. The general condition of the patient should be carefully assessed. His mental status, the stability of his cardiovascular system, and the absence of overt sepsis should be noted.

2. As in other patients with respiratory failure, the return of adequate respiratory mechanics should be evaluated. These include inspiratory force greater than 20 cm of water and adequate vital capacity, two to three times the predicted tidal volume.

3. Subsidence of edema should be evident. It is futile to attempt extubation while the swelling around the face and neck persists. External swelling is indirect evidence of intrapharyngeal and laryngeal edema.

4. An airleak around the endotracheal tube: This is one of the most reliable signs of a return to normalcy. The appearance of a sizable leak around the endotracheal tube with no change in cuff pressure is a good indication of lessening of airway edema.

5. Secretions: In the presence of sooty secretions, it is better to postpone extubation, since pulmonary toilet may be better accomplished with an endotracheal tube. The patient's own ability to bring up secretions and the presence of a strong cough reflex should also be evaluated.

6. Clearing of pulmonary infiltrates: Although an absolutely clear lung is not to be expected, prominent infiltrates are a contraindication to extubation.

7. Weaning: With the availability of intermittent mandatory ventilation (IMV), a gradual decrease in ventilatory assistance can be achieved. During this period, it is important to note the patient's own rate of breathing, a very fast rate being a predictor of impending respiratory failure. It is important, however, to realize that burned patients always breathe at a fast rate; a respiratory rate of 30 to 40 breaths per minute should not be considered unusual. The blood gases are also carefully followed in this critical period, and the degree of $CO_2$ retention is evaluated. If progressive deterioration occurs, weaning should be abandoned.

8. Timing: It is imperative that the extubation be performed at a time when help is and will continue to be available. Deterioration usually occurs within a

few hours after extubation, so ample time should be allowed to monitor the patient. It is probably best not to extubate either in the evening or on the weekend, when medical and nursing personnel tend to be at a minimum.

9. Planning: Extubation should not be attempted if the patient is to have surgery on the following day, since some deterioration of pulmonary function is expected. After surgery, extubation should be temporarily postponed until the patient's condition is stable.

## MANAGEMENT OF HEAD AND NECK BURNS IN THE RECONSTRUCTIVE STAGES

The initial effect of a burn is swelling; the delayed effect of a burn is scarring. Scars eventually contract to cause deformities. In other body areas, these deformities are functional and esthetic in nature; in the head and neck they may compromise the airway. A special challenge is thus presented to the anesthesiologist when these patients present themselves for surgery. Each case is different and each needs a different approach. Several generalizations can nonetheless be made.

### Preoperative Evaluation

In addition to the usual systemic preoperative evaluation, special attention should be given to the airway.

1. A complete history should be taken. Adequate information should be obtained from the patient, his family, or his friends regarding his breathing patterns, with particular attention to the presence of snoring. Snoring during sleep indicates a compromised airway and predicts the possibility of stridorous breathing during induction and recovery from anesthesia. Obstructive sleep apnea can sometimes occur in some patients during sleep.[61] Although significant chronic peripheral airway disease is uncommon in these patients, some are occasionally encountered with marked obstructive lung disease or bronchiolitis obliterans.[62, 63]

2. The ability to open the mouth should be ascertained with care. The extent to which the patient opens his mouth indicates the type of laryngoscope to be used and whether an oral airway can be inserted. The presence of teeth and their condition should also be noted.

3. The nares should be examined for patency. If a nasotracheal tube or a nasal airway needs to be inserted, the wider and more patent naris is used.

4. A fixed contracted neck makes intubation difficult, since extension of the head will not be possible. It is important to realize that scars frequently extend from the face to the neck and that, in this condition, the patient can open his mouth while the head is flexed but not during extension. The old dictum holds

true: If the space between the chin and the laryngeal prominence is less than two fingers wide, anticipate a difficult intubation, and if less then one finger wide, expect marked difficulty.

5. Radiographs, scans, and occasionally tomograms of the trachea are sometimes needed to detect deviation and/or stenosis of the trachea.

## Preoperative Medication

Anesthesia in these patients is usually induced by an inhalation technique. Narcotics are thus avoided, although sedatives can be safely prescribed to alleviate anxiety. Besides benzodiazepines, we prefer to use $H_2$-receptor blockers such as cimetidine or ranitidine to decrease stomach acidity and secretory volume as a prophylactic against acid aspiration. Anxiety increases gastric secretion. This, together with manipulation of the airway, including the frequent need for positive pressure with a face mask, tends to increase intragastric pressure and cause regurgitation of stomach contents into the tracheobronchial tree.

HYDRATION. It is advisable to start an intravenous (IV) infusion early, perhaps during the night before or early on the day of surgery. Adequate hydration allows the patient to tolerate the inhalation anesthetic better. Perhaps of more immediate importance, however, is that the sedative medication can be titrated through the IV line so that the patient arrives at the operating room in a comfortable and anxiety-free state.

## ANESTHETIC MANAGEMENT

Planning is of the utmost importance in these patients. One should have a thorough discussion with the surgical team to evaluate their expectations and plan accordingly. Difficulty can be avoided if the following considerations are kept in mind.

1. Planned inhalation induction: An inhalation induction is advantageous because the airway can be evaluated as the patient is anesthetized; if severe obstruction is encountered, the anesthetic can be discontinued and the patient allowed to wake up.

2. Antisialagogue: The administration of IV atropine or glycopyrrolate is extremely useful. It is very distressing if the patient has a mouthful of secretion during attempts at intubation.

3. Level of anesthesia: It is imperative not to attempt manipulation of the airway until a deep anesthetic level has been reached. If the patient is not adequately anesthetized during manipulation, coughing or laryngospasm may occur.

4. Oxygenation: Adequate oxygenation should be maintained during all attempts at intubation. Oxygenation can be monitored by pulse oximeter.

5. Manipulation of the tongue: In patients with severe contractures around the mouth, the tongue occupies a large area and can cause obstruction and thus limit one's ability to manipulate the laryngoscope. Pulling the tongue out with gauze or using a silk tongue stitch may prove very useful.

6. Stylet: It is better first to visualize and then shape the endotracheal tube on the stylet, rather than shaping it ahead of time.

7. Fiberoptic laryngoscope: In experienced hands, this is an extremely valuable instrument. However, in some patients previous scarring may make it difficult to discern anatomical features. Its use in very small children is also limited because of the lack of availability of smaller scopes.

8. Assistance from surgeons: If there is severe scarring at the neck, it is reasonable to start the anesthesia with a face mask. Once a satisfactory anesthetic level is established, the surgeon can incise the neck and partially release the contracture. Endotracheal intubation can then be attempted.[64]

9. Fixation of the endotracheal tube: If surgery will be near and around the endotracheal tube, it is advisable to include the endotracheal tube in the surgical field so that both the surgeon and the anesthesiologist can observe it. In some of these precarious situations, securing the endotracheal tube by a stainless steel wire to one of the teeth is extremely helpful.

10. Extubation: Extubation should be delayed until the patient is awake and meets accepted criteria for maintaining his own airway.

It is occasionally wise to proceed with surgery without attempting a traumatic intubation. Ketamine can be useful in some of these situations.[65] Such risks can be taken if surgery is minor and distant from the airays.

## SUMMARY

In summary, in managing patients with upper airway burns for two decades we have been impressed with the following observations:

1. In burns of the face and neck, upper airway obstruction occurs rapidly. Early endotracheal intubation is life-saving.

2. Almost all patients can be treated with nasotracheal intubation for even months without the need for tracheostomy.

3. Adequate functional equipment is a must.

4. Aggressive management is rewarding, but there is no room for error. The lives of these unfortunate patients depend on the experience of the people treating them.

## REFERENCES

1. Davies JWL: Toxic chemicals versus lung tissue—An aspect of inhalation injury revisited. J Burn Care Rehabil 7:213–222, 1986.

2. Herndon DN, Thompson PB, Linares JA, Traber DL: Respiratory injury: Part I. Incidence, mortality, pathogenesis and treatment of pulmonary injury. J Burn Care Rehabil 7:184–191, 1986.
3. Cahalane M, Demling RH: Early respiratory abnormalities from smoke inhalation. JAMA 251:771–773, 1984.
4. Moylan JA, Alexander LG: Diagnosis and treatment of inhalation injury. World J Surg 2:185–191, 1978.
5. Crapo RO: Smoke inhalation injuries. JAMA 246:1694–1696, 1981.
6. Levine BA, Petroff PA, Slade CL, Pruitt BA: Prospective trials of dexamethasone and aerosolized gentamicin in the treatment of inhalation injury in the burned patient. J Trauma 18:188–193, 1979.
7. Silverstein P, Dressler DP: Effect of current therapy on burn mortality. Ann Surg 171:124–129, 1970.
8. Sataloff DM, Sataloff RT: Tracheostomy and inhalation injury. Head Neck Surg 6:1024–1031, 1984.
9. Stephenson SFBC, Esrig BC, Polk HC, Fulton RL: The pathophysiology of smoke inhalation injury. Ann Surg 182:652–660, 1975.
10. Stone HHD, Rhame YD, Corbitt JD, et al: Respiratory burns: A correlation of clinical and laboratory results. Ann Surg 165:157–168, 1967a.
11. Trunkey DD: Inhalation injury. Surg Clin North Am 58:1133–1140, 1978.
12. Madden MR, Finkelstein JL, Goodwin CW: Respiratory care of the burn patient. Clin Plast Surg 13:29–38, 1986.
13. Fein A, Leff A, Hopewell PC: Pathophysiology and management of complications resulting from fire and inhaled products of combustion. Crit Care Med 8:94–98, 1980.
14. Silverman SH, Purdue GF, Hunt JL, Bost RO: Cyanide toxicity in burned patients. J Trauma 28:171–176, 1988.
15. Haponik EF, Munster AM, Wise RA, et al: Upper airway function in burn patients. Correlation of flow-volume curves and nasopharyngoscopy. Am Rev Respir Dis 129:251–257, 1984.
16. Cote CJ, Todres ID: The pediatric airway. In Ryan Todres ID, Cote CJ, Goudsouzian NG (eds): A Practice of Anesthesia for Infants and Children. Orlando, Grune and Stratton, 1985, pp 35–58.
17. Pruitt BA: Advances in fluid therapy and the early care of the burned patient. World J Surg 2:139–150, 1978.
18. Pruitt BA, Dowling JA, Moncrief JA: Escharotomy in early burn care. Arch Surg 96:502–507, 1986.
19. Goodenough RC, Burke JF: Care of burns. In Tinker J, Rapin M (eds): Care of the Critically Ill Patient. Berlin, Springer-Verlag, 1983, p 663.
20. Turbow ME: Abdominal compression following circumferential burn: Cardiovascular responses. J Trauma 13:535–541, 1973.
21. Venus B, Matsuda T, Copiozo JB, Mathru M: Prophylactic intubation and continuous positive airway pressure: The management of inhalation injury in burn victims. Crit Care Med 9:519–523, 1981.
22. Moylan JA: Inhalation injury. J Trauma 21(Suppl 8):720–721, 1981.
23. Moylan JA: Smoke inhalation and burn injury. Surg Clin North Am 60:1533–1540, 1980.
24. DiVincenti FG, Pruitt BA, Reckler JM: Inhalation injuries. J Trauma 11:109–117, 1979.
25. Mellins RB, Pack S: Respiratory complications of smoke inhalation in victims of fires. J Pediatr 87:1–7, 1975.
26. Whitener DR, Whitener LM, Robertson KJ, et al: Pulmonary function measurements in patients with thermal injury and smoke inhalation. Ann Rev Respir Dis 122:731–739, 1980.
27. Nishimuca N, Hiranuma N: Respiratory changes after major burn injury. Crit Care Med 10:25–28, 1982.
28. Moylan JA, Adib K, Burnbaum M: Fiberoptic bronchoscopy following thermal injury. Surg Gynecol Obstet 140:541–545, 1975.
29. Ramon PH, Wallaert B, Galizzia JP, et al: Tracheo-bronchial endoscopy in burns to the face. Rev Mal Respir 2:97–101, 1985.
30. Tan WC, Lee ST, Lee CN, Wong S: The role of fiberoptic bronchoscopy in the management of respiratory burns. Ann Acad Med 14:430–434, 1985.
31. Clark CJ, Reid WH, Telfer AB, Campbell D: Respiratory injury in the burned patient. The role of flexible bronchoscopy. Anaesthesia 38:35–39, 1983.

32. Martyn JAJ, Goldhill DR, Goudsouzian NG: Clinical pharmacology of muscle relaxants in patients with burns. J Clin Pharmacol 26:680–685, 1986.
33. Goudsouzian N, Young ET, Moss J, Liu LM: Histamine release during the administration of atracurium and vecuronium in children. Br J Anaesth 58:1229–1233, 1986.
34. Dwersteg JF, Pavlin EG, Haschke R, et al: High dose atracurium does not produce hypotension in the burned patient. (Abstract) Anesthesiology 65:A193, 1986.
35. Brown JM: Respiratory complication in burned patients. Physiotherapy 63:151–153, 1977.
35a. Mills A, Martyn JAJ: Evaluation of atracurium neuromuscular blockade in patients with thermal injury. Br J Anaesth 60:450–455, 1988.
36. Wootton R, Hodgson E: Physiotherapy in treatment of burns with inhalation involvement. Physiotherapy 63:153, 1973.
37. Mathru M, Venus B, Rao T, Matsuda T: Noncardiac pulmonary edema precipitated by tracheal intubation in patients with inhalation injury. Crit Care Med 11:804–806, 1983.
38. Dubick MN, Wright BD: Comparison of laryngeal pathology following long-term oral and nasal endotracheal intubation. Anesth Analg 57:663–668, 1978.
39. Roberts KW: New use for Swan-Ganz introducer wire. (Letter) Anesth Analg 60:67, 1981.
40. Tobias R: Increased success with retrograde guide for endotracheal intubation. Anesth Analg 62:366–367, 1983.
41. Bourk D, Levesque PR: A modification of retrograde guide for endotracheal intubation. Anesth Analg 53:1013–1014, 1974.
42. Stinson TW III: A simple connector for transtracheal ventilation. (Letter) Anesthesiology 47:232, 1977.
43. Lechman MJ, Donahoo JS, MacVaugh H: Endotracheal intubation using percutaneous retrograde guidewire insertion followed by antegrade fiberoptic bronchoscopy. Crit Care Med 14:589–590, 1986.
44. Zwillich C, Pierson DJ: Nasal necrosis: a complication of nasotracheal intubation. Chest 64:376–379, 1973.
45. Knodell AR, Beekman JF: Unexplained fever in patients with nasotracheal intubation. JAMA 248:868–870, 1982.
46. Eckerbom B, Lindholm CE, Alexopoulos C: Airway lesions caused by prolonged intubation with standard and with anatomically shaped tracheal tubes. A post-mortem study. Acta Anaesthesiol Scand 30:366–373, 1986.
47. Bendixen HH, Egberg LD, Hedley-Whyte J, et al: Respiratory Care. St Louis, CV Mosby, 1965, pp 114–137.
48. Berlauk JF: Prolonged endotracheal intubation vs tracheostomy. Crit Care Med 14:742–745, 1986.
49. Stauffer JL, Olson DE, Petty TL: Complications and consequences of endotracheal intubation and tracheostomy. Am J Med 70:65–76, 1981.
50. Grillo HC: Surgical treatment of postintubation tracheal injuries. J Thorac Surg 78:860–875, 1979.
51. Cooper JP, Grillo HC: The evolution of tracheal injury due to ventilatory assistance through cuffed tubes. A pathologic study. Ann Surg 169:334–338, 1969.
52. Grillo HC, Cooper JD, Geffin B, Pontoppidan H: Low pressure cuff for tracheostomy tubes to minimize tracheal injury. A comparative trial. J Thorac Cardiovasc Surg 6:898–907, 1971.
53. Carroll RG: Evaluation of tracheal cuff designs. Crit Care Med 1:45–46, 1971.
54. Deane RS, Shimozaki T, Morgan JG: An evaluation of the cuff characteristics and incidence of laryngeal complications using a new nasotracheal tube in prolonged intubations. J Trauma 17:311–315, 1977.
55. Boyd AD, Romita MC, Conlan AA, et al: A clinical evaluation of cricothyroidotomy. Surg Gynecol Obstet 149:365–368, 1979.
56. Lund T, Goodwin CW, McManus WF, et al: Upper airway sequelae in burn patients requiring endotracheal intubation or tracheostomy. Ann Surg 201:374–382, 1985.
57. Eckhauser FE, Billote J, Burke JF, Quinby WC: Tracheostomy complicating massive burn injuries. A plan for conservatism. Am J Surg 127:418–423, 1974.
58. Moncrief JA: Tracheotomy in burns. Arch Surg 188:34–37, 1978.
59. Eliachar I, Moscona R, Joachims HZ, et al: The management of laryngotracheal stenosis in burned patients. Plast Reconstr Surg 68:11–16, 1981.
60. Majeski JA, Schreiber JT, Cotton R, MacMillan BG: Tracheoplasty for tracheal stenosis in the pediatric burned patient. J Trauma 20:81–86, 1980.

61. Robertson CF, Zuker R, Dabrowski B, Levison H: Obstructive sleep apnea: A complication of burn to the head and neck in children. J Burn Care Rehabil 6:353–357, 1985.
62. Kirkpatrick MB, Bass JB: Severe obstructive lung disease after smoke inhalation. Chest 76:108–110, 1979.
63. Jaspar N, Bracamonte M, Sergysels R: Severe peripheral airway obstruction after inhalation burn. Intensive Care Med 8:105–106, 1982.
64. Waymack JP, Law E, Park R, et al: Acute upper airway obstruction in the postburn period. Arch Surg 120:1042–1044, 1985.
65. Jacobacci S, Towy RM: Anaesthesia for severe burn contractures of the neck. A case report. East Afr Med J 55:543–545, 1978.

# 5

# Acute Electrical Injuries

JOHN P. REMENSNYDER

Humans encounter electricity in a variety of forms every day, and carefully designed and protected electrical devices lend much to the comfort and convenience of modern life. However, electricity in its unprotected, naked form produces both death and devastating injury. Each year in the United States alone, over 1000 people die as a result of electrical contact, and roughly 3 per cent of the 250,000 burns treated annually in the United States are due to electricity.[1]

Low-voltage (less than 1000 volts) injuries most commonly occur in the home environment, producing patterns of injury which vary from the circumoral tissue destruction seen in the toddler who attempts to separate an electrical cord connection by pulling with his teeth to fatal electrocution in the bathtub if a hairdryer accidentally falls into the water. High-voltage (greater than 1000 volts) injuries occur more typically in the workplace, near high-voltage installations or from contact with high-tension power transmission lines. Patterns of high-voltage injuries include instant death, massive tissue loss, secondary ignition thermal injury, and associated fractures and CNS trauma.

Case series reported in the literature of high-voltage electrical injuries demonstrate a substantial mortality and morbidity. Mortality rates, including both adults and children, varied from 3 to 15 per cent for patients who arrived at a hospital for treatment (Table 5–1). A wide variety of complications occurred in an extraordinarily high percentage of cases. Major amputations constituted the single largest category of complications, being necessary in 25 to 68 per cent of patients treated. Total body surface burn involvement was usually relatively limited, with the exception of occasional large secondary clothing ignition burns.

From experience and the literature, a composite characterization (Fig. 5–1) emerges of the high-voltage electrically injured patient:

Young, less than 30 years of age
Male, almost exclusively
Competent, able/or working
Limited body surface area (BSA) involvement
Upper extremity more frequently injured than lower
Amputation commonly necessary

This chapter deals exclusively with high-voltage injuries emphasizing three aspects: (1) electricity—basic physics; (2) pathophysiology of electrical injury; and (3) clinical management—both acute and reconstructive.

TABLE 5–1. High-Voltage Electrical Injuries

| Authors | No. of Patients | Per Cent Mortality | Average Per Cent BSA | Percentage of Patients with Complications | Per Cent Patients Amputated |
|---|---|---|---|---|---|
| DiVincenti et al, 1969[2] | 53 | 18 | 20 | 75 | 38 |
| Hartford and Ziffren, 1971[3] | 16 | 6 | — | — | 38 |
| Salisbury et al, 1973[4] | 76 | 15 | 21 | — | 37 |
| Butler and Grant, 1977[5] | 40 | 13 | 11 | 76 | 65 |
| Solem et al, 1977[6] | 48 | 4 | 11 | 72 | 29 |
| Rouse and Dimick, 1978[7] | 42 | 5 | 23 | 71 | 48 |
| Quinby et al, 1978[8] | 22 | 5 | 16 | — | 68 |
| Wilkinson and Wood, 1978[9] | 28 | 14 | 22 | — | 43 |
| Hunt et al, 1980[10] | 102 | 3 | 15 | — | 25 |
| Holliman et al, 1982[11] | 68 | 7 | 13 | 78 | 35 |
| Luce and Gottlieb, 1984[12] | 31 | 0 | 19 | — | 35 |
| Parshley et al, 1985[13] | 43 | 5 | 8 | — | 40 |
| Gordon et al, 1986[14] | 49 | 6 | 17 | — | 24 |
| Hanumadass et al, 1986[15] | 16 | 0 | 21 | — | 63 |

— = Data not available

## PATHOPHYSIOLOGY

High-tension power lines criss-cross the modern landscape of industrialized nations and distribute electricity to home and industry. In the United States, long-distance power lines distribute alternating current utilizing voltages of up to 350,000 volts, which eventually is stepped down to 220 or 110-120 volts, 60

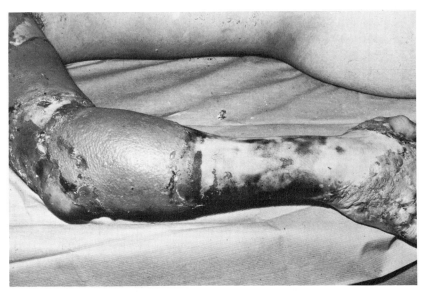

FIGURE 5–1. Severe deep conduction injury of the right arm of a 15-year-old boy who fell against a high-tension wire in a train tunnel.

Hz for domestic consumption. In the United Kingdom, electricity is distributed via the National Grid System beginning at 400,000 volts (400 KV), is gradually reduced during transmission to 275, 33, 11, 6.6, and 3.3 KV, and eventually reaches the consumer as a 240-volt, 50-Hz supply.[16] Virtually all industrial and domestic electricity is alternating current (AC), although direct current (DC) is still available in specialized circumstances. From the standpoint of human injury, at voltages of less than 1000, AC produces far more devastating effects than DC, while above 1000 volts AC and DC are equally dangerous.

Electrical burns are most usefully thought of as due to a conversion of electrical energy into heat, which causes direct tissue damage. The relation between voltages, resistance, and current is described by the familiar Ohm's Law:

$$I = \frac{E}{R}$$

where $I$ = current in amperes, $E$ = voltage in volts, and $R$ = resistance in ohms. Joule's law describes the relation between current and heat production: The rate at which heat is produced by steady current in any part of an electrical current is directly proportional to the resistance of the circuit, the square of the current, and the duration of the current. This may be expressed mathematically:

$$J = I^2 RT$$

where $J$ = the number of Joules of heat produced, $I$ = the current in amperes, $R$ = the resistance in ohms, and $T$ = the time in seconds. The variables of these two formulae interplay to produce the highly variable picture of clinical electrical injury. Despite the seemingly capricious nature of electrical injury, much becomes understandable by analyzing the two forms of electrical transmission in the human body: conduction and arc.

Injuries due to electrical conduction are by far the most common and cause the most extensive destruction. Schematically, the skin of the patient comes in contact with a voltage source and, if the resistance offered by the skin is overcome, current flows from the source into the body, through tissues of differing resistance and ultimately out through the skin again at a separate site as the current flows to ground. Skin offers high resistance to electrical current, especially when dry. The tough, calloused skin of the palm of a manual laborer may have a resistance of up to 1,000,000 ohms/sq cm, whereas normal dry palmar skin has a resistance of approximately 5000 ohms/sq cm and wet palmar skin only 1000 ohms/sq cm.[17, 18] The stratum corneum provides the majority of skin resistance and diminishes with prolonged voltage contact: Upon application of 50 volts to skin for 6 to 7 seconds, resistance diminishes, thus allowing current flow and hence exposing the deep tissues to the likelihood of electrical damage.[19] Once current enters the deeper tissues, it flows differently in different tissues according to their varying inherent resistance. Pack in 1924 determined the order of decreasing resistance in animal tissues: bone, fat, tendon, skin, muscle, blood, and nerve.[20] Later investigators have repeatedly confirmed these observations. One way of looking at the puzzling picture of deep conduction injury is to postulate that the differing tissue resistances to current flow produce greater or lesser amounts of heat (according to Joule's law) and hence variable amounts of thermal damage. The greatest damage generally is deep in the extremity, causing some to say that this is due to proximity to the bone, which, being of highest resistance, presumably generates the most heat during current passage. However, clinical experience does not always correlate well with this type of analysis. Also, tissues vary in susceptibility to thermal injury. For example, Baxter points out that even though nerve offers little resistance to current passage and hence little heat is produced, nerve tissue is exquisitely sensitive to even small degrees of thermal injury.[1] A more informative model of conduction injury derives from treating the body as a volume conductor with varying cross-sections in different anatomical areas. Cason points out that the total body acts as a volume conductor of 500 to 1000 ohms.[16] Pruitt and Mason make the argument succinctly:

> In high voltage trauma, heat is the principal mediator of tissue injury; the differences of tissue resistance are so small that the body acts as a volume conductor. Heat is generated in this conductor as a function of voltage drop and current flow per unit cross-sectional area, or current density. This dependence upon cross-sectional area accounts for the frequency of severe injury to the extremities and the variety of major injury to the trunk in high tension electrical injury. At points of contact, where the density is greatest, the skin is severely injured and chars.[21]

Points of current entry through the skin and exit sites show characteristic appearance, consistent with the notion of current density and hence heat. Entry wounds are characteristically depressed, leathery, irregular areas of intense tissue coagulation and necrosis, whereas exit wounds typically are more extensive and explosive in nature, almost as if the current must blast its way out of the body. The vast majority of entrance wounds involve the upper extremity, whereas most exit wounds are found in the lower extremity (Table 5–2). The electrical path from entrance to exit generally takes the shortest distance between the two points and may produce injury in any organ or tissue in the path of the current. Multiple exit wounds in some patients attest to the possibility of several electrical pathways in the body, thus placing virtually any structure in the body at risk

**TABLE 5–2. High-Voltage Electrical Injury Entrance and Exit Wounds**

| | Entrance | | | Exit | | |
|---|---|---|---|---|---|---|
| | *Per Cent Upper Extremity* | *Per Cent Lower Extremity* | *Per Cent Other* | *Per Cent Upper Extremity* | *Per Cent Lower Extremity* | *Per Cent Other* |
| Solem et al, 1977[6] | 88 | 2 | 10 | 6 | 78 | 16 |
| Burke et al, 1977[59] | 83 | 11 | 6 | 34 | 52 | 14 |
| Wilkinson and Wood, 1978[9] | 68 | 7 | 25 | 9 | 79 | 12 |
| AVERAGE | 80 | 7 | 13 | 16 | 70 | 14 |

from electrical insult. Observed damage to abdominal viscera, intrathoracic structures, and CNS areas remote from obvious extremity injury suggest multiple current pathways.

Injuries due to arcing of electrical current are less common but can cause intensive, localized tissue destruction. Arcing occurs when the current flows from the body to ground or above the surface to another part of the body. Under ordinary ambient conditions, high voltages may induce arc distances of 2 to 3 cm for every 10,000 volts, and an established arc may injure a person as far as 10 feet away.[22] Local arcs in the skin of flexed joints, such as wrist, knee, or axilla, produce small, depressed, coagulated lesions of great depth. Arc temperatures commonly are 2000 to 4000° C and may rise as high as 20,000° C; hence the injury produced, while discrete, is very deep and destructive.

Electrical injury is compounded by the "non-release" phenomenon due to sustained tetanic contraction of muscles in contact with alternating current. If a patient grasps a high-tension wire, the flexor muscles of the forearm go into a sustained contraction, making it impossible for the patient to release from the electrical source—hence the name "no-release" phenomenon. Such contractions are due to low-frequency current flow (amperage) of a magnitude above painful stimulus but less than the amperage required to produce tetany of respiratory muscles (Table 5–3). A patient escapes from the "non-release" phenomenon only if he becomes unconscious and falls away from the source, not infrequently falling a considerable distance from a height, thus sustaining secondary skeletal or CNS trauma. In attempting to free a person still in contact with a "live wire," great caution must be exercised so that the rescuer does not become part of the circuit or is not struck with an electrical arc. The victim must not be touched until the current source is either deactivated or pushed away from the patient by a non-conductor such as a length of dry wood.

## SPECIFIC TISSUE EFFECTS

The general tissue effects of electrical injury in each organ system translate into very specific, clinically important injuries. Some are acute and life-threat-

TABLE 5–3. Effects of Low-Frequency Electrical Current[19, 23]

| Current (milliamperes) | Physiological Effect |
|---|---|
| 1–2 | Sensory perception |
| 5 | Painful stimulus |
| 10–15 | Sustained muscular contraction |
| 30–100 | Tetany of respiratory muscles |
| | Ventricular fibrillation |
| 1000 | Sustained myocardial contractions |
| 5000 | Deep conduction injury |
| 10,000 | Massive irreversible CNS damage |

ening, whereas others may have an insidious onset months or even a few years after initial injury. Because the dividing line between acute and late specific tissue or organ injury is difficult to define, the acute and late effects are grouped together in discussing electrical injury in each organ system.

CARDIAC. Acutely, the most obvious and lethal effect of electrical injury is cardiac standstill and ventricular fibrillation producing instant death; most of these patients are never transferred to a hospital. Ten to 30 per cent of patients on entry show cardiac rhythm or electrocardiographic changes, including atrial fibrillation, supraventricular tachycardia, right bundle branch block, focal ectopic arrhythmias, and nonspecific ST-T segment changes.[24] These have been thought to be due to coronary artery spasm, coronary endarteritis, or direct myocardial injury. Proven myocardial infarction occurs infrequently, as does direct myocardial electrical damage.[5-28] Among the "folklore" beliefs current among electricians working on high-voltage lines is the belief that there is a very high incidence of late myocardial infarction among those who have sustained any form of conductive injury (H. Robinson, personal communication, 1978).

RENAL. Direct renal injury due to electrical insult is rare but may be significant in that it profoundly affects renal tubular transport.[29, 30] Much more common is acute renal failure due to a sudden elevation of serum free hemoglobin, myoglobin, and denatured proteins produced at the site of extensive muscle injury. A large hemochromogen load presented to the renal circulation coupled with a low-flow state of hypovolemia and/or hypotension can produce acute tubular damage leading to either oliguric or polyuric renal failure. Renal failure of this type has been reported in 3 to 15 per cent of major electrical injuries.[2, 6, 7, 11]

NERVOUS SYSTEM: CENTRAL, AUTONOMIC, AND PERIPHERAL. Massive cerebral, cerebellar, and brain stem destruction results from high-voltage, high-amperage electrical current causing instant death. These patients rarely are taken to a hospital, and hence little is known about the nature of this degree of CNS injury. Unconsciousness is common acutely, whereas convulsions and coma are uncommon. Christiansen[31] has defined in the acute injury transient lesions in the extrapyramidal tracts, anterior horns, cortex, and association areas which may produce varying levels of consciousness with or without respiratory and motor paralysis. These signs are usually transient with full recovery. Some patients may go on to permanent impairment, showing such diverse conditions as hemiplegia with or without aphasia, striatal syndrome, and brain stem dysfunction. These signs may occur as late as six to nine months after injury. Homonymous hemianopia and cerebellar ataxia as single entities following electrical injury have also been described.[32, 33]

Spinal cord damage occurs acutely following electrical injury, showing incomplete signs such as quadriparesis, paraparesis, or distal pain and paresthesias.[31, 34] Such signs are thought to be due to the direct effect of electrical current on cord structures. Interestingly, multiple vertebral fractures without spinal cord damage have been reported.[35] A particularly distressing syndrome is the delayed appearance of spinal cord signs which Panse first described in 1931 and termed "spinal atrophic paralysis."[36] The onset of Panse's syndrome may be insidious, occurring days to months after injury, with the predominating motor signs first noted during rehabilitation therapy: gait disturbance, muscle imbalance, impotence, or bladder dysfunction. If it is progressive, quadriplegia, hemiplegia, paralysis, or a state resembling amyotrophic lateral sclerosis may supervene,[34] and a discouragingly low percentage of patients show even incomplete recovery.[37] Farrell and Starr have theorized that delayed spinal cord damage due to electrical injury is similar to effects produced by ionizing radiation: progressive neuronal damage and cellular death due to direct cytological changes or progressive spinal cord ischemia secondary to endothelial cell damage and progressive obliteration of the nutrient arteries to the cord.[34]

Peripheral nerves are damaged along with all other structures in the massively damaged extremity. At the other end of the spectrum are peripheral neuropathies persisting late after injury. These are thought to be due to either direct electrical effect producing interruption of Schwann cell sheets and axonal fragmentation, progressive vascular obliteration and fibrosis of nerve, or compression effects of epineural scarring and contraction.[38–40]

Autonomic nervous system dysfunction following acute electrical injury produces reflex sympathetic dystrophy (causalgia); while not common, it may be extraordinarily refractory to usual forms of treatment such as continuous sympathetic block or surgical sympathetic ablation. Baxter reported that half of his observed cases occurred in extremities with regenerating incomplete peripheral nerve injuries and half in amputated extremities.[1]

**GASTROINTESTINAL.** Direct electrical injury to the abdominal wall may produce full-thickness destruction with evisceration requiring immediate repair. On the other hand, various intra-abdominal viscera may sustain injury manifest on a delayed basis as an acute abdominal emergency. Adynamic ileus and gastric atrophy commonly complicate the acute injury and predispose to aspiration pneumonia and electrolyte disturbances. Gastric or duodenal ulcers occasionally develop early after electrical injury either as a result of direct injury or secondary to stress.[1] Acute bowel perforation may follow direct abdominal wall injury or be delayed as long as two to three weeks post injury.[2] Various fistulae, such as duodenal, cecal, and vesicoenteric, may also occur in the days following electrical injury.[41–43] The gallbladder appears to be particularly susceptible to electrical injury, showing either necrosis and perforation[44] or a high incidence of cholelithiasis 12 to 18 months after injury.[1] Direct pancreatic injury produces acute pancreatitis with persistently elevated amylase or eventuates in a diabetic-like state requiring insulin.[45] Newsome et al reported a case of massive hepatic and retroperitoneal damage producing hepatic necrosis and an acute coagulopathy with Factor V, Factor X, and platelet deficits.[44] Baxter has described sudden severe potassium deficiency developing two to four weeks after injury in patients apparently doing well.[1] He found sudden serum potassium drops from normal levels to 1 to 2 mEq per liter in less than 48 hours, with accompanying respiratory arrest and arrhythmias.

PULMONARY. Respiratory arrest due to central nervous system injury causes instant death in electrical injury. However, several pulmonary conditions may complicate the course of the survivor of electrical insult. Direct electrical contact with the chest wall may cause direct pleural injury with subsequent hydrothorax requiring aspiration, lobar pneumonitis usually occurring within the first week after injury, or frank bronchial perforation with mediastinal compression.[29, 46] Pneumothorax occurs secondary to rib fractures, and post-traumatic respiratory distress syndromes may be complicated by pulmonary sepsis in up to 12 per cent of patients.[1]

OPHTHALMOLOGICAL. Direct electrical injury may produce direct globe injury or selective lesions of the cornea, fundus, and optic nerve while sparing the lens.[47] Photic maculopathy (retinopathy) similar to "arc-welders" or "eclipse-watchers" retinopathy has been observed and is thought to be due to flash.[48] The most common ophthalmological sequela of high-tension electrical injury is the development of cataracts, either unilateral or bilateral, from three weeks to three years after injury.[18, 49] The reported incidence climbs as high as 30 per cent in those patients in whom it is thought that the electrical current passed through the head, as evidenced by a wound of entry or exit in the scalp.

VASCULAR. Direct damage and obliteration of major arteries occur in the totally damaged extremity, but partially injured major vessels may produce secondary hemorrhage in open or freshly closed amputation sites. Hunt et al have shown sublethal major arterial damage in arteriograms from injured limbs showing narrowing, irregularity, and beading of the vessel wall.[50] Smaller nutrient arteries to large muscles are particularly susceptible to heat damage from electrical injury, whereas larger arteries are spared because their higher blood flow seems to be sufficient to dissipate potentially damaging heat. Skoog, using serial angiography, demonstrated progressive small arterial obliteration following electrical injury.[51]

MISCELLANEOUS. Fetal death and spontaneous abortion have been reported, as has the birth of a brain-damaged infant following electrical injury during late pregnancy.[52] Acute bone marrow aplasia on the third day following high-voltage injury has also been reported.[52]

## CLINICAL MANAGEMENT

High-voltage electrical injuries produce some of the most devastating wounds that one will encounter in trauma patients, calling upon the surgeon's utmost expertise in achieving the triple goals of management: (1) providing accurate *initial assessment* and effective *general resuscitative* measures; (2) dealing with the complex operative problems of *wound care and closure*, which may require repeated evaluation and several operations; and (3) foreseeing and achieving optimal *reconstruction* of the damaged parts.

## Acute Management

Accurate initial evaluation and estimates of the condition of a patient who sustains a major high-voltage electrical injury are critical to the successful preservation of life, limbs, and function. In the initial encounter, it is important to keep in mind that four types of damage may occur in electrical injuries, either singly or in any combination:

1. *Deep conductive* electrical injury producing extensive deep muscular injury, the extent of which is not always obvious at the first examination, as well as remote injury to parts of the central nervous system and the contents of the thoracic and abdominal cavities.

2. *Arc injury*, which produces limited, very deep burns, particularly across flexion areas such as wrist, elbow, axilla, and groin.

3. *Surface thermal burns* sustained from the flash ignition of clothing may involve an extensive body surface area and affect proximal parts of limbs, requiring later amputation and producing unstable scar in areas of future prosthetic applications.

4. *Associated injuries* occurring in a substantial number of patients who are convulsively thrown from an electrical source or fall from a height, producing intracranial trauma, spinal cord injury, long bone fractures, or thoracic or intra-abdominal trauma.

Establishment of a patent airway and adequate respiration takes first priority in such patients, who frequently are still unconscious when they arrive in the emergency ward. If endotracheal intubation is required, the possibility of cervical spine injury must be kept in mind. Tracheostomy is rarely indicated. Cardiac resuscitation occasionally is necessary, but most patients who have suffered cardiopulmonary arrest due to high-voltage injury do not reach the hospital.

After initial emergency airway and cardiac stabilization, a careful history of the accident and general medical status of the patient must be obtained, if at all possible, followed by a general physical examination, keeping in mind the four general categories of possible injuries. Initial abdominal and thoracic evaluation, supplemented by chest and other indicated radiographs, and an initial electro-cardiogram provide critical baselines for subsequent, repeated evaluations. A CT scan will yield useful information in the management of concomitant CNS injury. At the same time that the history and physical examination are being done, large-bore intravenous access lines must be placed, as well as a Foley catheter, in the extensively injured. Careful monitoring of vital signs and repeated physical examination of the patient in the acute period will pick up early signs of a developing CNS lesion or delayed visceral injury.

Specific initial assessment of the extent and depth of injury must be made. The surface extent of burn will help guide fluid resuscitation, and an evaluation of the depth and extent will guide initial operative intervention. The proximal limit of firm indurated edema, which develops rapidly in the first hours after electrical injury, constitutes a useful guide for the extent of underlying, hidden muscle damage and frequently indicates the level of subsequent amputation. Diminished peripheral nerve function serves as a clue to significant deep injury in otherwise normal-looking extremities. The circulatory status of involved extremities must be initally assessed, with a Doppler probe if necessary, and then followed carefully and repeatedly as edema and swelling supervene. Impaired circulation due to circumferential deep burn will improve with escharotomy done immediately in the emergency ward, incising the insensate, full-thickness burn throughout its full extent. Fasciotomies of deep muscle compartments may also be necessary to restore circulation but are best done immediately after leaving the emergency ward in the operating room where circumstances are more favorable for thorough and complete release of restricting fascia, assessment of deep injury, and control of bleeding.

General resuscitative and supportive measures must be vigorously instituted, accurately monitored, and constantly revised as needed with continuing patient re-evaluation. Fluid therapy must be begun promptly, with goals of restoring intravascular volume and replacing ongoing obligatory fluid losses due to fluid and protein leakage from the burn-damaged microvasculature. Ringer's lactate is a useful fluid for early resuscitation and should be given at rates to maintain urinary output at 50 to 100 ml/hr. Fluid replacement will be grossly underestimated if one bases estimates on the per cent of total body surface area (TBSA) involvement and a conventional burn formula. Conventional burn formulae call for crystalloid replacement in the first 24 hours at a rate of 2 to 4 ml/kg/per cent TBSA burn.[54, 55] Patients with deep conductive electrical injury will require 8 to 12 ml/kg/per cent TBSA—two to three times the usually estimated amounts—to effectively maintain fluid balance and renal output, particularly if blood and muscle pigments appear in the urine, a common finding in these patients.

Hemochromogens—free serum hemoglobin from destroyed red blood cells, myoglobin released from injured muscles, and other altered proteins—appearing in the urine and coloring it deep red or red-brown are an ominous sign. A massive pigment load presented to an ischemic renal vasculature will produce acute tubular nephropathy and renal failure. To prevent renal damage, blood pressure and circulatory volume must be maintained by running crystalloid infusion at rates to maintain urinary output at 100 ml/hour or greater until the urine clears. If necessary, mannitol, 12.5 gm/hour for several hours, will help maintain a high urinary output due to osmotic diuresis. Since metabolic acidosis is not uncommon in acute massive electrical injury and predisposes to tubular precipitation of hemochromogens and renal failure, alkalinization of the patient serves to protect the kidneys. Fifty ml of 7.5 per cent sodium bicarbonate (45 mEq) can be given several times in the first hours after injury—either as a bolus or added to the IV—up to a total of 300 to 400 mEq until an alkaline urine is established.

Cardiac monitoring is mandatory if myocardial damage is suspected or initial electrocardiograms show abnormalities. Serial measurements of cardiac isoenzymes will confirm or deny the presence of myocardial muscle necrosis: elevated levels of CK-MB, the cardiac-specific isoenzyme of creatine kinase, are diagnostic of myocardial damage, whereas normal levels of CK-MB rule out myocardial injury, even in the presence of grossly elevated levels of serum CK due to extensive skeletal muscle destruction. In addition, the LH-1 fraction of lactic dehydrogenase (LH) rises higher than the LH-2 fraction in the presence of acute myocardial damage, while under normal circumstances the LH-2 fraction exceeds the LH-1 fraction.[56]

Invasive sepsis looms as one of the most severe complications of high-voltage electrical injury, and both topical and systemic prophylaxis as well as antibiotics play a role in sepsis prevention. Tetanus toxoid booster or Hypertet should be given during initial treatment. Sulfamylon acetate (10 per cent) penetrates deeply and effectively, preventing both surface and deep bacterial growth and being particularly effective against clostridial organisms, which are always a potential threat to any patient with dead muscle. Penicillin systemically serves as an effective prophylactic measure against beta-hemolytic *Streptococcus*. Regardless of the prophylactic helpfulness of the above-mentioned agents, surgical debridement of dead and devitalized muscle and other tissue still remains the single most important therapeutic weapon in preventing and treating sepsis in the electrically injured patient.

## Wound Care

The four goals of operative management of major electrical injuries are:

1. Evaluation and re-evaluation of the wound and general condition of the patient
2. Prevention of further damage by releasing constricting burns or tight fascial compartments
3. Removal of dead and devitalized tissues, amputating extremities or parts thereof as indicated.
4. Early wound closure or coverage by appropriate means

Continued evaluation of the appearance, circulatory sufficiency, and neural function helps determine the need for and timing of operative intervention. Proximal, firm edema in an otherwise normal-appearing upper arm with electrical destruction of the hand repesents developing edema associated with injured and quite possibly dead muscle and as such constitutes an urgent indication for operative decompression and exploration. Arteriograms may be helpful in determing the presence of major arterial injury but give little help in determining the patency of critical nutrient arteries to muscles.[50] The technetium-99m pyrophosphate muscle scan has been reported to be accurate in locating deep, underlying muscle damage as well as in defining its anatomical extent. To maximize its usefulness, circulation to the extremity in question must be normal, with fasciotomies carried out if necessary before the scan. Nonperfused areas of dead muscle or "hot" spots of significantly injured muscle serve as reliable guides in operative planning.[10] At the time of operative exploration, serial frozen sections may be extremely helpful in deciding about questionable tissue, since the gross appearance of devitalized muscle may appear deceptively normal as surface hemoglobin and myoglobin become oxygenated on exposure to air. The histological appearance of fragmented and disrupted myocytes and the presence of hypereosinophilic fibers are diagnostic of irreversible muscle damage.[8]

Escharotomy and fasciotomy, if performed early, can prevent secondary ischemic necrosis in limbs with circumferential full-thickness burns or rapidly developing tight edema with circulatory shutdown. Simply incising a full-thickness burn throughout its extent will allow the skin and subcutaneous tissue to gape widely and may effectively restore circulation. This maneuver requires no anesthesia, since the eschar is insensate, and is easily done in the emergency ward if circulatory embarrassment occurs. If escharotomy fails to improve circulation, then fasciotomies are required and are best done in the operating room because accurate technique and subsequent hemostasis are essential. In the forearm the fascia overlying the superficial flexor muscles is opened as well as that covering the deep flexors. At the same time, the carpal tunnel should be opened as well as the fascial investment that holds the median nerve snugly against the deep surface of the superficial flexors. The extensor compartment may occasionally need fasciotomy. In the upper arm, fascia overlying the biceps-brachialis complex is incised as needed. In the lower extremity, the anterior tibial compartment is most commonly the site of compromise and should be widely released, even with minimal suspicion, to prevent secondary ischemic necrosis of this highly vulnerable muscle group. Unless circulation is easily restored by this maneuver, the two posterior muscle compartments should also be widely fasciotomized. Fasciotomies must be done promptly on suspicion of circulatory compromise and frequently are done as the preliminary step in operative exploration, debridement, and removal of devitalized tissue in the injured extremity.

Early, aggressive removal of all dead and devitalized tissue remains the keystone to the effective management of the electrically injured extremity (Fig. 5–2). Not only does early debridement serve to prevent infection, but the wound is prepared more rapidly for early closure. Timing of the initial operation depends upon the general condition of the patient and the results of wound assessment. With a stable patient, no other injuries of priority, and a demonstration or high suspicion of dead and devitalized tissue, operative exploration should not be delayed. Following appropriate fasciotomies and wide exposure, the muscles and structures of the involved limbs are explored systematically until unquestionably normal tissue is encountered. All destroyed and devitalized tissue is removed without regard for functional loss. Frozen section may help in questionable areas, and marginally viable tissue may be left for subsequent debridements. With loss of all or a high percentage of the essential structures in part of a limb, immediate amputation is indicated, with the stump being left open for secondary closure. Damaged major vessels must be ligated proximally in a normal segment and

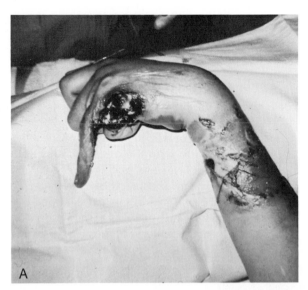

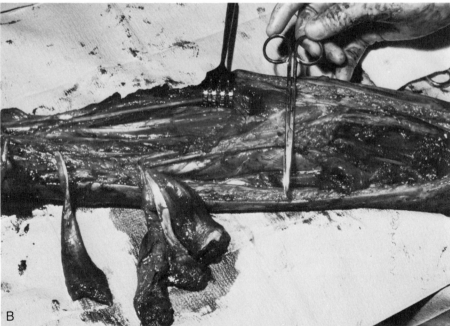

**FIGURE 5–2.** *A*, Status of the left hand and forearm of a 14-year-old boy 6 hours after contacting an electrical wire while climbing a tree. *B*, Exploration and debridement were carried out 8 hours and 48 hours after injury. At 48 hours, totally devitalized distal forearm and patchy necrosis of biceps and brachialis muscle (to the right of the scissors).

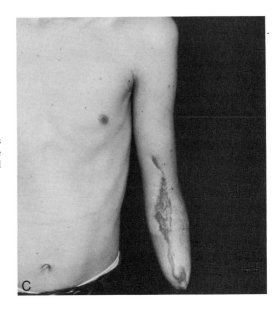

FIGURE 5–2 *Continued. C,* Six months after mid-forearm amputation. Note the skin graft necessary to close the proximal incision of exploration and debridement.

buried in viable muscle to prevent exposure, sepsis, and secondary hemorrhage. After the initial debridement, the open wound should be treated with dressings soaked in a topical antiseptic agent, splinted, and elevated. Repeated debridements are usually necessary in order to excise all devitalized tissue, which may not be completely evident until five or six days after injury. The patient should be returned to the operating room every two to three days for continued debridement and amputations as indicated until no further nonvital tissue remains in the wound. Only at this point is the wound ready for closure or coverage.

Coverage may be achieved most readily and easily by means of autogenous split-thickness skin grafts. If doubt remains as to the condition of the tissues, preliminary allografts should be applied; if they show early adherence and take, then autogenous grafts may be applied safely. Amputation sites should be closed primarily, when possible, preserving all possible length, leaving decisions as to stump revisions for a later date after primary healing. Closure of or grafting over still-devitalized tissue regularly results in rapid wound breakdown, necessitating re-debridement and coverage; hence, the importance of an accurate assessment of wound condition before proceeding with wound closure. If a substantial number of exposed muscles, tendons, and nerves are deemed viable at the initial or subsequent procedures, coverage within the first few days by a pedicle or free flap may preserve essential function in a way that no other coverage technique can achieve. Groin flaps are most useful in covering defects of the hand, wrist, and forearm and have the great virtue of being immediately available without preliminary delay. Flaps to exposed structures of the lower leg are more difficult. Local muscle or musculocutaneous or fasciocutaneous flaps provide useful coverage, but frequently the areas of these flaps are involved by the electrical injury. Increasingly, free flaps using microvascular transfer are being used for acute coverage of exposed vital structures in both the upper and lower extremities.[57]

## Amputations

Patients suffering deep conductive electrical injury require debridement of devitalized tissues; in a distressingly high percentage of patients this requires one or more amputations—both major and minor. Loss of fingers or toes produces relatively minor impairment, but loss of a hand, foot, or major portion of an extremity produces major disability requiring extensive rehabilitation and prosthesis fitting. Table 5–4 summarizes some of the reported experience with major amputations in high-voltage electrical injury. Of the 598 patients reported, 222 underwent one or more major amputations, or 37 per cent of all patients suffering high-voltage injury. Seventy-five per cent of the major amputations reported were in the upper extremity, while 25 per cent were in the lower. This correlates closely with the reported location of wounds of entrance and exit (see Table 5–2): the vast majority (80 per cent) of entrance wounds involved the upper extremity, whereas most of the exit wounds (70 per cent) were in the lower extremity. This may reflect the fact that the current in its initial entry into the body is concentrated with a high current density with consequently severe deep injury while the exit site is larger, more diffuse, and sometimes multiple—all factors favoring a reduced current density and hence less intense tissue damage.

There are four reasons for amputations in the course of caring for the

TABLE 5–4. Major Amputations with High-Tension Electrical Injury

| Authors | No. of Patients | No. of Patients Amputated | No. of Amputations | Upper Extremity | Lower Extremity | Percentage of Patients Amputated |
|---|---|---|---|---|---|---|
| DiVincenti et al, 1969[2] | 53 | 20 | 23 | 16 | 7 | 38 |
| Hartford and Ziffren, 1971[3] | 16 | 6 | 7 | 7 | 0 | 38 |
| Solem et al, 1977[6] | 48 | 14 | 15 | 10 | 5 | 29 |
| Quinby et al, 1978[8] | 22 | 15 | 19 | — | — | 68 |
| Rouse and Dimick, 1978[7] | 42 | 20 | 21 | 14 | 7 | 48 |
| Sinha et al, 1978[58] | 80 | 36 | 38 | 38 | 0 | 45 |
| Wilkinson and Wood, 1978[9] | 28 | 12 | — | — | — | 43 |
| Hunt et al, 1980[10] | 102 | 25 | 36 | — | — | 25 |
| Holliman et al, 1982[11] | 68 | 24 | 28 | 17 | 11 | 35 |
| Luce and Gottlieb, 1984[12] | 31 | 11 | — | — | — | 35 |
| Parshley et al, 1985[13] | 43 | 17 | 17 | 11 | 6 | 40 |
| Gordon et al, 1986[14] | 49 | 12 | 15 | 10 | 5 | 24 |
| Hanumadass et al, 1986[15] | 16 | 10 | 10 | — | 41 | 63 |
| | 598 | 222 | 229 | 123 | 41 | 37% |
| | | | | 75% | 25% | |

electrically injured patient: (1) during debridement and removal of dead and devitalized tissues in order to prevent infection and gain early wound closure; (2) guillotine amputation as an emergency measure for control of invasive, spreading sepsis; (3) removal of a partially salvaged limb which has become a painful, useless liability; and (4) revision amputation for functional improvement, usually a limited procedure carried out after initial healing. Timing of amputation is dictated by the condition of the injured limb, amputation being employed as a debriding procedure when the part shows so much destruction that there is no promise of saving useful function. The level of amputation is determined by essentially the same factors, and amputation during initial debriding procedures should be carried out at the level of viability without regard for optimal functional level.

Following major amputation during early debridement, the stump is most often left open for a few days to make sure no devitalized tissue is retained. However, prompt coverage once only vital tissue remains is essential to avoid invasive sepsis. Wound closure should be accomplished as simply as possible, usually by direct suture. Not infrequently the wound is so large that split-thickness skin grafts are needed to gain closure. Occasionally, local flaps must be used to cover exposed vessels or bone ends in the amputation stump.

Late problems plague patients with amputations following high-voltage injury. Prosthesis acceptance is variable, depending on the level. In the below-knee and forearm amputation groups, acceptance is generally high because prosthetic replacement at these levels is functionally very satisfactory. In patients with upper arm amputations or shoulder disarticulation, acceptance is generally low. The problem with prostheses for high amputations is that they provide little lateral resistance as a helping member, swinging to the side as the other hand is brought against it. Skin breakdown problems in scarred amputation stumps tend to follow the prosthesis acceptance pattern. In the high amputation groups, there are relatively few problems with stump breakdown for the simple reason that the prostheses are not much worn. Conversely, in forearm and below-knee amputations, skin breakdown problems are frequent because of constant prosthetic use in these very functional amputations. Usually relief of pressure or socket redesign can remedy such ulcers, although occasionally operative resurfacing is needed. A third late problem of these amputees is stiffness in proximal joints which appears to be a function of articular fibrosis due to the extensive nature of electrical injury, aggravated by the effects of prolonged healing and disuse. If such stiffness produces significant limitation of function, closed manipulation under anesthesia may be helpful.

## Reconstructive Surgery

Late reconstructive surgery consists of replacement and reconstruction of damaged functional parts. The two key goals of reconstruction are tissue replacement and maximizing of function in remaining partially damaged extremities.

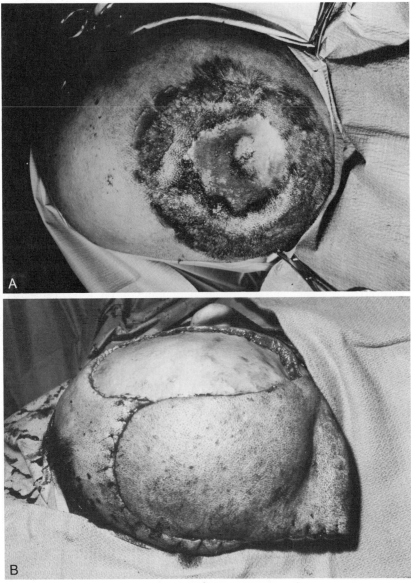

**FIGURE 5–3.** *A,* Wound of exit at the top of the head of a patient who contacted a high-tension source near a railway. Face is to the left. *B,* Scalp rotation flap to cover skull defect. Right temporoparietal flap based posteriorly was rotated to cover the defect, with a skin graft to the resultant defect. Orientation is the same as in *A.*

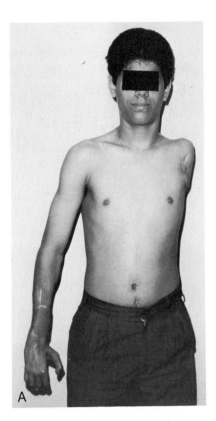

**FIGURE 5–4.** *A*, Sixteen-year-old boy who contacted a high-tension overhead wire while helping his father repair a TV antenna. Note shoulder disarticulation.

Figure 5–3 shows a patient who lost a large area of scalp and underlying full-thickness skull in an explosive wound of exit. A large rotation flap provided coverage for an acrylic cranioplasty. In this case replacement of the missing tissue represented functional restoration of the integrity of the skull. The second goal of late reconstructive surgery following electrical injury is to maximize function in the remaining extremity following amputation. Figure 5–4 shows a young man who required a shoulder disarticulation of the left arm after suffering a high-voltage injury. At the same time he suffered severe volar forearm damage in the opposite right arm. To restore function in the remaining right arm, the old scar was removed and replaced with a groin flap, which provided the coverage for later sural nerve grafts and tendon grafts. He illustrates the key point that major efforts must be made to restore every bit of function in the remaining extremity.

## SUMMARY

High-voltage electrical injury produces extensive devastating injuries, usually in healthy young adult males. Treatment requires a careful understanding of

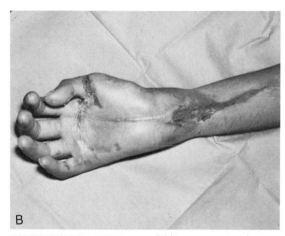

B

FIGURE 5–4 *Continued.* B, Extensive right volar forearm destruction and scarring. C, One year after groin flap to the right forearm, opponens transfer, and nerve and tendon grafts.

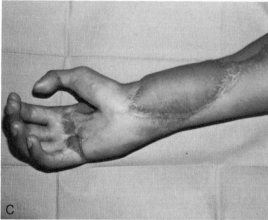

C

the special pathophysiology of electrical injury in order to provide accurate resuscitation, treat associated and secondary conditions, and adequately remove devitalized tissues while providing early coverage. Later treatment involves appropriate replacement of missing or destroyed tissue, prosthetic replacement for amputated parts, and optimizing of function in remaining partially damaged parts.

## REFERENCES

1. Baxter CR: Present concepts in the management of major electrical injury. Surg Clin North Am 50:1401–1418, 1970.
2. DiVincenti FC, Moncrief JA, Pruitt BA: Electrical injuries: A review of 65 cases. J Trauma 9:497–507, 1969.

3. Hartford CE, Ziffren SE: Electrical injury. J Trauma 11:331–336, 1971.
4. Salisbury RE, Hunt JL, Warden GD, Pruitt BA: Management of electrical burns of the upper extremity. Plast Reconstr Surg 51:648–652, 1973.
5. Butler ED, Gant TD: Electrical injuries, with special reference to the upper extremities. Am J Surg 134:95–101, 1977.
6. Solem L, Fischer RP, Strate RG: The natural history of electrical injury. J Trauma 17:487–492, 1977.
7. Rouse RG, Dimick AR: The treatment of electrical injury compared to burn injury: A review of pathophysiology and comparison of patient management protocols. J Trauma 18:43–46, 1978.
8. Quinby WC, Burke JF, Trelstad RL, Caulfield J: The use of microscopy as a guide to primary excision of high-tension electrical burns. J Trauma 18:423–431, 1978.
9. Wilkinson C, Wood M: High voltage electric injury. Am J Surg 136:693–696, 1978.
10. Hunt JL, Sato RM, Baxter CR: Acute electric burns: Current diagnostic and therapeutic approaches to management. Arch Surg 115:434–438, 1980.
11. Holliman CJ, Saffle JR, Kravitz M, Warden GD: Early surgical decompression in the management of electric injuries. Am J Surg 144:733–739, 1982.
12. Luce EA, Gottlieb SE: "True" high-tension electrical injuries. Ann Plast Surg 12:321–326, 1984.
13. Parshley PF, Kilgore J, Pulito JF, et al: Aggressive approach to the extremity damaged by electric injury. Am J Surg 150:78–82, 1985.
14. Gordon MWG, Reid WH, Awwaad AM: Electrical burns—incidence and prognosis in western Scotland. Burns 12:254–259, 1986.
15. Hanumadass ML, Voora SB, Kagan RJ, Matsuda T: Acute electrical burns: A 10-year clinical experience. Burns 12:427–431, 1986.
16. Cason JS: Treatment of Burns. London, Chapman and Hall, 1981, p 205.
17. Gaby RE: Electrical burns and electrical shock. Can Med Assoc J 17:1343–1345, 1927.
18. Jaffee RH: Electropathology. Arch Pathol 5:837, 1928.
19. Nichter LS, Bryant CA, Kenney JG, et al: Injuries due to commercial electric current. J Burn Care Rehabil 5:124–137, 1984.
20. Pack GT, Underhill FP, Epstein J, Kugelmass IN: Am J Med Sci 5:625–649, 1924.
21. Pruitt BA, Mason AD: High-tension electrical injury. (Letter to editor) Lancet 1:371, 1979.
22. Salisbury RE, Pruitt BA: Burns of the Upper Extremities. Philadelphia, WB Saunders Company, 1976, p 74.
23. Sevitt S: Burns: Pathology and Therapeutic Applications. London, Butterworth and Co, 1957, p 335.
24. Esses SI, Peters WJ: Electrical burns: Pathophysiology and complications. Can J Surg 24:11–14, 1981.
25. Burda CD: The electrocardiographic changes in lightning stroke. Am Heart J 72:521–524, 1966.
26. Imboden LE, Newton CB: Myocardial infarction following electrical shock. US Armed Forces Med J 3:497–502, 1952.
27. Kirchmer JT, Larson DL, Tyson RT: Cardiac rupture following electrical injury. J Trauma 17:389–391, 1977.
28. Purdue GF, Hunt JL: Electrocardiographic monitoring after electrical injury: Necessity or luxury. J Trauma 26:166–167, 1986.
29. Monafo WW, Freedman BM: Electrical and lightning injury. Boswick JA Jr, (ed): The Art and Science of Burn Care. Rockville, MD, Aspen Publications, 1987, p 244.
30. Taran VM, Podoprigora AP: A case of severe electric burns with kidney injury. Klin-Khir, March, 1982, p 65.
31. Christensen JA, Sherman TR, Balls GA, Wuamett JD: Delayed neurological injury secondary to high-voltage current, with recovery. J Trauma 20:166–168, 1980.
32. Gans M, Glaser JS: Homonymous hemianopia following electrical injury. J Clin Neuro Ophthalmol 6:218–223, 1986.
33. White JW, Deitch EA, Gillespie TE, McBeath JG: Cerebellar ataxia after an electric injury: Report of a case, review of the literature. J Burn Care Rehabil 4:191–193, 1983.
34. Farrell DF, Starr A: Delayed neurological sequelae of electrical injuries. Neurology 18:600–606, 1968.
35. Layton TR, McMurty JM, McClain EJ, et al: Multiple spine fractures from electrical injury. J Burn Care Rehabil 5:373–375, 1984.
36. Panse F: Die Schadigungen des Nervensystems durch technische Elektrizitat. Monatsschr Psychol Neurol 78:193–213, 1931.

37. Levine NS, Atkins H, McKeel DW Jr: Spinal cord injury following electrical accidents. J Trauma 15:459–463, 1975.
38. Critchley M: Electric injuries. Trans Med Soc London 59:19, 1936.
39. Ugland OM: Electrical injuries to peripheral nerves in animals. Acta Chir Scand 131:432–437, 1966.
40. Ugland OM: Electrical burn. Scand J Plast Reconstr Surg (Suppl 2), 1967.
41. Yang JY, Tsai YC, Noorhoff MS: Electrical burn with visceral injury. Burns 11:207–212, 1985.
42. Sinha JK, Roy SK: Perforation of the caecum caused by an electrical burn. Br J Plast Surg 29:179–181, 1976.
43. Miller FE, Peterson D, Miller J: Abdominal visceral perforation secondary to electrical injury: Case report and review of the literature. Burns 12:505, 1986.
44. Newsome TW, Curreri PW, Eurenius K: Visceral injuries: An unusual complication of an electrical burn. Arch Surg 105:494–497, 1972.
45. Bingham H: Electrical burns. In Ruberg R (ed): Advances in Burn Care. Clin Plast Surg 13:75–85, 1986.
46. Bowler CS, Gordon IJ: Perforation of a bronchus due to electrical injury. Br Med J 287:1346, 1983.
47. Adam AL, Klein M: Electrical cataract and review of the literature. Br J Ophthalmol 20:169–179, 1945.
48. Gardner TW, Ai E, Chrobak M, Shoch DE: Photic maculopathy secondary to short-circuiting of high-tension electric current. Ophthalmology 89:865–868, 1982.
49. Kazdan MS: Electrical cataract: A report of two cases. Can J Ophthalmol 4:104–105, 1969.
50. Hunt JL, McManus WF, Haney WP, Pruitt BA: Vascular lesions in acute electric injuries. J Trauma 14:461–473, 1974.
51. Skoog T: Electrical injuries. J Trauma 10:816–830, 1970.
52. Leiberman JR, Mazor M, Molcho J, et al: Electrical accidents during pregnancy. Obstet Gynecol 67:861–863, 1986.
53. Szabo K, Ver P: Bone marrow aplasia after high voltage electrical injury. Burns 10:184–187, 1984.
54. Baxter CR: Problems and complications of burn shock resuscitation. Surg Clin North Am 58:1313–1322, 1978.
55. Pruitt BA: Fluid and electrolyte replacement in burned patients. Surg Clin North Am 58:1291–1312, 1978.
56. Johnson CC, Bolton EC: Cardiac enzymes. Ann Emerg Med 11:27–35, 1982.
57. Wang XW, Bartle EJ, Roberts BB, et al: Free skin flap transfer in repairing deep electrical burns. J Burn Care Rehabil 8:111–114, 1987.
58. Sinha JK, Khanna NN, Tripathi FM, et al: Electrical burns: A review of 80 cases. Burns 4:261–266, 1978.
59. Burke JF, Quinby WC Jr, Bondoc C, et al: Patterns of high tension electrical injury in children and adolescents and their management. Am J Surg 133:492–497, 1977.

# 6

# Management of the Major Burn in the Intensive Care Unit

## ROBERT DEMLING

Dramatic physiological and biochemical changes occur in the post-resuscitation period related primarily to the onset of burn wound inflammation. Infection, both local and systemic, also becomes a major factor during this period. The patient with a large burn who was stable during the immediate post-resuscitation period frequently becomes unstable again when the hypermetabolic state becomes involved (beginning about day five). Infection is not necessary for this process.

## CHANGES IN BURN TISSUE

Macrophages and neutrophils begin infiltrating the wound at about day three or four, with numbers peaking at about seven to ten days. Macrophages and neutrophils are potent factories of interleukin-1 or endogenous pyrogen, cachectin or tumor necrosis factor, prostaglandins, leukotrienes, platelet-activating factor, and other vasoactive agents. Complement activation and oxygen radical production are also evident with the tissue inflammation. Inflammation, even without infection, can result in mediator-induced distant organ dysfunction. These wound mediators are also believed to be in large part responsible for perpetuation of the hypermetabolic state.[1-3] Many of these same mediators were also released immediately after the burn from mast cells, tissue macrophages, and injured endothelium. Proteases released from the inflammatory cells and from wound bacteria result in a separation of the burn eschar from the viable, now hyperemic, tissue beneath.

The persistent temperature and leukocytosis due to inflammation alone make the addition of an infection difficult to diagnose. Intermittent spiking fevers, usually initiated by burn wound manipulation, are the result of released pyrogens. There is no relationship between the degree of temperature spike and the presence of a wound infection. By six to seven days, bacteria are consistently present on the wound itself. Topical antibiotics can temporarily control but cannot eradicate bacterial growth in necrotic or ischemic tissue. There then begins an ongoing battle between wound bacteria and the host defenses in an attempt to prevent an invasive infection. Endotoxin and other bacterial products are released during this process, further stimulating the release of inflammatory mediators. This is an important concept when discussing treatment of burns, namely that burn wound inflammation and local infection alone can lead to distant organ failure. Circulating bacteria are not necessary to produce distant organ dysfunction and, in fact, cannot be documented in well over half of the burn patients who die of what appears to be sepsis-induced organ failure. The mortality of pulmonary, liver, or renal failure is extremely high in the burn patient, approaching 100 per cent due to the combination of the large focus on inflammation and infection, namely the burn wound. The mortality rate is nearly double that of the nonburn patient for sepsis-induced organ failure.

## POST-BURN PULMONARY DYSFUNCTION

### Pathophysiology

*Inhalation injury*–induced upper airway edema, caused by the heat-induced mucosal damage, begins to resolve between days two and four, as does the oral and facial edema from a concomitant burn injury. Airway mucosal irritation, however, persists for several days, leading to increased mucus production but decreased clearance due to the damaged ciliary action. The injured mucosa is therefore very prone to superinfection.[4]

The magnitude of the chemical injury to the smaller airways becomes much more clinically evident during this period. Increased mucus production is prominent. Characteristically, with a severe injury, the damaged mucosa becomes necrotic and begins to slough on day three or four. If not aggressively removed, the necrotic debris obstructs the smaller airways, causing distal atelectasis. The "shunt fraction," i.e., the portion of pulmonary blood flow to nonventilated areas, increases dramatically compared with that noted in the resuscitation period. A severe bronchorrhea is usually evident until the airway inflammation resolves. Subsequent bacterial colonization is inevitable because impaired airway clearance mechanisms are compounded by burn-induced immune suppression.

The hyperdynamic state results in an increase in pulmonary blood flow, but pulmonary vascular pressures remain relatively normal unless hypervolemia or superimposed sepsis occurs. There are, however, significant changes in ventilation, as $CO_2$ production is markedly increased, often doubled, in response to the increased metabolism and $O_2$ consumption. This results in an increase in minute ventilation two or three times the normal value for age and size. The increase is particularly prominent in the young adult. This significantly increases the work of breathing. If inadequate energy is provided, fatigue and $CO_2$ retention become evident, necessitating mechanical ventilatory support. Hyperventilation is further increased with the use of Sulfamylon as a topical antibiotic. Impaired chest wall excursion will, of course, continue due to pain and tissue edema if there are burns on the chest. Even after grafting, chest wall compliance can still be markedly decreased, particularly with use of meshed grafts after excision to fascia.

Pneumonia is a major pulmonary problem in the post-burn period. This process is particularly frequent in patients with an inhalation injury who have injured or actually denuded the airway mucosal barrier and is the major cause of death in the patient population. The pneumonic process is further accentuated by the immune deficiency state perpetuated by the continued presence of the inflamed or infected burn wound.

A less common but highly lethal complication is pulmonary dysfunction caused by burn wound sepsis. This adult respiratory distress syndrome (ARDS) is characterized by severe hypoxemia, decreased compliance, increased shunt, and pulmonary artery hypertension. The mechanism of injury has been quite perplexing in that frequently no bacteria or endotoxemia can be documented. Inflammatory mediators from the burn wound are a likely cause.

A deterioration in lung function can also be seen after debridement or excision procedures performed on inflamed and/or infected eschar. Any of the infection- or mediator-induced injuries will markedly complicate an already marginal situation as a result of the hypermetabolic state. Late respiratory failure in the burn patient has a mortality rate approaching 100 per cent and is now the leading cause of death in this population.[5]

## Treatment

As with the initial resuscitation period, maintenance of pulmonary function is of major importance during the post-resuscitation period owing to both the increased $O_2$ demands and $CO_2$ production. Infection risks to the lung are continually present because of the immunosuppressed state and any superimposed smoke damage.

### MAINTENANCE OF ADEQUATE ARTERIAL OXYGEN TENSION

Because of the near doubling of $O_2$ demands in the patient with major burns, an $O_2$ saturation of 95 per cent or greater is preferred, especially if this can be maintained at an $FiO_2$ below 0.5 so as to minimize any $O_2$ toxicity. Shunt fraction must be minimized by maintaining an adequate lung volume. Atelectasis from hypoventilation or secretion-induced small airways obstruction must be minimized.

### MAINTAIN ADEQUATE MINUTE VENTILATION

The increased $CO_2$ production characteristic of the post-burn hypermetabolic state requires a large increase in minute ventilation, sometimes two- to three-fold. The degree of increase depends upon the amount of wasted ventilation or dead space that is present as a result of any concomitant pulmonary dysfunction. If any operative procedures, i.e., excision and grafting, are to be performed, the anesthesiologist must be made aware of the need for increased ventilation in order to prevent severe hypercarbia.

Careful use of mechanical ventilation is required during this inflammation period, as the increased V/Q mismatch seen with positive-pressure ventilatory support, which may be tolerated in the early post-burn period, may not be tolerated in this stage of increased ventilatory demands. Any factor that increases $CO_2$ production, i.e., pain, excessive work, excessive carbohydrate calories, must be controlled.

### APPROPRIATE USE OF MECHANICAL VENTILATORY SUPPORT

Frequently, the increased work of breathing, particularly if a chest wall burn is present, requires some ventilatory assistance. A decrease in chest wall compliance from burns, either open or grafted, will markedly increase the work necessary to clear the extra $CO_2$ produced. Also, some positive end-expiratory pressure may be required to minimize atelectasis.

### CONTINUE AGGRESSIVE PULMONARY TOILET

Pneumonia is a major pulmonary problem during this period. Careful monitoring of the quantity and quality of sputum for detection of early infection remains an important factor in avoiding the development of a life-threatening pneumonia. In addition, aggressive chest physiotherapy, ambulation, and cough and deep breathing exercises must be continued until wound closure.

### CLOSELY MONITOR AND TREAT LUNG DYSFUNCTION, ESPECIALLY AFTER DEBRIDEMENT

A deterioration in lung function can also be seen after debridement or excision procedures performed on inflamed or infected eschar. Any of the infection or mediator-induced injuries will markedly complicate an already marginal situation as a result of the hypermetabolic state.

A more detailed description of airway and pulmonary pathophysiology and its treatment are discussed in Chapters 3 and 4.

## SYSTEMIC HEMODYNAMIC CHANGES

The local changes in the burn wound and the systemic hypermetabolic changes that occur beginning several days after injury are reflected by the development of a hyperdynamic circulatory state. Cardiac output increases to levels two- to three-fold above normal. Oxygen consumption increases from a normal value of about 125 ml/m²/min to values approaching 300 ml/m²/min. Urine output remains 1 to 2 ml/kg/hr as long as an increased solute load is present. Pulse rate again increases, as was seen in the initial hypovolemic phase, but now systemic vascular resistance is decreased. Systemic artery hypertension is not uncommon, particularly in patients with a relatively noncompliant vascular tree. Heart failure may well occur in patients with an impaired myocardium during this period if the increased cardiac work demands cannot be met by an increase in myocardial blood flow.

## Restoration of Blood Volume

Although cardiac output may be adequate during the resuscitation (0 to 24 hr) period, blood volume is frequently decreased, particularly in the patient with a large burn, owing to the large plasma-to-interstitial losses, edema being maximal at 24 to 36 hours. Restoration of blood volume is more feasible during the post-resuscitation period. Restoring plasma proteins toward normal if severe hypoproteinemia is present is also advantageous, as crystalloid needs will be decreased and improved gastrointestinal function will result. The latter process will be of considerable importance for nutritional support. Protein solutions should be used to replace volume loss and not be given in the presence of a normovolemic or hypervolemic state so as to avoid volume overload and its complications, especially during the fluid mobilization period.

Red blood cells are injured during the burning process and, again, as a result of mediator release from burned tissue. The increased fragility leads to a decreased half-life. Red cell hematopoiesis is also markedly impaired such that the combination of these processes leads to anemia beginning during the post-resuscitation period.[6] Red cell mass should be maintained as necessary to maintain a hematocrit of at least 30, given the increasing $O_2$ demands and the chronic nature of the impaired red cell production.

## Maintain Fluid and Electrolyte Balance

There is measurable increase in protein permeability in the vessels of burn tissue for days to weeks. The rate of fluid and protein loss into the burn interstitium is considerably less than during the first two days. However, loss of protein from the surface of partial-thickness burn is still substantial.

Evaporation from the surface of deep burns now becomes a major source of water loss that persists until the wound is closed.[7] The loss is measured in terms of water vapor pressure at the surface. In normal skin, the vapor pressure is 2 to 3 mm Hg, whereas on a full-thickness burn, where the eschar is soft and hydrated, pressure is about 32 mm Hg. Losses are comparable to those expected from an open pan of water with the same surface area. A reasonable estimate of this loss can be obtained from the following formula:

$$\text{Evaporation Loss (ml/hr)} = (25 + \% \text{ Body Burn}) \times \text{TBSA(m}^2).$$

Continued replacement of free water losses from evaporation and protein losses into burn tissue and from burn surfaces must be balanced against the intravascular fluid gains from edema resorption.[8]

Minimal amounts of sodium are usually required owing to the initial sodium loading and the fact that water evaporation is a major loss. Glucose administration is needed, as glycogen stores are now totally depleted. Once glucose administration and tissue utilization improve, large amounts of potassium need to be given as well. Replacement is particularly important once nutritional support is initiated.

During the post-resuscitation period, intravascular fluid is also gained from the absorption of edema fluid. The rate of absorption depends on the burn depth and subsequent lymphatic damage. Edema resorption is much more rapid in superficial burns, beginning at about day two or three, when lymphatics are intact but much slower after full-thickness injury. This is the period during which an elderly patient or one with impaired cardiac function can develop cardiogenic pulmonary edema, particularly if burns are partial thickness, as edema mobilization can be rapid. Avoidance of salt loading during this period and recognition of early signs of cardiac dysfunction avoids misinterpretation of decreasing perfusion as hypovolemia rather than hypervolemia. Small doses of diuretics are helpful to control this process.

The restoration of blood flow to the burn tissue after resuscitation results in the resorption of a large load of osmotically active particles, composed of solutes from disrupted cells and fragments of denatured proteins. The increased solute load frequently results in an obligate solute diuresis manifested by the increased output of high specific gravity urine.

Acute and perioperative fluid regimens have been described in more detail in Chapters 2 and 15.

## WOUND MANAGEMENT

Infection control and removal of burn eschar are the primary treatment approaches. Aggressive surgical excision and grafting are the treatments of choice in the first seven days.[9] As opposed to the first several days, when wound infection is minimal, aggressive manipulation of the burn wound after seven to ten days should be minimized to avoid bacteremia or endotoxemia.[10] A gentler approach is indicated. (See also Chapter 8.)

Surgical excisions of the burn wound during this phase are clearly more difficult beginning after seven days post burn. Many of the complications reported for excisional therapy are the results of excisions performed around the 14-day period.[11] These include increased pulmonary complications, septicemia, and massive blood loss. Excision during this period cannot be called "early." Excision in the first 10 days is very different from that after 10 days. Since the wound is always colonized by seven days, and possibly infected, perioperative antibiotics are indicated. A smaller area of excision, 8 to 10 per cent of TBSA, is also indicated in view of the extensive blood loss and absorption of mediators which will occur when operating on inflammatory tissue. Invasive wound infection can also be an indication for surgical removal, as antibiotics are not particularly effective in the presence of dead tissue. A bacteremia can certainly result from this maneuver and should be anticipated. An alternative approach at this stage is to gently remove the eschar on a daily basis and allow granulation tissue formation with subsequent skin grafting. The blood loss and bacteremic complications appear to be much less with this approach than with surgical excision of inflammatory tissue. Sufficient data have not been obtained in this area. As long as burn tissue is present, hypermetabolism and the risk of sepsis will persist.

Adequate management of wound pain and heat loss must be provided to avoid further stress-induced complications.


## HYPERMETABOLISM

Beginning at day five or six, there is a gradual increase in metabolic rate from a normal of 35 to 40 kcal/m²/hr to levels up to twice this value at about seven to ten days. The increase in metabolic rate after burns is far in excess of that seen after any other severe injury, including sepsis. The magnitude of increase is directly related to burn size. Young patients appear to generate a higher post-burn metabolic rate than do elderly patients.[12]

The hypermetabolic state is characterized by increased oxygen consumption, increased heat production, increased body temperature, and increased protein catabolism. Body temperature increases from a normal of 98°F (37°C) to 100 to 101°F (38 to 38.5°C). This process is believed to be due to a resetting of the hypothalamic temperature center due to the altered hormonal environment. Endotoxin can also cause the increased temperature by the same hypothalamic effect. The increased heat loss from the wound surface via evaporation is in part responsible for the increased heat production, and therefore excessive heat loss as a result of a cool environment will certainly accentuate the stress response.

The gluconeogenesis and hyperglycemia characteristic of the hypermetabolic state appear to be caused by a number of efferent mediators released as a result of the afferent stimulus. Plasma levels of catecholamines, cortisol, glucagon, and growth hormone are all increased post burn.[12] It appears that the burn response is a result of the interaction between all these hormones. Infusion of any one alone in human volunteers does not reproduce the stimulus to gluconeogenesis. However, the combined infusion of all three does, in fact, produce negative nitrogen balance.[13] Urinary catecholamine excretion is increased in proportion to the severity of injury and the metabolic rate. Insulin levels are also elevated, but the high levels of anti-insulin hormones appear to impair glucose transport into tissues, particularly into skeletal muscle. The decrease in tissue responsiveness to insulin may result in the necessity for exogenous insulin supplementation. In the early post-burn period, levels of thyroxine are normal but serum levels of $T_3$ are decreased. Thyroid hormone, however, does not appear to play a key role in this process, as thyroidectomized burned animals reach the same increase in $O_2$ consumption as those with an intact thyroid. Also, giving thyroid hormone increases metabolic rate to almost the same extent in the burn as in the nonburn animal.

## NUTRITION

Nutritional support to keep up with metabolic demands is best managed during this period by the enteral route, usually through a combination of a balanced tube feeding and voluntary intake. Parenteral supplementation through a peripheral vein may be necessary in the patient with a very large burn. Total parenteral hyperalimentation through a central vein is occasionally required if, for some reason, the gastrointestinal tract is not functioning adequately, as sometimes occurs in the ventilator patient or the patient with significant sepsis.

The objective of nutritional support is to provide both necessary nutrients to be used for calories and the necessary amino acids to be used for protein synthesis. A number of formulas are used to determine caloric requirements (see Chapter 10). The Curreri formula estimates daily calories by $25 \times$ wt(kg) + (40 $\times$ per cent body burn). Wilmore[12] utilizes a nomogram in which the increase in metabolic rate is estimated by the size of the body burn as well as by body weight. Protein (nitrogen) requirements are also calculated in a number of ways. A standard estimate of 2 gm of protein per kilogram of body weight can be used for all major burns. A more specific quantitative estimate is that based on the appropriate calorie-to-nitrogen ratio. A 150:1 calorie-to-nitrogen ratio has been the standard used for a number of years. Recent data in burn patients indicate that a 100:1 ratio may be preferable. This is based on the findings that a protein-rich diet is more effective in reversing the immune deficiencies seen in the post-burn period. Noninjured man normally consumes a diet with a ratio of about 250:1. In order to avoid use of the added protein as a substitute for gluconeo-genesis, sufficient glucose must be infused. Approximately 60 per cent of estimated calorie requirements needs to be given as glucose in order to effectively spare the nitrogen. Fat can be used as a calorie source for the remaining 40 per cent of nonprotein calories. Monitoring of triglyceride levels is necessary to avoid exceeding a value of 300 mg/dl 4 hours after cessation of the lipid infusion. Lipid clearance is not impaired in the majority of burn patients; in fact, lipid utilization may well be increased.

Since there is a large fluid requirement with large body surface burns, the majority of the calorie and protein requirements can be infused through a peripheral vein, particularly if a lipid emulsion is used. Enteral feedings utilizing a nasogastric tube can usually be initiated within four to five days after burn. The limiting factor to success, at least initially, is again the osmolarity of the solutions. Isosmolar solutions are reasonably well tolerated if begun slowly. Many of these standard solutions have a caloric density of 1 cal/cc but are low in protein (calorie:nitrogen ratio being over 200:1). Solutions with a higher protein content tend to be hyperosmolar, leading more frequently to diarrhea. Usually a gradual increase in the osmolarity of the solutions allows the eventual use of protein feeding.

Vitamin supplementation is also essential; in particular, vitamins A and C are known to be lost in increased quantities in the burned patient.

## SUMMARY: ICU MANAGEMENT

### I. Pulmonary
   A. Aggressive pulmonary toilet
   B. Avoid premature withdrawal of ventilatory support
   C. Need to compensate for increased $CO_2$ production
   D. Daily sputum smears looking for evidence of infection
   E. Initiation of antibiotics with first evidence of airways infection

### II. Fluids
   A. Low salt with glucose
   B. Adequate replacement
   C. Careful replacement of protein losses
   D. Replacement of red cells to maintain hematocrit greater than 30
   E. Initiation of nutrition: central or peripheral vein glucose, amino acids, lipids with transition to enteral feeding
   F. Maintenance of caloric nitrogen ratio 100:1
   G. Frequent rotation of intravenous catheters (every three to five days)

### III. Early Wound Closure
   A. Assure hemodynamic stability
   B. Perioperative antibiotics
   C. Maintain warm operating room environment
   D. Minimize operation time (usually 2 hours) with multiple team approach

### IV. Controlling wound infection
   A. Topical antibiotics twice a day
   B. Systemic antibiotics based on wound biopsy data or in perioperative period. Be careful to monitor levels.
   C. Aggressive debridement prior to established infection; then gentle wound manipulation
   D. Compulsive handwashing and other standard techniques to avoid bacterial cross-contamination

### V. Stress control
   A. Maintain optimal blood volume
   B. Maintain warm environment
   C. Maintain adequate pain control and sedation

## REFERENCES

1. Wilmore D, Aulick L, Mason A, Pruitt B: Influence of the burn wound on local and systemic response to injury. Ann Surg 186:444–450, 1980.
2. Harms B, Bodai B, Demling R: Prostaglandin release and altered microvascular integrity after burn injury. J Surg Res 34:274–280, 1981.

3. Herndon D, Wilmore D, Mason A: Serum mediated and cell dependent post thermal injury hypermetabolism. Br J Surg 66:894–900, 1979.
4. Demling RH: Fluid resuscitation after major burns. JAMA 250:1438–1442, 1983.
5. Zawacki B, Jung R, Joyce J: Smoke, burns, and the natural history of inhalation injury in fire victims. Ann Surg 185:100–109, 1977.
6. Euremus K: Hematologic changes in burns. *In* Artz C, Moncrief J, Pruitt B (eds): Burns: A Team Approach. Philadelphia, WB Saunders Company, 1979, pp 132–148.
7. Lamke L: Evaporative water loss from normal and burnt skin. Scand J Plast Reconstr Surg 5:17–22, 1971.
8. Demling RH: Fluid resuscitation after burns. Surg Clin North Am 67(10):15–30, 1987.
9. Demling RH: Improved survival after massive burns. J Trauma 23:179–184, 1983.
10. Sasaki T, Welch G, Herndon D: Burn wound manipulation induced bacteremia. J Trauma 19:46–51, 1979.
11. Peterson S, Umphred E, Warden G: The incidence of bacteremia following burn wound excision. J Trauma 22:274–279, 1982.
12. Wilmore D: The metabolic management of the critically ill. New York, Plenum Press, 1977.
13. Bessey J, Watters J, Aoki T, Wilmore D: Combined hormonal infusion simulates the metabolic response to injury. Ann Surg 3:264–281, 1984.

# Intensive Care Nursing of the Burned Patient

## MARJORIE McETTRICK-MALONEY

Burn nursing, despite the emotional and physical strain, is one of the most rewarding experiences. However, to most health professionals and lay people alike, burn nursing is not a popular specialty. What draws the young or seasoned nurse to take up the challenge? Burn nursing is not a required course in most nursing programs, nor is it a subject of primary concentration on the state licensure examinations. How then do nurses learn to care for one of the most disfiguring human conditions? What lures the intensive care nurse back each day to see another burned child or another family crisis or to perform another total body dressing on a 210-pound man? Is it the feeling of accomplishment at the end of the shift when they know that a patient is clean, comfortable, and well taken care of? Is it the weary smile of a young boy who says "thank you" on his way home after ten months in the sheltered world of the burn unit? Or is it the note of appreciation from a grieving family whose little girl has died but her eyes live on in another young child? Acute burn nursing has three prerequisites: knowledge of normal pathophysiology, an understanding of human behavior and relationships, and the willingness to constantly exceed the expected. It is a blend of intensive nursing, long-term rehabilitation nursing skills, and numerous hours of hard work and attention to the smallest detail.

This chapter is intended to be a functional guide for assessing the acutely burned patient and developing the subsequent nursing care plan for the acute phase. Emphasis will be placed on identifying the most common problems of the acute patient and the subsequent steps and nursing intervention.

The reconstructive and rehabilitative aspects of burn care are beyond the scope of this chapter. The reader will be encouraged to refer to specific chapters in this book for background information.

## INITIAL ASSESSMENT OF THE ACUTELY BURNED PATIENT

Although the burn injury itself presents as the most dramatic problem, it is essential to first assess the patient's basic life-sustaining systems (Fig. 7–1). As with any patient who has received an acute injury, time is of the essence. Movement and medical intervention must be purposeful and efficient. A system-

Date _____

Name _____ Age _____ Sex _____ Religion _____ Nickname _____

Diagnosis _____

T _____ P _____ R _____ BP _____ CVP _____ Weight _____ kg

Height _____ cm Head Circumference _____ cm

*Allergies _____ Person(s) interviewed _____

Legal Guardian _____

LABWORK DONE: CBC ( ) LYTES ( ) TP, OSM ( ) BS, BUN ( ) Creatinine ( ) PT, PTT ( )

 Platelets ( ) LFT's ( ) CPK ( ) HbCO$_3$ ( ) G$_6$PD ( ) Sickle Cell ( ) Clot ( ) UA ( )

BACTI CULTURES DONE: Wound ( ) Nose ( ) Throat ( ) Urine ( ) Stool ( ) Blood ( )

 Sputum ( )          PHOTOS TAKEN: ( )

1. PAST AND PRESENT HEALTH CARE

 Medical treatment prior to SBI admission _____

 _____

 _____

 Tetanus Toxoid given/date _____ Hx. of/Exposure to Chicken Pox/Other _____

 Medications at home/Meds today _____

2. INTEGUMENTARY

 Date/Time of Injury _____ Clothing _____

 % Burn/Describe skin condition _____

 _____

 _____

 Describe accident/First aid given _____

 _____

 _____

 WOUND CARE: Phisoderm body wash ( ) Nix shampoo ( ) Head Shave ( )

  Escharotomies _____

  Topical agents applied: _____

  Splints applied: _____

Parent _____ Airplane _____

Adm. Officer _____ Mode of Transport: Ambulance _____ MGH _____

Adm. packet given to parent/guardian: Yes ( ) No ( ) Deferred ( )

**Shriners Hospitals**                    **Burns Institute**
**for crippled children**        **Acute Nursing Assessment**
#2015-COL Rev. 5/88

**FIGURE 7–1.** Initial assessment form utilized at the Shriners Burns Institute Boston unit.

*Illustration continued on following page*

3. <u>RESPIRATORY</u>

Resp. problems/recent URI _____

If flame, enclosed or open space _____

Loss of consciousness with injury _____

Note presence of:   singed nasal hairs      _____         soot in mouth      _____
                   singed eyebrows/lashes  _____         soot in secretions  _____
                   singed hairline        _____         hoarseness       _____
                   coughing             _____         dyspnea         _____

Breath Sounds, secretions, CXR, other _____

_____

Mask/Treatment/% $O_2$ _____Intubated_____date_____

Location ETT_____Type/size of tube _____Length ETT_____cc's in cuff _____

Ventilator settings:  TV_____IMV_____PEEP_____PIP_____

4. <u>CIRCULATORY</u>

Edema: Location/describe _____

| Extremities: | Temp | Color | Sensation | Movement | Pulse Character |
|---|---|---|---|---|---|
| Rt. arm | | | | | radial<br>brachial |
| Lt. arm | | | | | radial<br>brachial |
| Rt. leg | | | | | pedal<br>popliteal |
| Lt. leg | | | | | pedal<br>popliteal |

Current IV/A-Line sites  —  date inserted      Old line sites  —  date D/C'd

_____    _____      _____    _____

_____    _____      _____    _____

_____    _____      _____    _____

5. <u>NUTRITION</u>

NGT_____date inserted_____type/size_____length _____

Diet/Tube Feedings prior to SBI _____

Hyperal _____Bowel sounds_____

Condition of oral cavity _____Any loose teeth _____

6. <u>ELIMINATION</u>

Foley_____date inserted_____size_____urine color_____Last BM_____

7. <u>NEUROLOGIC</u>

Describe L.O.C. _____

Pupils equal _____Round _____Reactive to light _____

Lacerations/Bruises on scalp _____

_____                            

Primary Nurse                     Date

_____         _____

Associate Nurse                 Date                Signature of Admitting Nurse

#2015-COL                   **ACUTE NURSING ASSESSMENT**

**FIGURE 7–1** *Continued*

based assessment will provide a basis for formulating the plan of care once the patient has been admitted to the burn or intensive care unit.

## Respiratory Assessment

As with other multiple-trauma patients, the first priority in thermal injury must be assessment and maintenance of the airway. Respiratory injury can be sustained as a result of flame and chemical burns via inhalation and also by direct contact with such burning agents as scalds.

Burn history should include the following:

Where the burn occurred—i.e., outside or in an enclosed space
Agents that could have been inhaled if the injury was sustained in an enclosed space
How long the patient was in the enclosed space
Any loss of consciousness or respiratory arrest
Distribution of the burn in relation to the respiratory system, i.e., face, chest, mouth, nares

**CLINICAL SIGNS.** On admission if any of the following signs is observed, it is highly likely that the patient sustained a respiratory insult.

Singed nasal hairs
Singed eyebrows/lashes
Singed hairline
Soot in the oral cavity
Soot in the secretions
Hoarseness/coughing
Dyspnea

The nurse must be alert to the fact that patients who have sustained burns about the face and neck but do not demonstrate such positive findings still have the potential for severe airway obstruction secondary to soft-tissue edema. Soft-tissue edema occurs rapidly, thereby increasing the potential for compromising the upper airway. Similarly, constricting full-thickness burn about the thorax or upper abdomen may present additional problems in maintaining adequate ventilation. Rapid surgical intervention in the form of escharotomies may be necessary to allow adequate pulmonary compliance and excursion.

### Nursing Interventions

The patient should be placed in a semi-Fowler's position to aid respiratory efforts unless otherwise contraindicated. This will decrease edema in the face, pharynx, and other structures above the level of the heart. Baseline arterial blood gases (ABG) should be obtained. Humidified oxygen at 30 to 50 per cent should be administered to aid oxygenation. Administration of 100 per cent oxygen is necessary if there is any question about exposure to carbon monoxide. A calming tone of voice and careful explanations should be used to help reduce the patient's anxiety. Prophylactic intubation may be necessary for patients who demonstrate significant facial and increasing laryngeal edema. Nasotracheal intubation is preferred for stability and patient comfort. A tracheostomy should be avoided whenever possible. The patient's pre-burn history should be obtained as soon as possible, with particular attention to recent upper respiratory infections, emphysema, allergies, asthma, or any other past respiratory problems.

## Cardiovascular Assessment

Owing to the sudden decrease in circulating volume as a result of the fluid shift from the intravascular space to the extravascular space, including the cells, the acutely burned patient is in a life-threatening situation. Four factors contribute to hypovolemia and burn shock in the immediate post-burn period[1]:

Increased capillary permeability
Increased sequestration of fluid in muscle cells
Increased evaporative water loss from the skin water barrier
Destruction of red blood cells due to the initial thermal insult

In burn shock there is a decrease in circulating volume and an increase in edema in areas affected by the burn. Red cells and other blood components are destroyed secondary to the heat of the injury rather than being lost, as in hemorrhagic shock. Fluid replacement must begin immediately after the burn has occurred.

The history of the burn injury must be ascertained and the following factors must be given immediate priority:

Exact time of injury
Significant medical events, loss of consciousness, or neurological trauma
    sustained as a result of a fall
Amount of fluid given since the burn injury occurred
Total body surface area (TBSA) involved and distribution of burns
Urine output since injury
Depth of burn wounds

There are numerous replacement formulas that are highly endorsed by individual burn units. The majority include the use of a combination of colloid and crystalloid to be administered within the first 24 to 48 hours. Initially, lactated Ringer's solution is the replacement fluid of choice. The author does not intend to endorse one formula over another but rather to emphasize the nursing interventions pertaining to fluid administration.

### Nursing Interventions

Pulse and blood pressure should be obtained immediately and repeated every 15 minutes, or more frequently as indicated, to monitor the patient's cardiovascular status. When burns involve the extremities, then pulses, temperature, circulation, sensation, and movement (CSM) of the affected areas should be monitored closely. Doppler ultrasonography is a useful diagnostic tool when palpation of pulses becomes difficult or uncertain. Constriction of the blood flow secondary to edema and constricting eschar has the potential for causing necrosis of tissue distal to the burn injury. For this reason, nursing efforts should be made to elevate the involved extremities to reduce swelling (if not contraindicated). If adequate perfusion is not being maintained, as evidenced by minimal or absent pulses, negative capillary refill, and CSM, then escharotomies need to be performed immediately by the surgical staff.

Preferred sites for the administration of fluid include central venous lines placed in the antecubital spaces, internal jugular, and/or subclavian region. Nursing considerations are directed toward maintaining integrity of the intravenous (IV) sites and accurate administration and recording of the fluids. If the patency of the line is questionable, it must be dealt with immediately, as fluid replacement is of the utmost importance. Lines should be sutured in place to ensure proper placement, as tape has less of an affinity for moist, burned tissue. The IV site should be observed for redness, swelling, and excoriation. Betadine ointment or a similar antiseptic agent should be applied and covered with a sterile gauze; the site should be cleansed and the dressing changed as needed. Commercially available transparent adhesive sheets are useful in securing the lines if the surrounding tissue is unburned. Unnecessary motion of the catheter in the vein and surrounding tissue increases the potential for infection at the site. The use of passive restraint may also be necessary to keep the lines in place.

The nurse should observe the patient for signs of hypovolemia during the initial fluid replacement:

Decreased urinary output
High urine specific gravity
Fall in blood pressure
Low central venous pressure
Rising blood urea nitrogen

A pre-burn history should be obtained as soon as possible after the patient has been stabilized. The history would include approximate pre-burn weight and past medical history with particular attention to the history of heart disease, use of diuretics, diabetes, blood dyscrasia, and kidney problems. A positive finding in any of these areas may affect fluid replacement efforts.

## Integumentary Assessment

The American Burn Association's Criteria of Burn Injury Severity establishes the following guidelines for the classification of burns.

**Minor burns.** Second-degree burns of less than 10 per cent TBSA in children. Less than 15 per cent second-degree burns in adults or less than 2 per cent third-degree burns not involving eyes, ears, face, or genitalia in a child or adult.

**MODERATE BURNS.** Ten to twenty per cent second-degree or up to 10 per cent third-degree burns in children. In adults, 15 to 25 per cent second-degree burns or less than 10 per cent third-degree burns not involving special care areas.

**SEVERE BURNS.** Twenty per cent or greater second-degree or greater than 10 per cent third-degree burns in children. Greater than 25 per cent second-degree or greater than 10 per cent third-degree burns in adults. All burns involving face, hands, genitalia, eyes, ears, and feet. All inhalation injuries and electrical burns.

The depth of burns is universally categorized as follows:

### FIRST-DEGREE BURNS

| | |
|---|---|
| Cause: | Flash, flame, ultraviolet (sunlight) |
| Surface appearance: | Dry, no blisters, minimal or no edema |
| Color: | Erythematous |
| Pain level: | Painful |
| Histological depth: | Epidermal layers only |
| Healing time: | Two to five days with peeling; no scarring; may have discoloration |

### SECOND-DEGREE PARTIAL-THICKNESS BURNS

| | |
|---|---|
| Cause: | Contact with hot liquids or solids<br>Flash flame to clothing<br>Direct flame or chemical |
| Surface appearance: | Moist blebs, blisters |
| Color: | Mottled white to pink to cherry red |
| Pain level: | Very painful |
| Histological depth: | Epidermis, papillary, and reticular layers of dermis. May include fat domes of subcutaneous layer. |
| Healing time: | *Superficial:* Five to 21 days with no grafting.<br>*Deep partial:* With no infection, 21 to 35 days. If infected, converts to full thickness. |

### THIRD-DEGREE FULL-THICKNESS BURNS

| | |
|---|---|
| Cause: | Contact with hot liquids or solids<br>Flame, chemical, electrical |
| Surface appearance: | Dry with leathery eschar until debridement. Charred blood vessels visible under eschar. |
| Color: | Mixed white, waxy pearl. Dark khaki, mahogany. Charred. |

| | |
|---|---|
| Pain level: | Present but of different type and intensity compared to partial thickness. Hair pulls out easily. |
| Histological depth: | Down to and including subcutaneous tissue. May include fascia, muscle, and bone. |
| Healing time: | Large areas require grafting, which may require months. Small areas may heal from edges after weeks. |

Calculation of the TBSA is usually based on two prominent methods: the Lund and Browder Chart and the Rule of Nines developed by E. J. Pulaski and E. W. Tennison. See Figure 7–2 for an example of a burn diagram calculation sheet. An accurate initial estimate of the TBSA is essential for the correct calculation of replacement fluids administered during the first 48 hours of treatment.

### Nursing Interventions

The patient's clothing should be removed immediately if it has not already been removed at the scene to prevent further damage due to the heat contained in the fabric. The patient's clothes should be set aside carefully for possible investigation of fabrics worn or agents used to ignite the fire. Burn diagrams depicting the distribution and depth of the injury should be completed grossly; details can be drawn later. The body should be washed with a warmed, mild soap solution to remove soot and devitalized skin. The scalp should be examined closely for burns or exit points (in the event of an electrical injury). Topical agents should be applied as ordered by the physician. Large quantities of topical agents are not necessarily better for wound healing. Application varies with the individual manufacturer. If the patient is being transferred to a burn facility, he should be wrapped in dry sterile gauze. This allows the receiving facility to adequately assess the per cent and depth of injury without distraction or recleaning the wound to remove cream-topical agents.

## Thermostability

Most often the patient presents with a core body temperature below normal. This is especially true if the patient has been transported in cold saline towels from the accident scene to the emergency room. Because the skin is the largest organ of the body and its primary function is to protect the body from infection and maintain temperature, external efforts must be employed to assist the body in these areas when a moderate to severe burn is sustained. The greater the TBSA, the greater the heat loss.

### Nursing Interventions

The triage area should be warmed as much as possible, and examination of the patient should be efficient. Care should be taken to alternately cover the

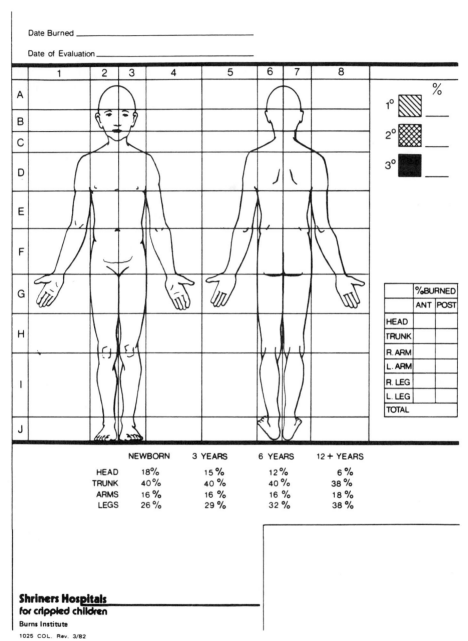

Date Burned _____

Date of Evaluation _____

|  | 1 | 2 | 3 | 4 | 5 | 6 | 7 | 8 |
|---|---|---|---|---|---|---|---|---|
| A | | | | | | | | |
| B | | | | | | | | |
| C | | | | | | | | |
| D | | | | | | | | |
| E | | | | | | | | |
| F | | | | | | | | |
| G | | | | | | | | |
| H | | | | | | | | |
| I | | | | | | | | |
| J | | | | | | | | |

$1°$ ⬚  %  ____
$2°$ ⬚  ____
$3°$ ⬛  ____

|  | %BURNED | |
|---|---|---|
|  | ANT | POST |
| HEAD | | |
| TRUNK | | |
| R. ARM | | |
| L. ARM | | |
| R. LEG | | |
| L. LEG | | |
| TOTAL | | |

|  | NEWBORN | 3 YEARS | 6 YEARS | 12 + YEARS |
|---|---|---|---|---|
| HEAD | 18% | 15% | 12% | 6% |
| TRUNK | 40% | 40% | 40% | 38% |
| ARMS | 16% | 16% | 16% | 18% |
| LEGS | 26% | 29% | 32% | 38% |

**Shriners Hospitals**
**for crippled children**
**Burns Institute**
1025 COL. Rev. 3/82

**FIGURE 7–2.** Burn diagram sheet used at the Shriners Burns Institute Boston unit to calculate the burn distribution, depth, and degree.

torso, limbs, and head with dry sterile towels during examination. Wet dressings should be withheld until the patient's temperature has reached 100 to 101°F and is expected to remain at that level. Once the patient is warmed by the application of dry dressings or blankets or a temperature-controlled environment, the core body temperature will rise. Temperature rebounds to 101 to 102°F should be expected. This is due to the body's natural defense mechanisms and fluid resuscitation efforts. Efforts to externally cool the patient should not be employed unless the temperature is in excess of 104°F. Needless cooling can further compromise the patient's ability to adjust to the massive fluid volume changes he will experience during the first 48 hours.

## Genitourinary Assessment

Soft-tissue swelling in the genital area is significant in moderate to severe burns. Whether or not the burn involves the genital region, edema of the surrounding tissue can be sufficient to constrict urinary flow. This makes catheterization more difficult as time passes in the acute resuscitation phase. For this reason an appropriate-size Foley catheter needs to be inserted as soon as possible to maintain accurate measurements of output. Too large a catheter may cause ulceration of the urethra when placement is prolonged. Feeding tubes are useful for small children when conventional catheters are too large. Urine output of 1 cc/kg/hour in children and 30 cc/hour in adults must be maintained in the initial 48 hours. Concentrated urine, as evidenced by a specific gravity greater than 1.025, is an indication of insufficient fluid replacement. Serum and urine electrolytes should be monitored every 2 to 4 hours to determine the patient's response to fluid replacement. After successful fluid replacement, normal serum sodium (135 to 145 mEq/L) and potassium (3.5 to 4.5 mEq/L) levels are restored. The presence of blood in the urine, detected either visually or by dipstick, indicates that the red cells have been destroyed and are releasing hemoglobin into the circulation. It may also be indicative of the release of myoglobin from destroyed muscle mass. This heralding sign must be brought to the physician's attention immediately. An osmotic diuretic such as mannitol is usually ordered and administered until the urine is clear and specific gravity has returned to a more normal range. Intravenous fluids are also increased to maintain optimal perfusion through the kidneys to prevent acute renal tubular necrosis.

## Gastrointestinal Assessment

Patients who have sustained burns of 20 per cent or greater TBSA are at risk for developing a paralytic ileus as a result of gastric dilatation. During the initial hours, patients are usually kept NPO. The presence or absence of bowel sounds should be noted. A nasogastric tube may be necessary to decompress the stomach and aid in the administration of antacids to neutralize increased gastric acidity.

## Special Considerations

Circumstances involving children and burn injury must be evaluated carefully. Although most burn injuries involving children are accidental, the potential for abuse should not be overlooked. The majority of children who sustain burns as a result of abuse or neglect are less than five years old,[2] and these burns are usually the result of immersion. The areas commonly involved include the feet, buttocks, and hands. When children have burns of suspicious etiology or when the distribution of burn does not correlate with the description of the accident, the assessment of the patient must include a search for any evidence of abuse. The presence of old bruises and fractures may be additional evidence of long-standing abuse. A full bone series should be obtained when abuse is suspected.

## Approach to the Patient

Careful explanation of medical procedures within the parameters of age and developmental level is necessary to gain the patient's cooperation during the initial hours of stabilization. A calm and controlled demeanor and environment, with careful consideration for the person who is the patient, is as essential as other medical and nursing interventions. Once the initial assessment has been made and the patient is medically stable, it is often helpful to the patient (especially if it is a child) to have a familiar person providing support during the remaining admission activities. The ground rules and specific supportive statements, as well as what the person will be seeing, should be discussed prior to including the person in this process.

## Electrical Injuries

The reader is encouraged to review the chapter on electrical injuries (Chapter 5) for detailed information.

## PLANNING NURSING CARE

Nursing care of the burned patient is complex and time-consuming and requires strict attention to detail. The nursing plan is based on assessment of the data, nature and severity of the injury, and potential and actual problems that occur during the patient's hospitalization. Thus, the care plan is ongoing and reflects the patient's progression from illness to wellness. This can be a very lengthy process.

The primary nurse is in the best position to draw together all the facets of care of the burn patient to form a consistent and individualized plan of care. The nursing plan and the patient needs are communicated to the interdisciplinary team for their input. The primary nurse is not only in the position of managing the patient's care on a 24-hour basis but is also helping the patient and family to understand and accept the outcomes of this devastating injury.

Six preliminary care plans, common to most burn patients, are outlined in this section. They are intended to be a functional guide to which individualized nursing actions may be added to form a complete nursing care plan.

## Infection

Once fluid resuscitation has been accomplished and the patient is in a state of relative fluid and electrolyte balance, focus is on combatting infection. Infection is a determinant in patient survival. It occurs in all burn wounds, but the spectrum of organisms, their sensitivity, and their resistance patterns vary. Antibiotic use and medical treatment of burn wounds differ from one burn unit to another, as do the choice of topical agents and protocols for wound closure. The overall goal of the various methods is to minimize infection and promote wound healing.

Nursing considerations relative to infection control are universal. Nursing efforts must be vigilant with regard to infection control in the following aspects of patient care:

*Handwashing between patients is first and foremost.

*Utilizing barrier technique when performing dressing changes and routine procedures to prevent the transfer of organisms from one extremity or body part to another. Whenever possible, the clean areas should be attended before dirty ones. Movement in the opposite direction is likely to contaminate the clean areas. Changing gloves when moving from one wound area to another and completing one extremity dressing before beginning another are small but important steps in preventing cross-contamination. Care must be taken in the handling and disposal of contaminated dressing materials and instruments, not only because of the risks to the nurse of AIDS and hepatitis if they are improperly handled, but also because they are a source of environmental contamination.

*Proper attire should be worn by all personnel and visitors in contact with the patient.

*Comparative wound assessment must be made at each dressing change. Assessment includes color, odor, drainage, and evidence of healing.

*The patient's immediate area should be clean and uncluttered.

*All surfaces (e.g., countertops, floor) should be kept clean by using an appropriate germicidal solution to reduce likely sources of infection.

*Patient items should be labeled and reserved for single patient use only.

*Shared items such as go-carts, wheelchairs, walkers, and toys should be thoroughly cleaned before and after each patient use.

The reader is encouraged to review chapters 2, 6, 18, and 19 which deal with infection and wound treatment for more detailed information.

The nursing care plan relative to infection control should include at least the following elements:

**PATIENT PROBLEM.** Potential for infection secondary to altered skin integrity as a result of burn injury.

**EXPECTED OUTCOME.** Promote wound healing and minimize wound infection.

**NURSING ACTIONS**

1. Obtain and record vital signs every hour until stable. Report variations in trends.

2. Observe for trends indicative of sepsis:
   —Low-grade temperature
   —Sinus tachycardia
   —Low blood pressure
   —Oliguria
   —Minimal or absent bowel sounds
   —Disorientation
   —Increased bleeding from wounds
   —Petechiae

3. Administer prescribed antibiotics with attention to the following:
   —Compatibility with other antibiotics administered
   —Infuse antibiotics over the recommended period of time to ensure efficacy and minimize side effects.
   —Follow blood levels to ensure that prescribed dose is effective.

4. At each dressing change observe the wounds and document the character of the wounds.

5. Culture wound surfaces and any questionable tracts or pockets.

6. Make recommendations to increase or decrease the frequency of dressing changes based on wound observation.

7. Wash unburned skin with mild soap and warm water with each dressing change. Protect unburned and healed skin from topical agents using moisturizer or petroleum gauze.

8. Perform line care every 2 to 3 hours to all indwelling lines according to unit procedures. Observe site for symptoms of localized infection and loose or broken sutures.

9. Culture removed catheter tips.

10. Track wound, blood, sputum, and urine cultures.

11. Maintain room temperature at a constant level, usually between 25 and 30°C or 75 and 80°F. Avoid extremes of temperature.

## Respiratory

Inhalation injury is a leading cause of morbidity and mortality in burn patients. The very young and the elderly are at special risk. Respiratory injury can be divided into three areas:

*Airway Damage.* Edema forms as a result of exposure to heat, gases, steam, or chemicals. This injury can result in significant airway obstruction because of bronchospasm and sloughing of respiratory epithelium, requiring an artificial airway to maintain ventilation.

*Alveolar Damage.* Fire conditions produce toxic gases. When these gases make contact with alveolar epithelium, they produce chemical burns in the respiratory tract and alveoli. The pulmonary-capillary endothelium is destroyed by decreased surfactant production. The end result is diminished compliance and oxygenation. The clinical picture is analogous to the adult respiratory distress syndrome (ARDS).

*Carbon Monoxide Poisoning.* Carbon monoxide is present in all fire conditions and binds to the hemoglobin molecule. This results in decreased oxygen-carrying capacity and profound tissue hypoxia that can be fatal.

Patients who have sustained a circumferential or full-thickness trunk burn should be carefully and frequently assessed. If they are ventilated, peak inspiratory pressures and tidal volume should be measured hourly. If they are not intubated, chest excursion, respiratory rate, and blood gases are useful parameters. The level of analgesia directly correlates with respiratory effort. Pain and anxiety elevate respiratory rate, thereby decreasing the effective alveolar ventilation. The intravenous route is the preferred route for administration of medications, particularly during the acute phase, because absorption by way of the gastrointestinal tract and subcutaneous absorption may be impaired due to altered blood flow.

The appropriate nursing plan of care is dependent upon the location and nature of the respiratory insult. The following is recommended as a general starting point:

PATIENT PROBLEM. Inadequate ventilation related to airway obstruction.

EXPECTED OUTCOME. Patient maintains an adequate airway and tissue oxygenation as evidenced by clear breath sounds in all lobes, absence of clinical signs of hypoxia, satisfactory ABGs, minimal use of accessory muscles for respiration, and absence of pulmonary congestion on chest radiograph.

NURSING ACTIONS

1. Monitor respiratory parameters at least hourly, including:
   —Respiratory rate
   —Depth
   —Patterns
   —Level of consciousness
   —Peripheral perfusion
   —Heart rate
2. Elevate head of bed 45 degrees or higher (if not contraindicated).
3. Administer warm humidified oxygen as ordered to aid in oxygenation and prevent mucosal drying.
4. Perform chest physical therapy (CPT) every 4 hours and prn.

5. Maintain artificial airway:
   —Sedate patient and/or use passive restraint to prevent accidental extubation.
   —Firmly secure endotracheal tube by using twill tape or other means.
   —Resecure tube as needed to adjust to changing facial edema.
   —Avoid prolonged pressure on the nares to prevent nasal necrosis. Use a small bandage roll to support junction of the endotracheal tube and ventilator tubing.
   —Check cuff pressures every shift per unit procedure.
6. Monitor adequacy of ventilation:
   —ABG as clinical condition warrants
   —Carboxyhemoglobin level as ordered
   —Hourly peak inspiratory pressure and tidal volume measurement
   —Monitor cardiac output, degree of shunting and pulmonary capillary wedge pressure (PCWP) if Swan-Ganz catheter is in place.
7. Assist with weaning the patient from the ventilator.
   Criteria for weaning:
   —Vital capacity 10 to 15 ml/kg
   —Normal respiratory rate for age
   —Normal heart rate for age
   —Normal blood pressure for age
   —Normal hemoglobin
   —Acceptable blood gases
   —Stable fluid and electrolyte balance
8. Extubation should be scheduled for early in the day after dressing changes have been completed, thus minimizing the stress on the pulmonary system which occurs with pain during dressing changes.

## Fluid and Electrolyte Balance

Marked fluid shifts occur in the first 48 hours of burn treatment. The patient is at great risk of developing hypovolemic shock from the massive shift of fluids from the vascular space into the interstitial and extracellular spaces and from loss of plasma protein through the weakened capillary membranes.

Serum potassium levels are initially elevated (4.0 mEq/L) because of hemolysis and tissue necrosis. Serum sodium and chloride levels may be within the normal range. The hematocrit is usually elevated primarily to hemoconcentration because of extravasation of plasma water.

Once the patient begins to diurese, usually during the 48- to 72-hour period as evidenced by a urine output two to three times greater than previously recorded, another potentially life-threatening imbalance occurs. Potassium formerly retained is now being lost, as demonstrated by a decline in serum potassium and by an increase in urine potassium (>.40 mEq/L). Potassium must be monitored closely and replaced judiciously so as to avoid potential cardiac arrhythmia. Serum sodium and chloride may increase or decrease during the diuretic phase. Overly aggressive fluid replacement, particularly during the first few days of injury, can result in an overexpansion of the extracellular space resulting in edema of burned and nonburned areas, including the lungs. Pulmonary edema can also be a result of pulmonary capillary damage secondary to inhalation injury. The nurse should be aware of the potential for fluid overload and electrolyte imbalance. The signs and symptoms of fluid overload are:

Increased peripheral edema (not burn-related)
Decreased specific gravity
Increased urine output
Increased or decreased serum sodium level

Diuretics and fluid restriction are usually employed to assist the kidneys in ridding the body of this excess fluid.

During all phases of fluid replacement, the nurse must accurately record hourly intake (e.g., crystalloid, plasma, medications, boluses) and output (urine, gastric aspirates, blood samples, emesis, and stools). Additional fluid replacement may be indicated to compensate for the decreased cardiac output due to ventilatory support, for fever, and for evaporative and insensible water losses.

Basic nursing interventions pertaining to fluid and electrolyte balance are outlined below:

**PATIENT PROBLEM.** Alterations in fluid and electrolyte balance secondary to burn.

**EXPECTED OUTCOME.** Stable fluid and electrolyte balance evidenced by serum and urine electrolytes within normal limits, adequate urine output, absence of diarrhea, clear chest radiograph, normal blood pressure and heart rate for age, and appropriate psychological orientation.

### NURSING ACTIONS

1. During fluid replacement monitor adequacy of intravascular volume. Monitor at least hourly:
   —Urine output
   —Mean arterial pressure of 80 to 100 mm Hg, CVP 5 to 10
   —Heart rate
   —PCWP, PA pressure where indicated
2. Titrate intravenous fluids as ordered to maintain the above parameters.
3. Document hourly intake and output (I&O).
4. Obtain serum urine osmolarity every 4 hours and prn. Obtain total protein and albumin daily and prn.
5. Ensure patency and security of Foley catheter and intravenous lines to prevent inaccurate I&O data.
6. Observe for signs of fluid and electrolyte imbalance (hypokalemia, overload, hypernatremia).

7. Adjust intravenous fluids to oral nasogastric intake to maintain appropriate fluid balance.

## Nutrition

The burn patient is in a hypermetabolic state until he is nearly healed. Consequently, the demands for protein and other essential nutrients cannot be underestimated. A direct correlation between delayed wound healing and a lack of appropriate nutrients has been well documented. The primary goal of most nutritional programs is to provide the body with more quality calories than usually required in a state of relative well-being. This is especially important in the case of second- and third-degree burns that involve 30 per cent or greater TBSA. It is preferable to allow the patient to take calories by mouth when possible. Nasogastric, duodenal, and intravenous support, however, are usually necessary to assist the patient in attaining the expected 24-hour requirements. Pre-burn weight, dietary habits, food preferences, elimination patterns, and food allergies should be ascertained by the nurse or dietitian. Repeated surgical procedures to remove the eschar and establish wound closure will significantly interrupt the nutritional plan. Refer to Chapter 10 on nutrition for further specifics.

Nursing interventions pertaining to the nutritional aspects of the burned patient are outlined as follows:

**PATIENT PROBLEM.** Alteration in nutritional needs secondary to burn injury.

**EXPECTED OUTCOME.** Patient will achieve expected daily caloric requirements with appropriate blend of fats, carbohydrates, and protein.

### NURSING ACTIONS

1. Obtain admission height and weight.
2. Weigh twice weekly and prn.
3. Obtain diet history from patient or family member.
4. Maintain an accurate daily calorie count.
5. Report diarrhea or absence of stool, indicating a need to change or alter the patient's nutritional regimen or oral medication schedule.
6. Encourage the family to bring favorite food items from home.
7. Schedule dressing changes and other painful procedures so as not to interfere with meals.
8. Provide quiet, pleasant surroundings for mealtimes.
9. Encourage the patient to feed himself as much as possible.
10. Offer small, high-protein snacks.
11. Discourage "empty calories" such as soft drinks and candy.
12. If enteral feedings are used to provide total calories or as a supplement to oral intake, the following should be considered:
    —Hourly feedings should be administered via slow continuous infusion.

—The concentration as well as the hourly volume should be increased gradually.

—Enteral preparations should be delivered at room temperature.

## Emotional Care of the Burned Patient and Family

The psychological impact of a burn injury on the patient, family, and friends can be devastating (see Chapters 17 and 20). Relationships and coping mechanisms are strained during hospitalization. The skills of all members of the interdisciplinary team are needed to provide the family and patient with the emotional support and guidance needed to cope with what lies ahead.

The nurse's primary focus in this aspect of patient care is to learn how the patient dealt with stress, separation, and hospitalization prior to this injury. Family dynamics and how they impact on the patient should also be assessed. Additionally, the nurse must identify the patient's individual strengths and sources of strength (e.g., religion) within the family and environment.

Painful procedures become the norm for the burn patient. Taking time to allow the patient to make choices when there are choices is beneficial in developing a trusting relationship. Encouraging the patient to participate in his dressing changes, when possible, can significantly decrease his level of anxiety and response to pain.[3] This has proved to be significant in patients as young as 18 months.[4]

Quiet periods tend to draw out the patient's most intense emotions and fears. The nurse's presence and verbal and nonverbal responses at these times are important. It is necessary for the nurse to skillfully guide the conversation, display a confident and caring approach, and, most importantly, be an attentive listener. There are often no substantive answers to questions about the future, but the nurse can offer support and realistic expectations based on his or her clinical knowledge and experience. The following care plan addresses these issues:

**PATIENT PROBLEM.** Alteration in coping secondary to hospitalization and separation from family.

**EXPECTED OUTCOME.** Premorbid family relationships will be maintained and supported.

### NURSING ACTIONS

1. Assess patient's and family's understanding of current situation and previous methods of coping with stressful situations.

2. Identify important and supportive persons in the patient's family and social group.

3. Explain all procedures to the patient as age, condition, and developmental level allow.

4. Encourage the patient and family to ask questions. Allow for quality time to talk with them in an area away from interruption as much as possible.

5. Conduct family meetings as needed to discuss the patient's progress and/or needs.

6. Collaborate with other team members to discuss patient status, needs, and overall direction.

7. Encourage the patient's participation in planning such daily events as meal times, dressing changes, visiting, and rest times.

8. Encourage spouse and family members to take breaks from hospital visiting and vigils.


## OPERATIVE NURSING CONCERNS AND INTERVENTIONS

Owing to the nature and severity of burn injury, most patients require numerous surgical debridement and grafting procedures during the acute phase of their hospitalization. Although the patient gains familiarity with the operating room staff and procedures, the anxiety and fear remain. The operating room staff need to be cognizant of the patient's fear and resultant behaviors.


### Preoperative Nursing Interventions

1. Establishment of a relationship with the patient before transport to the operating room. This should be done the day before in the form of a preoperative visit. Explanation of what the patient will see, smell, and hear, as well as who will be in the operating room (primary nurse, favorite toy), is important.

2. Review the patient's overall condition, complications, and special procedures to be performed while the patient is under anesthesia, e.g., head shave, physical therapy, skin biopsy.

3. Reassure the patient that the circulating nurse will be present during induction of and emergence from anesthesia.


### Intraoperative Nursing Interventions

1. Maintenance of body temperature
   —The operating room, induction room, and transfer and holding areas should be as warm as possible.
   —A warming blanket should be placed on the operating table.
   —An overhead warmer should be placed over the patient.
   —Uninvolved extremities should be covered as much as possible with warm blankets and sterile plastic bags.
   —The head should be covered with stockinette.
   —Prep and irrigating solutions should be warmed.
   —Body temperature is continuously displayed by a temperature-monitoring probe, usually attached by the anesthesiologist.

2. Aseptic technique
   —Maintenance of sterile field and barrier technique
3. Patient safety
   —Adequate staff for transfer
   —Grounding for electrocautery; ensure that the body is not in contact with metal table parts.
   —Postoperative check of grounding site
4. Prevention of injury
   —Position patient appropriately for planned surgical procedure to prevent nerve injury.
   —Adequate padding and support
   —Advise surgical team not to lean unnecessarily on patient.
   —Correct application of tourniquet (if used)
   —Proper application of splints: adequate padding, correct positioning, properly secured
5. Communication to receiving unit
   —Status reports are appreciated by the receiving unit personnel. Additional equipment can be obtained if advance notice is given.
6. Communication to family
   —A status report should be passed on to anxious family members waiting in the lobby or at home, since surgical procedures last many hours.

## Postoperative Nursing Interventions

1. Nursing report from the circulating operating room nurse to the receiving nurse, including:
   —Procedure performed, location of donor sites, dressings, and location of temporary wound coverings
   —Estimated blood loss
   —Amount and type of replacement fluids
   —Urine output
   —Anesthesia used
   —Recent arterial blood gases, vital signs, and other pertinent laboratory values
   —Intraoperative complications
   —Special procedures performed such as line changes
2. Patient stabilization in recovery area
   —Room should be warmed.
   —Warm blankets should be available.
   —Vital signs should be taken immediately and then as per hospital routine.
   —Evaluate cardiovascular and respiratory status.
   —Operative sites should be elevated and observed closely for bleeding.
   —Administer pain medication on time.

—A familiar object or face will enhance the patient's recovery from anesthesia.

—Activity and noise should be kept to a minimum.

—Repeated surgical procedures prolong the patient's recovery time and require vigilant postoperative observation and care.

3. Family preparation

—The family should be prepared for the physical appearance of the patient and the equipment they will see postoperatively.

## REFERENCES

1. Salisbury R: Manual of Burn Therapeutics: An Interdisciplinary Approach. Boston, Little, Brown & Company, 1983, p 10.
2. Wachtel T: Current Topics in Burn Care. Rockville, MD, Aspen Publications, 1983, p 180.
3. Kavanaugh CK: Psychological intervention with the severely burned child: Report of an experimental comparison of two approaches and their effects on psychological sequelae. J Am Acad Child Psychiatry 22:145–156, 1983.
4. Lasoff EM, McEttrick MA: Participation versus diversion during dressing changes: Can nurses' attitudes change? Issues Compr Pediatr Nurs 9:391–398, 1986.

## BIBLIOGRAPHY

Charnack EL, Meehan JJ: Postburn respiratory injuries in children. Pediatr Clin North Am 27(3):661–676, 1980.
Hudak C, Lohr T, Gallo B: Critical Care Nursing. Philadelphia, JB Lippincott, 1982.
Hummel R (ed): Clinical Burn Therapy. Boston, John Wright, 1982.
Jacoby FG: Nursing Care of the Patient with Burns. St. Louis, CV Mosby, 1976.
Kavanaugh CK: Psychological intervention with the severely burned child: Report of two experimental approaches and their effects on psychological sequelae. J Am Acad Child Psychiatr 22:145–156, 1983.
Lushbough M: Critical care of the child with burns. Nurs Clin North Am 16(4):635–647, 1981.
McLaughlin E, Crawford J: Burns. Pediatr Clin North Am 32(1):61–75, 1985.
Salisbury R (ed): Manual of Burn Therapeutics, An Interdisciplinary Approach. Boston, Little, Brown & Company, 1983.
Shapiro B, Harrison R, Kacmarek R, Cane R: Clinical Application of Respiratory Care. Chicago, Year Book Medical Publishers, 1985.
Wachtel T, Kahn V, Frank H: Current Topics in Burn Care. Rockville, MD, Aspen Publications, 1983.
Zawacki B, Jung R, Joyce J, Ricon E: Smoke, burns, and the natural history of inhalation injury in fire victims: A correlation of experimental and clinical data. Ann Surg 185(1):100–110, 1977.

# 8

# Rationale for Acute
# Surgical Approach

SUSAN E. BRIGGS

Early excision and grafting of the burn wound as soon as the patient is hemodynamically stable remain the keys to survival for patients with major thermal injuries. Colonization of the nonviable and necrotic burn wound eschar with bacteria and fungi presents a major risk of infection in all burned individuals. Prompt excision and coverage of the burn wound, either with temporary or permanent coverage, lessen the risk of infectious complications, including death. Prior to definitive coverage of the burn wound, topical antimicrobial agents, synthetic dressings such as Biobrane, and biological dressings such as cadaver skin play important roles as adjuncts to treatment (Fig. 8–1).

## PATIENT SELECTION

Early excision and grafting of a small burn were first described by Lustgarten in 1891, but the concept did not gain widespread acceptance until Janzekovic in 1970 reported excellent results with early excision and coverage of burns of varying depths.[1, 2] Postulated benefits of early excision and grafting are (1) decrease in the incidence of systemic sepsis originating from the burn wound, (2) decrease in mortality from burn wound sepsis, and (3) decrease in hospital stay.

One of the physician's most difficult tasks is to estimate accurately the depth of the burn and the time required for healing in order to determine the best method of treatment. There are no reliable devices or laboratory tests for determining burn depth, and the diagnosis must be based on clinical expertise. The etiology of the burn, age of the patient, appearance of the wound, and sensory nerve examination are all important clues to the depth of the thermal wound and its potential for healing. The time required for wounds to heal depends on numerous factors such as the thickness of the skin, the number of viable dermal skin appendages, the general health of the patient, and the presence or absence of infection. Most burns cannot be accurately assessed in the emergency room, as thermal injuries require time to reveal the extent of tissue necrosis. Scald burns secondary to nonviscous liquids generally require three to five days to show the extent of tissue injury. In chemical burns and

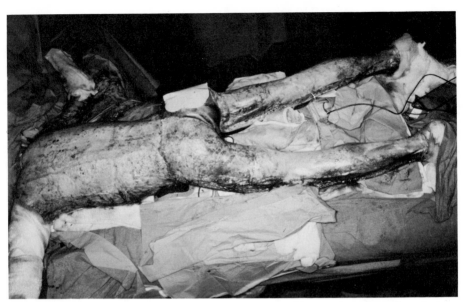

**FIGURE 8–1.** Temporary coverage of 95 per cent TBSA thermal burn with synthetic skin substitute (Biobrane) following early excision of wound.

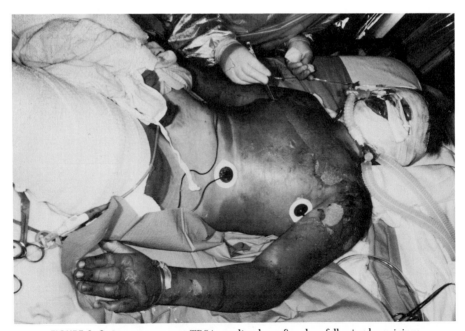

**FIGURE 8–2.** Seventy per cent TBSA gasoline burn five days following burn injury.

burns with viscous liquids such as grease, it may take as long as 7 to 10 days before the extent of injury becomes apparent (Fig. 8–2).

Burns involving only the superficial dermis generally heal within three weeks without significant functional or cosmetic deformities. Primary excision and grafting in such burns do not reduce morbidity or mortality, do not improve appearance or function, and substitute the discomfort of donor sites for the pain of the burn.[2–4]

Early excision of the burn wound with either temporary coverage of the wound or grafting with autogenous tissue is the procedure of choice for most mid- to deep dermal burns of significant size and for all full-thickness burns. Inhalation injury with associated thermal burns is not a contraindication to early excision and grafting of the burn wound. In fact, those with inhalation injury are most likely to succumb to fatal septicemia from wound or pulmonary sepsis, and early surgical excision should be performed as soon as the patient is hemodynamically stable.

Unfortunately, many burns, especially scald burns, may be indeterminate in depth, so that the decision whether or not to proceed with early excision and grafting is less clear (Fig. 8–3). Excision of deep burns over joints, tendons, and bones may produce wounds that are difficult to cover surgically.

A number of general principles may be helpful in determining the depth of the burn wound and its potential to heal.

1. Burns in infants, small children, and the elderly are usually deeper than anticipated. In particular, scald burns in these groups should not be assumed to be second-degree burns based on etiology (Fig. 8–4). In infants under two years of age, most scald burns are a combination of second- and third-degree burns.

2. Immersion and contact burns are rarely superficial burns.

3. Burns from viscous liquids such as fat or soup are usually deeper than nonviscous scald burns.

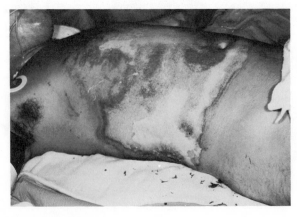

**FIGURE 8–3.** "Mixed" second- and third-degree gasoline burn of chest.

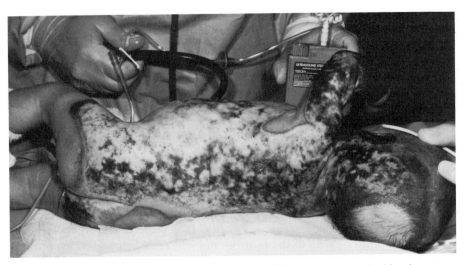

**FIGURE 8–4.** Full-thickness 70 per cent TBSA scald burn in a two-month-old male.

4. Chemical, gasoline, and electrical burns should be assumed to be third-degree burns until proven otherwise (Fig. 8–5).

5. Most burns of the palms and soles heal spontaneously, with the exception of contact burns.

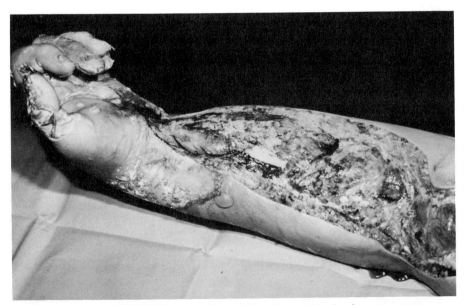

**FIGURE 8–5.** Full-thickness electrical burn of the hand.

## EXCISION AND GRAFTING TECHNIQUES

The primary reasons for graft failure are inadequate excision of burn eschar or granulation tissue, infection, and mechanical loss from factors such as motion or bleeding.[4-6] The goal of surgical therapy in burns is to select a method of treatment which provides excision and coverage of the burn wound before the patient becomes septic and minimizes the chance of graft loss in a particular patient. The techniques of surgical excision depend upon the depth of the burn wound, the total body surface area (TBSA) involved, the health and age of the patient, the presence of associated injuries, and the presence or absence of inhalation injury.

Excision of the burn eschar should be performed as early as possible in the patient's hospital course. The advantage of early excision must be balanced against the patient's hemodynamic instability. It is preferable to proceed with early excision and coverage of the burn wound within 72 hours. The hyperemic response to inflammation in the burn wound is a significant factor after 72 hours, and surgical excision is then associated with greater blood loss.[3, 5]

Patients with uncomplicated second- and third-degree burns of less than 40 per cent TBSA may be considered for tangential excisions within the first week following injury. In patients with inhalation injury or significant cardiopulmonary disease, the key principle is to minimize operating time and decrease blood loss to avoid the need for excess fluid replacement. In such groups of high risk patients, fascial excision is utilized more frequently. Fascial excision is also used frequently in patients with significant TBSA burns. The key objective in such burns is to diminish overall burn size to avoid overwhelming sepsis. Large anatomical areas (trunk and upper extremities) are excised first, while small anatomical areas (hands and feet) are excised last. Facial burns are debrided aggressively but are not excised early in order to allow maximal healing and to preserve as much soft tissue as possible for the best cosmetic result.

### Tangential Excision

Sequentially layered excision of the burn eschar to viable bleeding points, even to subcutaneous fat, is the preferred method of excision in smaller burns (Fig. 8–6). The major benefit of tangential excision is cosmetic, as the technique allows preservation of all unburned tissue. In particular, the goal of tangential excision of burn eschar is to preserve unburned subcutaneous fat, which provides contour and form to the human body, especially in regions such as the face, hands, and upper chest. The burn eschar can be removed by any of a variety of cutting instruments, ranging from blades such as the Goulian and Watson knives to hand- and power-driven dermatomes (Fig. 8–7). Donor harvesting is an example of tangential excision. Topical vasoconstrictors such as thrombin or epinephrine should not be applied to the wound until the excision is completed, as bleeding is the most reliable sign of the adequacy of the tangential excision.

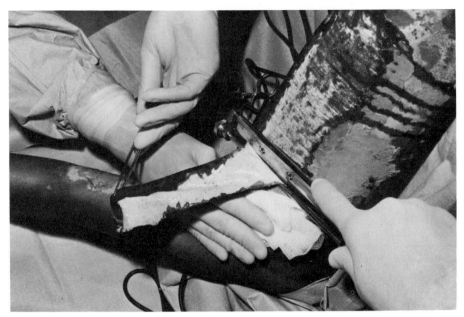

**FIGURE 8–6.** Tangential excision of the arm.

**FIGURE 8–7.** Padgett dermatome utilized for tangential excisions and donor sites.

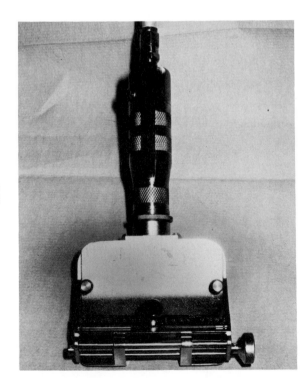

The major disadvantage of tangential excision is the excessive blood loss accompanying the excision. This factor limits the feasibility of this technique in large TBSA burns or infected burns of significant caliber in which removal of the burn eschar rapidly, often in a single operative session, is imperative. Patients with significant inhalation injury or cardiopulmonary dysfunction often cannot tolerate the fluid replacement necessary to compensate for the extensive blood loss of a tangential excision and are better treated with fascial excision of the burn eschar, even in smaller TBSA burns.

A second disadvantage of tangential excision is the greater potential for inadequate excision of the burn eschar, especially in edematous wounds in which bleeding is often less accurate as a gauge of the adequacy of excision than in the nonedematous wound. If possible, the most dependent portion of the wound should be tangentially excised first to avoid obscuring of one's operative field by blood while completing the tangential excision. The third major disadvantage is the time-consuming nature of the process, especially when larger TBSA burns are excised in patients who are unstable hemodynamically. Fascial excision is often preferable to minimize anesthetic time and blood loss.

Tangential excision is an extremely valuable and cosmetic technique of surgical excision of the burn wound. Face and hands are high-priority areas for tangential excisions. The chest and upper extremities are greater priorities for tangential excision than are the lower extremities in stable patients. Fifteen per cent TBSA may usually be tangentially excised in a single operative session with acceptable blood loss. The very young and the elderly often tolerate less TBSA tangential excision than do other groups.

## Fascial Excision

Fascial excision is the technique of removing the epidermis, dermis, and subcutaneous fat by excising the burn in the anatomical plane above muscle fascia.[2, 3] This technique removes the subcutaneous fat even if it is not burned. Excision to fascia is generally reserved for patients with large TBSA burns and for patients who are hemodynamically unstable or at high risk for operative complications (Fig. 8–8).

The major disadvantage of fascial excision is cosmetic deformity. By removing the subcutaneous tissue, the body loses its normal form and contour. Obviously many major burns extend deep to the fat and require fascial excision by virtue of the anatomy of the burn. Large burns (greater than 70 per cent) that are deep second-degree or full-thickness burns also may require fascial excision in order to remove all the burn eschar early in the patient's hospital course to avoid septic complications.

The major advantages of fascial excision are several. The burn excision is technically easier, as the fascia is a definable surgical plane, and the excision is performed more rapidly than with a tangential excision. The chest and back are the easiest fascial planes to excise. The upper extremities are next in order of

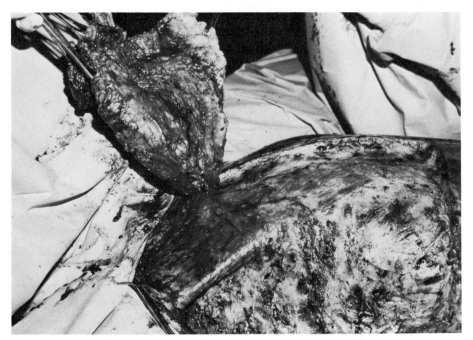

**FIGURE 8–8.** Fascial excision of chest full-thickness thermal burn.

ease of excision. The lower extremities and gluteal regions are more difficult. Inadequate excision of burn eschar is less likely with fascial excision because of the well-defined anatomical plane. The major advantage of fascial excision is the dramatic decrease in blood loss, since the fascial plane is relatively avascular. The major portion of the blood loss is from adjacent unburned tissue.

Fascial excision may be performed with cutting or cautery instruments. The electric cautery with the coagulation setting is the preferred method at our institution.

One last theoretical advantage of fascial excision is that fascia is better vascularized than fat for skin grafting.[2, 3] In infected burns and high-risk patients, this may well be an important factor, especially in elderly patients. In the vast majority of patients, this consideration does not play an important role in the choice of excision technique.

## CHOICE OF SKIN GRAFTS

A major consideration in the grafting of burn patients is the choice of skin graft. The first consideration must be the advantages and disadvantages of sheet versus meshed grafts in a particular patient. The ultimate decision is based on the availability of skin and the condition of the wound bed. Sheet grafts offer

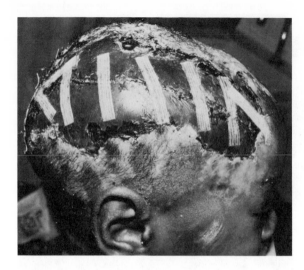

**FIGURE 8–9.** Sheet graft of scalp burn following tangential excision.

significantly better cosmetic results than meshed grafts. The major disadvantage of sheet grafts in acute burns is lack of drainage in a heavily contaminated burn (Fig. 8–9).

Additionally, mechanical factors such as motion or hematoma formation are less well tolerated with sheet grafts than with meshed grafts. Two anatomical regions (the face and hands) should be considered for sheet grafts if at all possible, especially if tendons are exposed on the hands. Sheet grafts prevent dessication of the exposed tendons better than meshed grafts.

Meshed autografts may be expanded 1:1½, 1:3, 1:6, or 1:9 to conserve available donor tissue (Fig. 8–10). The greater the expansion, the longer the

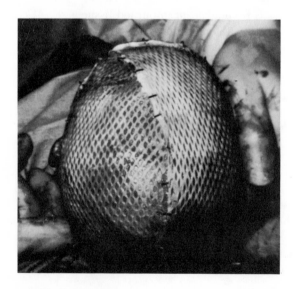

**FIGURE 8–10.** Meshed (1:1½) autograft of scalp burn following tangential excision.

time necessary for the interstices of the graft to contract and provide complete coverage of the wound. The longer the areas within the interstices remain open, the more hypertrophic scar tissue forms. For this reason, various authors have attempted to cover widely expanded autografts with biological or synthetic dressings until the wound is completely healed. In clean wounds, this technique may be valuable. However, in heavily contaminated wounds, the necessity for drainage through the interstices of the meshed graft remains the most important reason for choice of a meshed graft.

Unexpanded, meshed 1:1½ grafts offer the advantage of a better cosmetic result as well as the potential for drainage of the burn wound. Another consideration in skin grafting is the thickness of the donor graft. The thicker the graft, the better the cosmetic result, the less scar contracture, and the longer the time for healing by capillary ingrowth. In large burns, contaminated burns, and high-risk patients, the key considerations are preservation of donor tissue and rapid healing of the grafts to prevent sepsis. Therefore, in acute burns, thinner grafts are taken than in elective reconstructive situations. In particular, if the donor site must be utilized many times because of lack of available unburned tissue, very thin grafts should be harvested to allow rapid re-epithelialization. In the adult, grafts are generally harvested at 1/12,000 of an inch. In children, the thickness of the donor graft is variable depending on the age of the child. The more contaminated the wound, the earlier the burn dressing should be changed following excision and grafting. Coverage of the graft with a single layer of coarse mesh allows early change of the primary dressing and adequate drainage without dislodging the graft.

## CONCLUSION

Early surgical excision and grafting remain the keys to survival in major thermal injuries. Burn care must be "individualized" to facilitate healing in as short a time as possible while maximizing the cosmetic and functional results for the patient. Young children, elderly patients, and individuals with associated traumatic injuries and major thermal burns greater than 80 per cent TBSA represent the greatest challenges in burn care, and the search for the perfect skin substitute still remains an elusive goal.

## REFERENCES

1. Artz CP, Moncrief JA: The Treatment of Burns. Philadelphia, WB Saunders Company, 1969.
2. Boswick JA Jr (ed): The Art and Science of Burn Care. Rockville, MD, Aspen Publishers, Inc, 1987.
3. Heimbach DM, Engrav LH: Surgical Management of the Burn Wound. New York, Raven Press, 1984.
4. McDougal WS, Slade CL, Pruitt BA Jr: Manual of Burns. New York, Springer-Verlag, 1978.
5. Peacock EE Jr: Wound Repair. Philadelphia, WB Saunders Company, 1984.
6. Ruberg RL (ed): Advances in burn care. Clin Plast Surg 13(1):1986.

# 9

# Toxic Epidermal Necrolysis

JOHN A. GRISWOLD and JOSEPH A. MOLNAR

It is necessary to begin with an historical review in order more accurately to develop a description of terms. The first recorded observations of epidermal blistering and slough due to a systemic disease state were made in 1866 by Von Hebra.[1] He wrote of a diffuse group of annular and papular erythematous rashes that progressed to skin loss. The disease was named erythema multiforme (EM) and divided into minor and major forms to delineate severity of disease. Other terms were added depending on the appearance of the initial bullous lesions. Those with annular rings were called erythema annulare centrifugum. Those eruptions that consisted only of bullae were called erythema bullosum, and those with elevated edges surrounding the blisters were called erythema marginatum. All of the terms appear to describe varying degrees of the same process—a systemic response that leads to loss of squamous epithelium. In 1922, Stevens and Johnson described a syndrome of eruptions and subsequent epithelial loss accompanied by fever, inflammation of buccal mucosa, and severe purulent conjunctivitis.[2] This disease, given the name Stevens-Johnson syndrome, described the same process that Von Hebra observed but also noted involvement of other areas of squamous epithelium. Allen Lyell introduced the term *toxic epidermal necrolysis* (TEN) in 1956, describing the process as an acute generalized sheet like loss of epidermis which resembles a scald injury.[3] This article and a subsequent paper described the process as an epithelial slough at the dermal-epidermal junction (Fig. 9–1).

During the 1960s and early 1970s, there were several publications that implicated *Staphylococcus* as the cause of TEN.[4, 5] Biopsy studies of patients and experimental animals have proven that this skin infection occurs high in the epidermis itself without cell death or visible inflammation. It is now termed staphylococcal scalded skin syndrome (SSSS) (Fig. 9–2) and is a milder form of epidermal loss induced by staphylococcal toxin. It is easily treated with antistaphylococcal antibiotics and results in a much lower morbidity and mortality. Healing is more rapid owing to the superficial epidermal involvement without the danger of secondary infection often seen with TEN.[6]

An experience in North Africa was reported in 1968 in which a population was given a long-acting sulfonamide to control an epidemic of meningitis. An outbreak of epidermal slough developed ranging in degree from erythema multiforme minor described by Von Hebra to severe forms of TEN described by Lyell.[7] Obviously the nomenclature is confusing, including several eponyms and

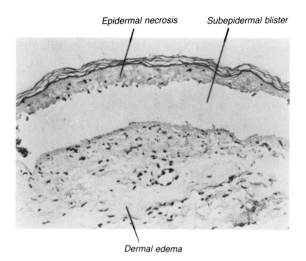

Epidermal necrosis    Subepidermal blister

**FIGURE 9–1.** Toxic epidermal necrolysis. (Hematoxylin-eosin; × 150.) Note the subepidermal blister, epidermal necrosis, and dermal edema.

Dermal edema

terms for what appear to be various degrees of the same pathophysiological process. At a recent international conference, Lyell suggested that there is no real difference between these diseases and that all should be encompassed under the term TEN.[8]

## ETIOLOGY

The major etiological categories are drug-induced, infectious, and idiopathic (Table 9–1). In a number of series the etiology is not known in 20 per cent of cases.[9] No history of drug administration, chemical contact, or infectious process can be identified. Fumigants and insecticides have been named as possible offending agents in several patients with TEN.[10] The drug group first incriminated in causing TEN was older long-acting sulfonamides such as sulfisoxazole.[11] Since then a number of antibiotics have been implicated—penicillins, tetracyclines, cephalosporins, and erythromycin. The second largest drug group consists of anticonvulsants, especially phenytoin and phenobarbital. Other drugs that have been implicated are chlorpropamide, allopurinal, aspirin, clofibrate, and several of the nonsteroidal anti-inflammatory agents. It is somewhat difficult to be sure of all the antibiotics mentioned, since some may have been used for prodromal symptoms and therefore started after the syndrome began.

The most common infectious organisms associated with TEN are *Mycoplasma pneumoniae* and herpes simplex virus.[11, 12] As mentioned above, staphylococcal infections once thought to be a cause of TEN have now been shown to cause an entirely different entity. Since a large number of patients have upper respiratory tract symptoms just prior to the onset of epidermal involvement, infection, possibly viral, may play a larger role in the etiology than currently thought.

There has been some investigation into immune function and its relationship

Acantholytic cell    Stratum corneum

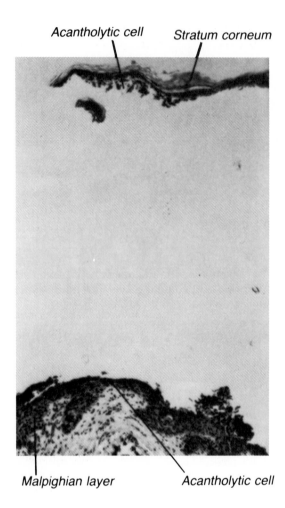

**FIGURE 9–2.** Staphylococcal scalded skin syndrome. (Hematoxylin-eosin; × 75.) Note sloughing of skin just below the stratum corneum in the superficial epidermal layers.

Malpighian layer         Acantholytic cell

**TABLE 9–1. Etiologic Agents of Toxic Epidermal Necrolysis**

1. Drug-induced
    Antibiotics
    Anticonvulsants
    Anti-inflammatory agents
2. Infections
    *Mycoplasma pneumoniae*
    Herpes simplex
3. Fumigants and insecticides
4. Idiopathic

to the development of TEN.[7, 13] The possibility of immune complexes being responsible for cutaneous lesions has been examined. However, immunofluorescence studies in a small number of patients give conflicting results. Neutrophil function in several patients from our series at the University of Washington has been studied which shows normal chemotaxis and adherence capabilities but markedly depressed phagocytic ability. This probably does not reflect an etiological connection but may help explain the increased risk to these patients of the subsequent development of infection.

The possibility that this disease process is an allergic response has been discussed frequently. It is true that in a number of reports the majority of patients have some type of positive allergy history. It may be that the infecting organism or drug produces an antigen-mediated allergic reaction specific to a patient, but this has yet to be proven. With the consistent prodromal respiratory tract symptoms, Lyell suggests that drugs may act synergistically with other drugs or infecting organisms unique to each individual to produce the syndrome.[7]

## PATHOPHYSIOLOGY

As previously mentioned, a prodromal phase usually can be identified in most patients if a careful history is taken. This consists of low-grade fever, malaise, coughing, vomiting, and symptoms suggestive of an upper respiratory tract infection. The symptoms can last from one to 14 days prior to any cutaneous manifestations.[13, 14] Some have documented stomatitis and conjunctivitis one to two days prior to the onset of the skin lesions.[15]

There have been multiple descriptions of the lesions as they first appear. In general, erythematous macules are first seen which quickly become edematous and papular with what some describe as target lesions. Over the next 24 to 96 hours the papular erythema becomes blistered and coalesces. In areas that have not blistered the epidermis easily separates from the dermis with pressure (positive Nikolsky's sign) (see Fig. 9–1).[9, 13] At this point the patient appears to have a very uniform superficial second-degree burn, an important observation guiding therapy to be discussed later.

Microscopically, separation is seen at the basement membrane, where necrosis of the basal cell layer begins the blister formation. The more superficial epidermal layers show signs ranging from vacuolization to extensive necrosis.[13] There has been much debate over dermal changes and how the disease should be classified. Findings are varied. Lyell in his most recent article uses Achten and Ledoux-Corbusier's term of "dermal silence," since minimal involvement is seen.[7] Others have noted varying degrees of lymphocyte or monocyte vascular invasion with immunoglobulin deposits in vessel walls and disruption of the endothelium.[9, 13, 16] Electron microscopy shows necrosis of the basal cell layer with aggregation of keratin and tonofibrils in cells of the more superficial layers which correspond to "eosinophilic bodies" seen on light microscopy.[13]

TEN and its variants seem to be diseases involving squamous epithelium. Other areas besides exposed skin can be involved. These include mucous membranes of the mouth and vagina, the urethra and anus, and the esophagus and conjunctiva. Statistics regarding the incidence of acute ocular involvement in TEN vary from 25 to 90 per cent. Most pathological descriptions consist of a nonspecific inflammatory reaction of the conjunctiva with perivascular lymphocytic infiltration.[17, 18] The conjunctivitis reduces the number of or destroys completely the goblet cells that are necessary for the normal distribution of tears over the cornea.[19] Signs and symptoms of conjunctival involvement have been well described. There are erythematous patches with a discharge that is purulent or pseudomembranous. Adhesions (synechiae) can quickly form between the tarsal and bulbar conjunctiva owing to loss of epithelium. The cornea may ultimately become involved with the possibility of maceration, perforation, or significant scarring. The patients experience significant photophobia and blepharospasm.

The oral mucosa is often significantly involved. There is mucosal erosion over most of the oropharynx and usually extending into the hypopharynx. The lips are usually crusted and bleed easily on manipulation. The mouth is held open, and drooling is prominent owing to pain on swallowing. This is a major deterrent to oral nutrition. The pain on breathing as air moves across the raw mucosa significantly adds to pulmonary difficulties. The patients tend to take very shallow breaths, leading to atelectasis, and most refuse to cough. The esophagus may be involved owing to its squamous epithelial lining. Only a few esophageal complications have been reported, usually stricture. Bleeding from the gastrointestinal tract invariably comes from the stomach and not the esophagus.

Pulmonary involvement has been cited by some owing to the increased risk of pneumonia in these patients along with poor ventilation. There are no specific studies showing true tracheobronchial injury by bronchoscopy. It is true that multiple studies at autopsy have implicated respiratory complications as the ultimate cause of death, including pneumonitis, bronchopneumonia, and bronchiolitis.[20] Since squamous epithelium does not line the tracheobronchial tree and TEN is a disease of squamous epithelium, it may be that the respiratory problems are secondarily related to pain on breathing and swallowing owing to oropharyngeal involvement, pain on respiration from chest wall involvement, and risk of aspiration due to difficulty swallowing.

There is some debate as to fluid and electrolyte requirements. All authors agree that fluid and electrolyte balance needs to be maintained, but the amount required and the means of calculation differ. In the past many physicians believed that these patients experienced significant fluid loss similar to that of burn patients. In fact, the group from Créteil, France, who have a unique situation as the referral for most TEN cases in that country, recommends that fluid loss be estimated just as is done for burn patients of similar body surface area involvement.[21] This differs from the experience at the University of Washington. Despite the burnlike appearance of TEN, massive fluid requirements have not been observed as with patients with superficial second-degree thermal burns. It appears that acute phase reactants involved in fluid shifts in burn patients are not released in patients with TEN.[6] This has been a consistent finding throughout the series in Seattle, which also may reflect the successful therapy to be discussed later.

## MANAGEMENT

### Controversy in Treatment

*Steroids* have been a mainstay of therapy of TEN in the past, used with the hope of halting the allergic or inflammatory response thought to be the cause of the disease. It has already been mentioned that there is no consistent histopathological evidence for inflammatory infiltration, and pure allergic etiology has yet to be proven. Several authors believe that the extension of the necrolysis has been arrested by the use of steroids. The problem comes from the fact that the natural history of TEN is variable, and the unpredictability of the disease sheds doubt on claims that steroids have altered the disease course. No prospective or randomized trials using steroids could be found in the literature to give scientific support for their use. Rasmussen did attempt a controlled study using steroids; he could find no decrease in the progression of TEN with steroids but found instead a significant morbidity due to the complications of their use.[22] Lyell himself states in his most recent article that the indications for the use of steroids, in his opinion, are vague at best.[7] There have been several case reports of patients who continue to progress to significant skin loss in spite of high-dose steroids.[13, 23] TEN has also developed in patients already receiving high-dose steroid therapy. There are reports of longer hospital stays for children treated with steroids and marked increase in the rate of complications.[15] Kim et al found an 80 per cent mortality in patients treated with steroids, compared to 20 per cent in those who did not receive steroids.[24] Other series have documented these findings.[23] The high risk of subsequent infection in patients with TEN adds even further weight against the use of steroids.

*Antibiotics* have also been used empirically in the past from the time of admission. These were usually combined with systemic steroids. There are a few

### TABLE 9–2. Management of Toxic Epidermal Necrolysis

1. Immediate removal of sloughing epidermis and application of xenograft in the operating room.
2. Meticulous eye care from the beginning.
3. Enteral feeding at slightly higher than basal requirements.
4. Air-fluidized therapy bed.
5. Intensive supportive care in ICU setting.
6. Empirical use of steroids and antibiotics is to be avoided.
7. Central lines and Foley catheters are to be avoided when possible.

centers that still recommend their use prophylactically. The risk of emergence of highly resistant strains of bacteria with the use of prophylactic antibiotics in this disease is significant. The consensus now appears to support the use of antibiotics only when infection is present and a specific organism is documented. A possible exception is the use of topical antibiotics in treating the ocular conjunctival slough. Corneal perforation can occur quickly owing to bacterial colonization of the denuded conjunctiva.[14, 19]

*Treatment of the skin wound* from epidermal slough is also a controversial point. Various modes are suggested such as the use of drying agents like calamine lotion over blisters or saline over denuded areas.[14] Some recommend potassium permanganate baths several times a day to remove necrotic tissue, followed by the application of silver nitrate dressings[7] or the use of silver sulfadiazine (Silvadine) applications.[13]

As has been discussed, the skin wound that develops is exactly the same as a uniform superficial second-degree burn. This is a perfect setting for a "biological" dressing. If the exposed dermis can be protected from desiccation and heavy bacterial colonization, rapid resurfacing by proliferation of epithelium from skin appendages will occur. Silver sulfadiazine, silver nitrate, and mafenide acetate (Sulfamylon) are the most commonly used topical antimicrobial creams or solutions. They minimize desiccation and reduce bacterial colonization somewhat, but they have been shown to delay epithelial proliferation and thus slow wound healing.[25] Biological dressings such as porcine xenograft or cadaver allograft are used routinely in superficial second-degree burns. If applied early before significant bacterial colonization, they will adhere to the dermis, decreasing the risk of infection and reducing evaporative losses across the wound. Rapid re-epithelialization is associated with the use of these biological coverings with minimal to no scarring or altered pigmentation. The pain experienced by these patients is markedly reduced by the dermal protection and the elimination of one to several daily dressing changes.

In 1978, Demling et al in a case report suggested the use of biological dressings to provide the proper healing environment before infection sets in.[26] Since that time this approach has been used at the University of Washington on a significant number of patients with excellent results. Porcine xenograft is now used exclusively. Cadaver homograft was compared but showed no superior qualities. Synthetic dressings such as collagen mat with Silastic covering (Biobrane®) has also been tried but did not adhere well, especially in patients with large body surface areas involved. This therapy has all but eliminated wound infections, markedly decreased the pain experienced by these patients, and cosmetically gives excellent results with no scarring and temporary pigment differences only at junctures of the pieces of xenograft or where the xenograft did not adhere.[6]

## An Approach to Management

A description of the treatment protocol used at the University of Washington follows (Table 9–2).[6] Upon referral to the burn unit at the University, a brief evaluation is made to ensure adequate hydration and stable vital signs and to rule out any other ongoing process. The patient is then taken to the operating room. After satisfactory anesthesia on a transport stretcher, the patient is turned to the prone position on an operating table that is covered with a heating blanket. It is extremely important to avoid hypothermia during the operation. The patient's core temperature can drop 3°C per hour despite heating the operating room and warming intravenous and topical solutions. In the prone position the patient's wounds are washed with a cloth moistened in normal saline. No detergents or ointments are used. The loose skin and blisters are debrided. Areas with a positive Nikolsky's sign are vigorously wiped to remove epithelium that is in the early stages of sloughing. Porcine xenograft is then meticulously applied to all areas of exposed dermis and stapled in place. The patient is then moved to the supine position on a prewarmed air-fluidized bed (Clinitron®) and the same procedure is repeated on the anterior surface. Air-fluidized therapy is used to keep the xenograft dry and to facilitate adherence. With a team of several surgeons the entire process can be completed in 60 to 90 minutes. At this time an ophthalmological examination is performed by the ophthalmological service to begin removing any conjunctival synechiae with a glass rod. This is continued on a daily basis. The patient is taken to the intensive care area of the burn unit immediately upon completion of the procedure.

Our institution's experience with TEN has led to some specific anesthetic recommendations.[27] In the past, anesthesiologists have attempted to manage the patient in the manner of burn patients owing to the pathological similarity to superficial burns. It is true that special care must be taken to keep the patient normothermic; as with burn patients, it has been recommended that succinylcholine be used with caution owing to the potential for hyperkalemia.[27] Similarly, some individuals have been found to be resistant to nondepolarizing muscle relaxants. However, unlike burns, blood loss with TEN is minimal, and thus massive intraoperative fluid resuscitation is not necessary. Finally, despite some reports to the contrary, there is no specific contraindication to endotracheal intubation with TEN, since the trachea and vocal cords are not involved.

As mentioned before, massive fluid resuscitation as with burn patients is not needed in TEN patients, but special attention is required for fluid and electrolyte balance. The use of an air-fluidized bed may increase the patient's daily evaporative water loss by 5 to 6 liters. If steroids had been started prior to referral, their administration is stopped or quickly tapered unless the patient was taking steroids for other chronic medical problems. In this case they are kept at pre-TEN doses. Enteral alimentation is started immediately through a nasogastric feeding tube. Owing to the oropharyngeal mucositis the majority of patients are not able to maintain nutritional intake voluntarily. Oxygen consumption and carbon dioxide production measurements done on TEN patients at the University of Washington have been in the high-normal range, in contrast to patients with burns of similar size, which produce a metabolic rate nearly twice normal. If sepsis is avoided, the gastrointestinal tract functions normally. Weight and positive nitrogen balance can be maintained on enteral feeding with caloric intake appropriate for body size.

Intensive pulmonary toilet is started immediately postoperatively. Pneumonia is a common complication in TEN patients due to aspiration of sloughed mucosa and shallow breathing due to chest wall and oropharyngeal pain with resulting atelectasis. Systemic antibiotics are used only for specific infections. Physical therapy is begun 24 hours postoperatively, with care to minimize shearing of the xenograft from the dermis. Meticulous eye care is begun immediately. Every hour crusts are removed from lid margins, and lubricating eye drops and topical antibiotic ointments are applied. Oral care is provided similarly, removing crusts and sloughing mucosal lining. Intravenous catheters, especially central lines, are avoided whenever possible, since they are a significant portal of entry for bacteria and the patient can be monitored easily without invasive techniques. Pain is controlled using an elixir of methadone, hydroxyzine, and acetaminophen. Once the dermis is covered with xenograft, pain is decreased and management is not a problem. Bladder catheters are also avoided or removed as soon as adequate urine output is documented.

The xenograft is inspected several times a day. Small areas that become dislodged are replaced in the intensive care unit. If large areas are lost, the patient is returned to the operating room for reapplication. As the wounds heal beneath, the xenograft becomes brittle and desiccates. These areas are trimmed each day. The patient is transferred to the acute burn care ward once the majority of wounds are healed and there is no sign of sepsis.

To date we have treated 33 patients at the University of Washington. The average length of hospital stay was 19 days, with an average of 14 days spent in ICU. There were 27 survivors and six deaths. Of these six three had significant concomitant diseases. One elderly woman, who had significant steroid-dependent chronic obstructive pulmonary disease, was transferred to us late in her course with pneumonia and sepsis. Another elderly patient had significant atherosclerotic disease and subsequently developed complete abdominal aortic occlusion, and a 9-year-old boy developed sepsis from an infected ventriculovenous shunt. The average TBSA involved was greater than 60 per cent, much larger than in other reported series. There has been no long-term morbidity in any of the survivors.

## SUMMARY

Toxic epidermal necrolysis is a specific syndrome separate from staphylococcal scalded skin syndrome and requires histological diagnosis. The etiology is unclear but may be infectious or drug-related. The process is confined to squamous epithelium, including mucous membranes, esophagus, and conjunctiva, but the trachea and vocal cords are spared. Management does not include steroids, empirical antibiotics, or massive fluid resuscitation but requires early debridement in the operating room with the placement of xenograft and the initiation of ocular care. Anesthetic management concentrates on maintenance of normothermia and avoidance of succinylcholine. Postoperative morbidity and mortality are minimized with attention to ocular and pulmonary care and enteral nutrition.

## REFERENCES

1. Von Hebra F: Erythema exudative multiforme. *In* Fragg CH (ed): On Diseases of the Skin, Vol I. London, New Sydenham Society, 1866, p 285.
2. Stevens AM, Johnson FC: A new eruptive fever associated with stomatitis and ophthalmia. Am J Dis Child 24:526–533, 1922.
3. Lyell A: Toxic epidermal necrolysis: An eruption resembling scalding of the skin. Br J Dermatol 68:355–361, 1956.
4. Koblenzer PJ: Acute epidermal necrolysis (Ritter von Rittershain-Lyell). Arch Dermatol 95:608–617, 1967.
5. Rycheck RR, Taylor PM, Gezon HM: Epidemic staphylococcal pyoderma associated with Ritter's disease and the appearance of phage type 3B/71. N Engl J Med 269:332–341, 1963.
6. Heimbach DM, Engrav LH, Marvin JA, et al: Toxic epidermal necrolysis: A step forward in treatment. JAMA 257:2171–2175, 1987.
7. Lyell A: Toxic epidermal necrolysis (the scalded skin syndrome): A reappraisal. Br J Dermatol 100:69–86, 1979.
8. Lyell A: TEN—historical perspective. Paper presented at the Symposium of Toxic Epidermal Necrolysis. Créteil, France, Oct 4–5, 1985.
9. Crosby SS, Murray KM, Marvin JA, et al: Management of Stevens-Johnson syndrome. Clin Pharm 5:682–689, 1986.
10. Radimer GF, Davis JH, Acherman AB: Fumigant-induced toxic epidermal necrolysis. Arch Dermatol 110:103–104, 1974.
11. Carroll OM, Bryan PA, Robinson RJ: Stevens-Johnson syndrome associated with long-acting sulfonamides. JAMA 195:179–181, 1966.
12. Bell WE, Riegle EV, Golden B: Erythema multiforme exudativum (Stevens-Johnson) syndrome in association with *Mycoplasma pneumoniae*. Clin Pediatr 10:184–187, 1971.
13. Rasmussen J: Toxic epidermal necrolysis. Med Clin North Am 64:901–920, 1980.
14. Avaiyo OE, Flowers FP: Stevens-Johnson syndrome. J Emerg Med 2:129–135, 1984.
15. Ginsberg CM: Stevens-Johnson syndrome in children. Pediatr Infect Dis 1:155–158, 1982.
16. Revuz J, Penso D, Roryeau JG, et al: Toxic epidermal necrolysis: Clinical findings and prognosis factors in 87 patients. Arch Dermatol 123:1160–1173, 1987.
17. Duggan JW, Gaines SR: The ocular complications of erythema exudativum multiforme. Am J Ophthalmol 34:184, 1951.
18. Howard GM: The Stevens-Johnson syndrome: Ocular prognosis and treatment. Am J Oththalmol 55:893–900, 1963.
19. Arstkaitis MJ: Ocular aftermath of Stevens-Johnson syndrome. Arch Ophthalmol 90:376, 1973.
20. Boe J, Dalgaard JB, Scott D: Mucocutaneous-ocular syndrome with intestinal involvement. Am J Med 25:857–867, 1958.
21. Ravuz J, Roryeau JG, Guillaume JC, et al: Treatment of toxic epidermal necrolysis: Créteil's experience. Arch Dermatol 123:1156–1158, 1987.
22. Rasmussen JE: Erythema multiforme in children: Response to treatment with systemic corticosteroids. Br J Dermatol 95:181–186, 1976.
23. Halebian PH, Corder VJ, Herndon D: A burn center experience with toxic epidermal necrolysis. J Burn Care Rehabil 4:176–183, 1983.
24. Kim PS, Goldforb IW, Gaisford JC, et al: Stevens-Johnson syndrome and toxic epidermal necrolysis: A pathophysiologic review with recommendations for treatment protocol. J Burn Care Rehabil 4:91–100, 1983.
25. Burleson R, Eiseman B: Effect of skin dressings and topical antibiotics on healing of partial thickness wounds in rats. Surg Gynecol Obstet 136:958, 1973.
26. Demling RH, Ellerbe S, Lowe NJ: Burn unit management of toxic epidermal necrolysis. Arch Surg 113:758–759, 1978.
27. MacIntyre P, Pavlin E, Dwersteg J, et al: Toxic epidermal necrolysis: Anesthetic implications including possible resistance to atracurium. Submitted.

# 10

# Nutritional Support of the Burn Patient

STACEY J. BELL and GEORGE L. BLACKBURN

As discussed in this chapter, nutritional guidelines for burned patients have changed significantly since the middle of the century.[1-2] The National Research Council on therapeutic nutrition then recommended caloric intakes in the range of 35 kcal/kg and protein intake of 2 to 4 gm/kg daily.[3] Emphasis was on nitrogen intake rather than calories because of the enormous losses through the urine and skin.

Physicians caring for the thermally injured patient have historically recognized the need for nutritional support. Early accounts by Levenson and others[4] recognized that this type of massive injury would induce weight loss, excessive nitrogen losses, and hypermetabolism within a few days. These authors describe nutritional concerns for burned patients, including victims of the Coconut Grove Night Club fire in Boston. Although anorexia was present in most patients, its severity was positively correlated with the extent of injury. All patients were encouraged to consume calorically dense food that included a rich source of complete proteins. If the patient was unwilling to consume ample amounts of food orally, a nasogastric tube and/or peripheral intravenous catheter was inserted to augment caloric and protein intake.

The metabolic response to burn injury and the ensuing nutrient requirements are reviewed in this chapter. Current standards of nutritional management are presented, with particular emphasis on severe burns of more than 30 per cent of the total body surface area (TBSA). Detailed descriptions of the practical issues of administering total parenteral nutrition and tube feeding diets are included.

## METABOLIC RESPONSE TO INJURY

### Ebb Phase

The human body has an extraordinary ability to respond appropriately to a massive trauma. Cuthbertson[5] aptly characterized the initial period following injury (in this case the burn) as the *ebb* or shock phase. In severe burn trauma, this phase may extend from hours to days, during which proper fluid resuscitation is critical to survival. A unique series of events occurs during the ebb phase, and these events are co-ordinated to help the body adjust to the insult. Most notably, there is a dulling effect on what is often excruciating pain.

A diminution of blood flow occurs almost immediately to compensate for continued blood losses typically present with trauma. Core temperature decreases despite diminished peripheral circulation. Additionally, urine output is reduced or completely absent. It is enhanced by fluid therapy utilizing one of several strategies.[6] Of nutritional concern are the increased urinary losses of nitrogen, magnesium, potassium, sulfur, and phosphate. Potassium is routinely replaced via resuscitation fluids; however, deficits in the remaining nutrients accrue until nutritional support is initiated. Given that these metabolites are components of muscle tissue and that these losses are positively correlated with the loss of methyl histidine and creatinine, it is likely that the early responses to injury are largely due to muscle catabolism.

The composition of the systemic circulation alters in several ways. First, an alteration in plasma proteins is manifested by a fall in albumin and a rise in acute-phase C-reactive proteins and alpha$_1$ acid glycoproteins. Metabolic acidosis may be present.

Alterations of the delicate hormone substrate milieu accompany the most striking metabolic changes. There is a dramatic rise in circulatory catecholamines, cortisol, and growth hormone.[5, 7] These counterregulatory hormones, together with monokines, stimulate the mobilization of stored protein and energy in support of key pathways necessary for host defense and recovery (i.e., a redistribution of body cell mass and fat mass). The rises in norepinephrine and growth hormone, in particular, suppress insulin release to promote lipolysis and ketogenesis, which become primary energy sources. As a result of the decreased metabolic rate, a more favorable environment is present for $O_2$ supply and demand, thus supporting the principal objective of the ebb period, hypothermia. Hyperglycemia is present only during convalescence, and it resolves during the

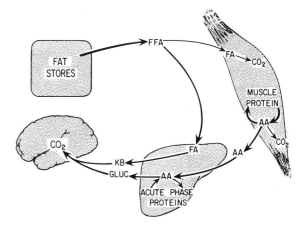

**FIGURE 10–1.** Metabolic response to injury, the interrelationship of fat, muscle, and liver in meeting energy requirements. FFA = Free fatty acids; AA = amino acids; KB = ketone bodies; GLUC = glucose. (Adapted from Blackburn et al: Nutrition in the Critically Ill Patient. Anesthesia 47:181–194, 1977; with permission.)

flow phase. Concomitantly, the release and production of glucagon are stimulated. This new hormonal balance is, in fact, compatible with survival, and the absence of these hormonal and substrate changes may lead to death.

Metabolic alterations are best understood as a redistribution of macronutrients from such labile reserves as skeletal muscle and adipose tissue to more active tissues such as liver and bone marrow (Fig. 10–1).[8] Endogenous fat counteracts the caloric deficit, while the skeletal muscle mass provides amino acids to support the increased visceral protein synthetic rates and to provide carbon precursors for hepatic and renal gluconeogenesis. Micronutrients are also redistributed.[9] In particular, there are increases in the uptake of zinc (enzymatic cofactor) and transferrin (a tissue iron–sequestering mechanism that reduces the amount available to support pathogenic microorganisms).

## Flow Phase

### Hypermetabolism

The ebb phase is rapidly replaced by a flow phase when adequate burn resuscitation is accomplished. Characteristic of the early acute period of the flow phase is hypermetabolism, during which the energy needs of a burn patient may reach twice the predicted basal rate[10] (Fig. 10–2). Energy regulation in the burn patient is influenced by the increased heat gradient to maintain thermal neutrality in the face of open wounds, temperature and humidity levels, and, to some extent, pain medications.[11-13] It appears that part of the increased metabolism is a response mechanism to a higher temperature set point, dictated by the hypothalamus. The exact hypothalamic influence remains unclear, however, as metabolic rate responds to elevated body temperatures independent of hypothalamic control. In any event, Wilmore and others[13] demonstrated that burned patients selected higher comfortable temperatures than did normal controls. Thus, maintaining the patient in a warm environment during the convalescent period may reduce the degree of hypermetabolism and improve patient comfort.

### Substrate Metabolism

With stabilization of the patient, including the provision of such exogenous fuel substrates as lactate and glucose during fluid resuscitation, surges of the counterregulatory hormones subside and insulin release is stimulated. A favorable environment for nutritional support, including glucose and amino acid feeding, is then present. These substrates, ideally provided via the gastrointestinal tract in the absence of clinical contraindication (discussed later), permit restoration of the body cell mass. Protein synthesis and catabolism are each elevated during the flow phase[14] so that if adequate substrates are not provided exogenously, endogenous stores are utilized, and this leads to protein malnutrition. The goal of early feeding therefore is to support protein sparing by minimizing the catabolism of muscle, gut mucosa, and connective tissue stores during synthesis.

Of the potential endogenous energy and protein stores, fat is in the most

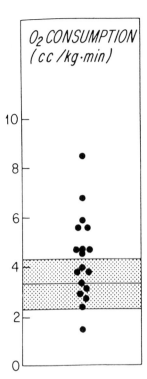

FIGURE 10–2. Resting oxygen consumption in burn patients as compared to mean + 2 SD for normal volunteers. (From Wolfe RR, Durkot MJ, Allsop JR, et al: Glucose metabolism in severely burned patients. Metabolism 28:1031, 1979; with permission.)

abundant supply.[5] Typically, a 70-kg man contains 8 to 12 kg of protein, 100 to 200 gm of carbohydrate stored as glycogen in liver and muscle, and 16 to 20 kg of fat. Most appropriately, the body adapts to using fat as its main energy source, as evidenced by increased lipolysis (elevated serum free fatty acid and triglyceride levels) after a burn injury. Although regulation is initially controlled by hormonal influence, provision of exogenous sustrates may retard the process during the flow phase.

## NUTRITIONAL REQUIREMENTS

Knowledge of the individual substrate requirements of burned patients has expanded in the past decade. The use of indirect calorimetry has essentially and single-handedly precipitated a dramatic decrease in the total amount of calories provided. Additionally, sensitive isotopic tracer techniques (with both radioisotopes and stable isotopes) have been used to determine synthetic and catabolic rates of protein and the oxidation rates of glucose and lipid. Hence, a clearer picture of optimal substrate requirements after thermal injury is now available.

Male
BEE (Kcal) = 66 + (13.7 × W) + (5 × H) − (6.8 × A)

Female
BEE (Kcal) = 665 + (9.6 × W) + (1.7 × H) − (4.7 × A)

where: W = weight in kg, H = height in cm, and A = age in years.

**FIGURE 10–3.** Harris-Benedict equation. (From Harris JA, Benedict FG: Biometric Study of Basal Metabolism in Man. Carnegie Institute, 1919.)

## Energy Requirements

Of all hospitalized patients, those with severe burns have the greatest increase in metabolic demand. Thus, many clinicians attempt to provide them with excessive caloric regimens. Recent studies using indirect calorimetry indicate that an upper limit to the required calories exists, and it is approximately twice the predicted basal energy expenditure (BEE)[10, 14–20] (Fig. 10–3). Provision of calories at twice the predicted BEE should supply adequate energy to meet the needs of even the most massively burned patient (Fig. 10–4).

Saffle and others[15] at the Intermountain Burn Center in Utah measured energy expediture in 29 burned patients twice weekly by indirect calorimetry. The average resting energy expediture (REE) for burns exceeding 30 per cent TBSA was 147 per cent of the predicted basal needs. A similar study corroborated

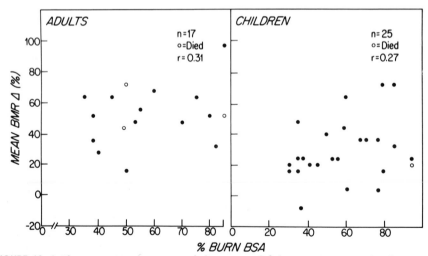

**FIGURE 10–4.** The average increase in metabolic rate in adult burn patients treated with excisional therapy is less than 100 per cent. The small increase in metabolic rate in children may reflect the fact that they were maintained in a warm, humid environment. (From Wolfe RR, Molnar JA: Meeting the special nutritional requirements of the burn patient. Nutr Ther News 3:1–6, 1981; with permission.)

Saffle's work.[16] Here the measured energy expediture (MEE) for 35 patients ranged from 1275 to 3410 kcal, which equated to an average of 122 per cent above basal levels. When admission second- and third-degree burn size, ranging from 10 to 75 per cent, was correlated with MEE, the results were significantly and positively correlated ($r = 0.72$).

It is important to note that only one study separated the data on children from those on adults.[17] These investigators reported that, on the average, children required slightly fewer calories than adults (1.29 versus 1.55 above predicted BEE). The reason for the discrepancy may be that the children were housed in thermally controlled nursing units where the average temperatures remained above 80°F (Fig. 10–4).

Room temperature, humidity, and control of pain are essential concerns for all burned patients. Similarly, provision of adequate free water and electrolytes, colloid, and blood and control of acid-base balance are essential for utilization of nutritional support therapy.

In each of the aforementioned studies, it is clear that the once-popular concept of "if some is good, more is better" is incorrect. Some incremental increase in caloric prescription over the MEE is required, but these amounts are likely to be small, since such routine daily events as physical work, dressing change, and fever add minimal caloric expenditure. To determine the caloric goal of burned patients, it should be understood that all patients, adults as well as children, should receive no more than twice the predicted BEE and no less than 150 per cent of the BEE. For adults and children, the use of the Harris-Benedict equation[20] to predict BEE automatically incorporates relevant patient characteristics such as age, sex, height, and weight. Since weights are often difficult to obtain in the presence of bulky dressings or splinting materials or are unreliable if the patient has edema, the ideal body weight of Table 10–1 should be incorporated into the Harris-Benedict equation. For elderly patients[22] (65 years and older), the data from Table 10–2 are appropriate, and for children the fiftieth percentile from the standard growth curve[23] is best used.

## Alterations of Metabolic Rate

Although hypermetabolism is the inevitable response to injury, the degree of the response is variable. The extent of injury, premorbid health, nutritional state, and age are observable characteristics that affect the degree of hypermetabolism. In addition, Mochizuki and collaborators[24] postulated that the provision of enteral calories within two hours of injury could lessen the typical metabolic response to a burn. Animals were given a 30 per cent TBSA burn and fed a standard diet within two hours or at 72 hours post burn. Energy expenditure averaged 109 per cent of premorbid levels for the early feeding group, whereas the other group had increases simulating those of patients (144 per cent of pre-burn values). Although the animal model was used, these results should and have stimulated further research.

TABLE 10–1. Ideal Body Weight of Adults 18 to 64 Years* (in Kilograms)

| Standing Height (cm) | Men | Women |
|---|---|---|
| 142.2 | NA† | 44.8 |
| 144.7 | NA | 45.9 |
| 147.3 | NA | 47.3 |
| 149.8 | NA | 48.6 |
| 152.4 | NA | 50.0 |
| 154.9 | 53.4 | 51.4 |
| 157.4 | 55.0 | 52.9 |
| 160.0 | 56.4 | 54.5 |
| 162.5 | 57.7 | 56.6 |
| 165.1 | 59.3 | 58.4 |
| 167.6 | 61.1 | 60.2 |
| 170.1 | 63.2 | 62.0 |
| 172.8 | 65.0 | 63.9 |
| 175.2 | 66.8 | 65.7 |
| 177.8 | 68.9 | 67.5 |
| 180.3 | 70.9 | NA |
| 189.9 | 72.9 | NA |
| 185.4 | 75.0 | NA |
| 188.0 | 77.3 | NA |
| 190.5 | 79.5 | NA |

*From Bell SJ, Hegarty MT, Burke JF: Step-wise guide to determine the nutritional needs of the pediatric and adult burned patient. Unpublished manual, January 1984.

The ideal body weights represent the average for the two extreme weights listed under the middle-frame portion of the Metropolitan Tables.[21]

The data presented in the Metropolitan Tables are frequently used without the corrections for height with shoes (1″ men, 2″ women) and weight with clothing (over 3 lb women, 6 lb men). The data presented in this table are corrected to reflect weight without clothing and height without shoes.

†Not available.

Wound closure is the ultimate means of allowing the metabolic rate to subside to a normal range.[25] Treatment using early primary excisional therapy or conservative hydrotherapy may affect the rate of change of the metabolic rate. Recent serial measurements of REE[26] revealed no significant differences in patients treated by the two different methods.

### Carbohydrate Requirements

The combination of isotopic tracer methodology and indirect calorimetry (measuring $O_2$ consumption and $CO_2$ production) has drastically modified the amount of carbohydrate provided to all patients. Traditionally, vast quantities (>700 gm) of glucose were provided as a means of sparing endogenous protein breakdown for gluconeogenesis. Extra carbohydrate was provided, but it produced numerous complications including impaired liver function,[27] since excess carbohydrate is used for lipogenesis. Under usual circumstances, lipogenesis is not harmful, but persistent hyperinsulinemia in response to carbohydrate infusion prevents mobilization of the fat. Deposition of lipid occurs in the liver and the amount may be significant enough to impair or prevent diaphragmatic excursion. Burke and others[28] theorized that this phenomenon may have contributed to the mortality that occurred in eight burned children who were fed an average of

## TABLE 10–2. Ideal Body Weight (in Kilograms) of Elderly Persons*

| Standing Height (cm) | 65 to 69 Years | | 70 to 74 years | | 75 to 79 Years | | 80 to 84 Years | | 85 to 89 Years | | 90 to 94 Years | |
|---|---|---|---|---|---|---|---|---|---|---|---|---|
| | Men | Women | Men | Women | Men | Women | Men | Women | Men | Women | Men | Women |
| 147.3 | NA† | 48.2 | NA | 45.5 | NA | 44.5 | NA | NA | NA | NA | NA | NA |
| 149.8 | NA | 48.6 | NA | 46.4 | NA | 45.0 | NA | 40.5 | NA | 40.0 | NA | NA |
| 152.4 | NA | 49.1 | NA | 46.8 | NA | 45.9 | NA | 42.7 | NA | 40.9 | NA | NA |
| 154.9 | 51.8 | 50.0 | 50.5 | 47.7 | 50.0 | 46.4 | NA | 44.1 | NA | 42.3 | NA | NA |
| 157.4 | 52.9 | 50.5 | 51.4 | 48.6 | 50.5 | 47.7 | 49.1 | 45.0 | 48.2 | 43.6 | NA | 43.2 |
| 160.0 | 53.2 | 51.4 | 51.8 | 50.0 | 51.4 | 48.6 | 49.5 | 46.4 | 49.1 | 45.0 | NA | 43.2 |
| 162.5 | 54.1 | 52.3 | 53.2 | 50.9 | 51.8 | 50.0 | 50.0 | 48.2 | 50.5 | 46.4 | NA | 43.6 |
| 165.1 | 55.0 | 53.6 | 54.1 | 52.3 | 52.7 | 50.9 | 51.4 | 49.5 | 51.8 | 48.2 | 47.3 | 45.0 |
| 167.6 | 55.9 | 55.0 | 55.5 | 53.6 | 53.6 | 51.8 | 52.3 | 50.9 | 52.7 | 50.0 | 48.2 | 46.8 |
| 170.1 | 56.8 | 56.4 | 56.4 | 55.0 | 54.5 | 53.2 | 53.6 | 52.3 | 53.6 | 51.8 | 49.5 | NA |
| 172.8 | 57.7 | 57.7 | 57.3 | 56.4 | 55.9 | NA | 54.5 | NA | 55.5 | NA | 50.9 | NA |
| 175.2 | 59.1 | 59.5 | 59.1 | 58.2 | 57.3 | NA | 55.9 | NA | 56.8 | NA | 52.3 | NA |
| 177.8 | 60.9 | NA | 60.0 | NA | 59.1 | NA | 57.7 | NA | 58.2 | NA | 54.1 | NA |
| 180.3 | 62.7 | NA | 61.4 | NA | 60.5 | NA | 59.5 | NA | 60.0 | NA | 55.9 | NA |
| 182.9 | 64.5 | NA | 62.7 | NA | 62.3 | NA | 61.8 | NA | NA | NA | NA | NA |
| 185.4 | 66.4 | NA | 64.5 | NA | 63.6 | NA | NA | NA | NA | NA | NA | NA |

*The ideal body weight represents the lowest weight for the 20th percentile of the average weight at each inch of height.
†Not available.

TABLE 10–3. Autopsy Findings in Patients Treated with Very High Glucose Infusions*

| Patient | Sex | Age | Per Cent TBSA Burned† | Muscle Atrophy | Hypercal‡ for 3 Weeks Before Death | Rate of IV Glucose (mg/kg/min) | Liver Weight at Autopsy (Per Cent Above Normal) |
|---|---|---|---|---|---|---|---|
| 1 | M | 11 | 80 | 0 | yes | 13.5 | 254 |
| 2 | F | 14 | 66 | 0 | yes | 14.8 | 246 |
| 3 | F | 10 | 86 | 0 | yes | 9.3 | 164 |
| 4 | M | 13 | 54 | 0 | yes | 10.8 | 309 |
| 5 | F | 16 mo | 47 | 0 | yes | 17 | 291 |
| 6 | M | 10 mo | 39 | 0 | yes | 17 | 324 |
| 7 | M | 3 | 85 | 0 | yes | 13.1 | 440 |
| 8 | F | 4 | 70 | 0 | yes | 14.3 | 331 |

*From Burke JF, Wolfe RR, Mullany CJ, et al: Glucose requirements following burn injury. Ann Surg 190:274–285, 1979, with permission.
†TBSA = total body surface area.
‡Total parenteral nutrition.

three times the now accepted amount of glucose (Table 10–3). Despite adequate nutritional support, as evidenced by at least three weeks of total parenteral nutrition (TPN) and absence of muscle atrophy, the patients expired. Postmortem examination revealed extremely enlarged livers that may have contributed to their demise.

The potential toxicity of glucose is also manifested in pulmonary function. The process of triglyceride synthesis produces per mole of fat over four times the amount of $CO_2$ that would be produced from oxidation of a mole of glucose (Fig. 10–5).[29] Expiration of $CO_2$ may become problematic, particularly in the presence of pulmonary compromise such as is common in burned patients with inhalation injuries.

The optimal carbohydrate dose should prevent, or minimize as much as possible, gluconeogenesis and should be oxidized rather than stored as triglycerides. Burke[28] and others elegantly demonstrated, by using isotopic tracers, that infusion of 4.7 to 6.8 mg/kg/min allowed both these attributes to prevail in pediatric and adult burned patients. Figure 10–6 shows that the respiratory quotient (RQ) surpasses the normal, fed range (0.84), and when glucose provision exceeds the desired infusion rate, RQ rises, presumably owing to lipogenesis. Moreover, the percentage of glucose oxidized to $CO_2$ and water leveled off when glucose was infused at rates higher than approximately 7 mg/kg/min (Fig. 10–7). Serendipitously, the authors noted optimal rates of protein synthesis (5.2 gm/kg/day) when glucose was infused at the desired rate. Hence, carbohydrate needs of burned patients should approximate 4.7 to 6.8 mg/kg/min, and in clinical practice we have used 5.0 mg/kg/min as the goal.

## Protein Requirements

Although carbohydrate needs are quite well established, less is known about protein needs. Whereas the fate of carbohydrate may be readily traced, protein is more difficult to follow. It is possible to measure whole body rates of protein

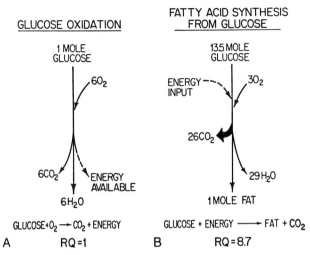

**FIGURE 10–5.** Glucose oxidation provides energy with $O_2$ consumption and $CO_2$ production in equal molar concentrations (RQ = 1). Fat synthesis releases more than eight times as much $CO_2$ for each mole of $O_2$ consumed and is an energy-consuming process. Hence, RQ>1. (From Wolfe RR, O'Donnell TF Jr, Stone MD, et al: Investigation of factors determining the optimal glucose infusion rate in total parenteral nutrition. Metabolism 29:892–900, 1980; with permission.)

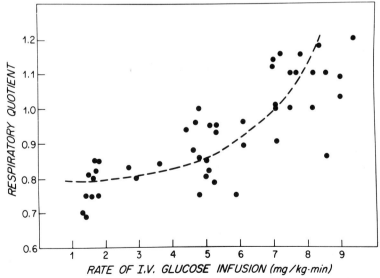

**FIGURE 10–6.** As parenteral glucose infusion rates exceed 5 mg/kg/min, the respiratory quotient rapidly increases, suggesting increasing lipogenesis. (From Burke JF, Wolfe RR, Mullany CJ, et al: Glucose requirements following burn injury. Ann Surg 190:274–285, 1979; with permission.)

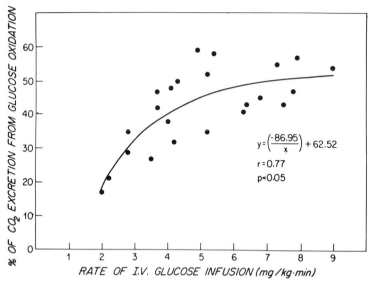

**FIGURE 10–7.** The percentage of $CO_2$ oxidized from glucose reaches a plateau after the infusion rate of dextrose in burned patients exceeds 5.0 mg/kg/min. (From Burke JF, Wolfe RR, Mullany CJ, et al: Glucose requirements following burn injury. Ann Surg 190:274–285, 1979; with permission.)

synthesis, yet the methodology of determining compartmentalization—visceral versus peripheral—of those rates is not available. Nitrogen balance studies are subject to error and are therefore supected of being unreliable.[30] Moreover, these balances simply show the relationship between what is fed and lost over time, rather than pinpointing direct utilization. Despite these limitations, it is possible to estimate optimal protein needs from two key studies.

Wolfe and others[31] conducted whole body protein turnover studies in eight burned patients fed a high-protein diet of 2.2 gm/kg/day and subsequent low-protein regimen of 1.4 gm/kg/day. While the nitrogen balance increased with higher protein intake, net whole body synthesis did not improve, and synthesis and catabolism both increased, implying that there was no net beneficial effect from dietary protein.

In direct contrast to these data, Alexander and collaborators[32] found that, in burned children, it was advantageous to give protein as 134 gm/M²/day over 105 gm/M²/day, as evidenced by measurements of opsonic index, C3, IgG, transferrin, total protein, number of bacteremic days, and survival. This study was later criticized[32] (see appendix of article) for its lack of equality between the two groups. The control group had significantly more days of parenteral nutrition and fewer calories from an oral diet than did the study group. Thus, it is conceivable that the control group was sicker.

Even in light of these conflicting reports, Molnar and Burke[33] caution against prescribing excessive amounts of dietary protein, as it has been implicated in hypercalciuria, increased hypoxic ventilatory response, and increased metabolic rate. They suggest providing pediatric and adult burned patients with 1.5 to 2.5 gm/day of protein.

## Fat Requirements

Fat is considered vital only for supplying essential fatty acids (EFA). Given the constraints placed upon glucose, however, it becomes necessary to administer fat as a nonprotein caloric source. Exact needs for burned patients are unknown, but a minimum of 2 per cent of the total calories should come from EFA.

Interestingly, when fat is provided as intravenous long-chain fatty acids, approximately 26 to 36 per cent is directly oxidized for energy in burned patients.[34] The remainder is stored as triglyceride and creates a metabolic burden on the liver to form very low density lipoproteins. Moreover, animals with femur fracture given intravenous long-chain fats became septic, whereas those provided a 50:50 mixture of long- and medium-chain triglycerides did not.[35] The concern is that lipid high in linoleic acid (e.g., soybean, safflower oil) may accentuate immunosuppression, presumably through production of prostaglandins of the 2-series. Although EFA and calories are required by the burned patient, the exact amount or type of fat required has to be determined.

These same phenomena do not occur when the fat source is present in enteral diets, particularly as medium-chain triglycerides. Critically ill patients, however, may benefit from low-fat diets (40 gm/day) because fat may be a contributory factor in diarrhea.[36] Mochizuki and collaborators[37] additionally concluded from animal data that during the acute phase of burn injury the

### TABLE 10–4. Estimation of Macronutrient Requirements*

| Macronutrient | Formula | Exceptions | Example: 70-kg Man on Oral Diet |
|---|---|---|---|
| Calories | 2 × BMR (kcal) | Children under 20 kg receiving solely parenteral nutrition: Required kcal = 1.75 × BMR | 2 × 1700 kcal = 3400 kcal |
| Protein | 1.5–2.5 gm/kg/ day | Children under 20 kg receiving solely parenteral nutrition: Required protein = 3 gm/kg/day | 2.5 × 70 kg = 175 gm protein = 700 kcal |
| Carbohydrate | 5 mg/kg/min | None | 5 mg × 70 kg × 1440 min/ day = 1000 mg/gm 504 gm CHO = 2016 kcal |
| Fat | Remainder of kcal | Intravenous fat, maximum allowed: Children: 4 gm fat/kg/ day Adults: 2.5 gm fat/kg/day | Total kcal − (CHO kcal + protein kcal) = fat kcal 3400 − (700 kcal + 2016 kcal) = 684 kcal = 76 gm fat |

*From Bell SJ, Molnar JA, Mangino JE, Burke JF: Manual of Nutritional Support for Adult and Pediatric Burn Patients, 1982 (unpublished). Copy may be obtained through Shriners Burns Institute, Boston Unit.

optimal enteral lipid content after burn injury ranges from 5 to 15 per cent of the nonprotein calories.

Hence, the lipid data are paradoxical. Given the constraints on carbohydrate and protein, fat needs to be provided in sizeable quantities; for example, a 70-kg man would need 20 per cent of his total calories, or 76 gm, as fat. Evidence suggests that both parenteral and enteral lipid administration is often excessive and perhaps harmful. It is clear that more work is required, not only to determine exact fat requirements, but also to determine optimal fatty acid chain length.

## Summary of Macronutrient Guidelines

Table 10–4[38] records the suggested guidelines for macronutrients set forth by the Massachusetts General Hospital and Shriners Burns Institute. As stated earlier, calculation for each substrate is based on the patient's ideal body weight. The energy, carbohydrates, and protein needs are determined first, with fat making up the remainder of the caloric deficit. This protocol appears to be useful in meeting macronutrient and caloric requirements while avoiding the toxic effects of carbohydrate.

## Micronutrient Requirements

In contrast to the extensive knowledge base about macronutrient requirements for burned patients, micronutrient needs are virtually unknown. As the metabolic response to injury results in an alteration of metabolism of vitamins, minerals, and trace elements, requirements for these presumably increase, but the amount of the increase is unknown.

Bell and others[39] have described three general principles for guiding micronutrient prescription for pediatric and adult burned patients. The exact prescriptions are listed in Table 10–5.

Certain micronutrients are known to have major toxic side effects if given in excessive quantities. Consequently, the American Medical Association Nutrition Advisory Group[40, 41] guidelines for parenteral administration and the Recommended Dietary Allowances (RDA)[3] for enteral administration were adapted for use of those vitamins or other elements that have great toxic potential.

Secondly, they[39] advise providing several times the recommended amount of therapeutically beneficial micronutrients to burned patients. In particular, vitamin C[42] and zinc[43] have little inherent toxic potential and are thought to promote wound healing. These nutrients are provided in amounts of up to six times the RDA, both parenterally and enterally.

Finally, those nutrients that are nontoxic and conceivably have increased rate of depletion through wound loss, increased uninary excretion, or catabolism are supplemented at twice the RDA. Vitamin B complex is included in this group.

**TABLE 10–5. Micronutrient Protocols for Parenteral and Enteral Diets**

| | Vitamins | | | |
|---|---|---|---|---|
| | *Adult Burned Patients* | | *Pediatric Burned Patients* | |
| *Specific Vitamin* | *Parenteral** | *Enteral†* | *Parenteral* | *Enteral* |
| Fat-Soluble | | | | |
| Vitamin A (RE) | 750–772 | 569–1139 | 991 | 569–1139 |
| (Retinal equiv.) | | | | |
| Vitamin D (ng) | 6.25–6.45 | 5–10 | 5 | 5–10 |
| Vitamin E (TE) | 1.25–1.28 | 7–14 | 10 | 7–14 |
| (Tocopherol equiv.) | | | | |
| Vitamin K‡ | 0 | 0 | 0 | 0 |
| Water-soluble | | | | |
| B Complex | 2 × AMA guidelines§ | 2 × RDA** | 2 × AMA guidelines | 2 × RDA†† |
| Vitamin C (mg) | 200–300 | 100 | 100 | 100 |
| Folic acid (mg) | 1.5 | 1.0 | 0.25 | 0.2 |
| Vitamin $B_{12}$ (mg) | 0 | 3.5–7.0 | 5 | 3.5–7.0 |

*Sources: MVI and MVI-12, Armour Pharmaceutical Co., Blue Bell, PA.
†Sources: Adult, Standard Multivitamin and whole egg powder
  Child: Flintstones vitamins, Elkhart, IN, and whole egg powder
‡Vitamin K is not routinely administered.
§From Reference 39, with permission.
**Berroca C, Roche Laboratories, Nutley, NJ.
††B complex with C, Squibb Lab, Princeton, NJ.

| | Minerals | | | |
|---|---|---|---|---|
| | *Adult* | | *Child* | |
| *Mineral* | *Parenteral** | *Enteral†* | *Parenteral* | *Enteral* |
| Sodium (mg) | Added as needed, based on serum values | | | |
| Potassium (mg) | Added as needed, based on serum values | | | |
| Calcium (mEq) | 9–13.5 | 10–20‡ | 9–27 | 40–60 |
| Magnesium (mEq) | 16–24 | 4–8‡ | 8–24 | 12–33 |
| Phosphorus (mM) | 26–50 | 26–60‡ | 9–27 | 26–60 |
| Iron (mg)§ | 0 | 0 | 0 | 0 |

*Sources: calcium gluconate; magnesium sulfate; and sodium or potassium as phosphate or acetate.
†Sources: calcium gluconate; magnesium sulfate; and Neutra-Phos or Phospho-Soda.
‡Supplemented based on serum values.
§Not routinely supplemented because adequate iron is provided through blood product transfusions.

| | Trace Elements | | | |
|---|---|---|---|---|
| | *Adult* | | *Child* | |
| *Element** | *Parenteral†* | *Enteral‡* | *Parenteral* | *Enteral* |
| Zinc (mg) | 2–3 | 100§ | 2.5 | 50§ |
| Copper (mg) | 1–1.5 | 0.24–0.48 | 0.5 | 0.20–0.48 |
| Chromium (mg) | 0.01–0.015 | 0.035–0.07 | 0.005 | 0.03–0.07 |
| Manganese (mg) | 0.4–0.6 | 0.15–0.3 | 0.25 | 0.1–0.3 |
| Iodine (mg) | 0.056–0.084 | 0.19–0.38 | 0 | 0.15—0.38 |

*Selenium and fluoride are not routinely added because of their high potential for toxicity and low potential for deficiency.
†Source: MTE concentrate, Lyphomed, Chicago, IL, and Armour Pharmaceutical Co., Blue Bell, PA.
‡Sources: Whole egg powder contains some trace elements, but $ZnSo_4$ is added to approximate our recommendations.
  Chromium and manganese may be supplemented.
§Added as $ZnSO_4$: 100 mg $Zn_4$ = 440 mg $ZnSO_4$.

## NUTRITIONAL SUPPORT

### Parenteral Nutrition

Generally speaking, the enteral route of feeding is the preferred one; it is physiologically closer to normal, safer, and less costly. However, TPN must often be implemented because of the absence of a functioning bowel as a result of post-traumatic and postoperative ileus. Given the unique requirements of the burned patient (see Table 10–4), it is not often possible to provide standard TPN formula, such as 250 gm detrose and 42 gm protein per liter, to the patient and readily meet his need. Hence, a modular approach to feeding, whereby individual patient requirements are satisfied, is desirable, and since macronutrients such as carbohydrate, protein, and fat are sold separately it is easy to administer them exactly.

Table 10–6[39] demonstrates the amounts of each substrate required by a 70-kg adult and a 15-kg child based on the nutrient prescription in Table 10–4. All the macronutrients and micronutrients except intravenous fat were traditionally

**TABLE 10–6. Modular Parenteral Diets for Burned Patients***

| Nutrient | Source | Daily Quantity | |
| --- | --- | --- | --- |
| | | *Adult (70 kg) (2500 cc)* | *Child (15 kg) (1000 cc)* |
| Calories Provided | | 3400 kcal | 1147 kcal |
| Protein | Crystalline amino acids (10%) | 1750 cc | 450 cc (Children under 20 kg receiving solely parenteral nutrition. Required protein - 3 mg/kg/day) |
| Carbohydrate | $D_{50}W$ | 1008 cc | 216 cc |
| Fat | Intravenous fat emulsion (20%)† | 495 cc‡ | 300 cc (maximum 4 gm/ kg/day) |
| **Vitamins** | | | |
| Water-soluble | Berocca-C§ | 2 ml Berocca-C 1500 mg vitamin C 1.5 mg folic acid | 1 ml Berocca-C 0.2 mg folic acid |
| Fat-soluble | MVI-12** | 10 ml | 10 ml |
| **Minerals** | | | |
| Sodium | NaCl | Additions as needed | Additions as needed |
| Potassium | KCl or K acetate | per laboratory monitoring | per laboratory monitoring |
| Calcium | Ca gluconate | 13.5 mEq $Ca^{2+}$ | 9 mEq $Ca^{2+}$ |
| Phosphorus | $NaPO_4$, $KPO_4$ | 33.5 mM $PO_4^{2-}$ | 9 mM $PO_4^{2-}$ |
| Magnesium | $MgSO_4$ | 24 mEq $Mg^{2+}$ | 8 mEq $Mg^{2+}$ |
| Zinc | $ZnSO_4$ | 2.5 mg | 2.5 mg |

*From Bell SJ, Molnar JA, Burke JFG: Guidelines for the nutritional support of the burned patient. Pharm Pract News 13:1–21, 1986, with permission.

†Use of a solution containing 39% branched chain amino acid (BCAA) supplementation is desirable in order to assure intake of 35 to 50 gm BCAA (leucine, isoleucine, and valine in 1:1:1 molar ratios), particularly if the patient is hypermetabolic from infection and in negative nitrogen balance (i.e., greater than −2 gm/day).

‡Patient reaction to IV fat varies; thus patients receiving IV fat should be carefully selected.

§Roche Laboratories, Nutley, NJ.

**UVS Pharmaceutical Corp., Tuckahoe, NY.

combined in an administration bag. Fat was provided through the same central vein by a piggy-back device or by peripheral access. It has recently become possible to combine the entire array of dietary components in one bag, thereby facilitating the modular approach to providing TPN.[44]

## Enteral Nutrition (Tube Feeding)

In contrast to the intravenous route, there is less flexibility in providing modular diets by the enteral route, primarily because tube feeding formulas are available only with fixed nutrient percentages. It would be necessary to stock numerous formulas in order to meet the wide range of needs. As an alternative, single modules of carbohydrate (glucose polymer), protein (egg), and fat (corn oil) have been combined with required micronutrients to make the optimal formula (Table 10–7).[17] Confirmation of the adequacy of this modular formula was later made with a view to producing positive nitrogen balance and allowing for compliance with nutrient goals.[45] The modular diet is no more costly than comparable enteral formulas. If modular formulas are not a possibility, it is

**TABLE 10–7. Modular Tube Feeding for Burned Patients**

| Nutrient | Source | Daily Quantity | |
| | | *Adult (70 kg)* | *Child (15 kg)* |
|---|---|---|---|
| Calories | | 3400 kcal* | 1500 kcal |
| Protein | | | 79 gm |
| | Whole egg | 220 gm | 0 gm |
| | Egg white | 89 gm | 114 gm |
| Carbohydrate | Polycose† | 501 gm | |
| Fat | Corn oil | None—adequate fat in whole egg | 75 ml |
| **Vitamins** | | | |
| Water-soluble | Whole egg solids plus | 2 ml Berroca-C‡ | 1 capsule |
| Fat-soluble | supplements | 500 mg ascorbic acid | B complex with C§ |
| | | 1 mg folate | 0.5 mg folate |
| | | No additions | Pediatric multivitamin three times per week** |
| **Minerals** | Whole egg solids plus following supplements: | | |
| Sodium | Sodium chloride | Additions as needed | 14 mEq |
| Potassium | Potassium chloride | per laboratory | 11 mEq |
| Calcium | Calcium gluconate | monitoring | 40 mEq |
| Phosphorus | Phospho-Soda | | 26 mM |
| Magnesium | Magnesium sulfate | | 13 mEq |
| Zinc | Zinc sulfate | 440 mg | 220 mg |

*From Harris JG, Benedict FG: Biometric study of basal metabolism in man. Washington, DC, Carnegie Institute, 1919, with permission.
†Ross Laboratories, Columbus, OH.
‡Roche Laboratories, Nutley, NJ.
§Squibb, Princeton, NJ.
**Miles Laboratory, Elkhart, IN.

prudent to provide patients with a so-called high-protein diet, with greater than 15 per cent of calories from protein, or to use a standard formula with an additional protein source such as whey protein.

## Nutritional Assessment

In order to guarantee that nutrient needs are met, it would be advantageous to have clinical tools with which to assess the efficacy of the regimen. Despite the fact that there are countless nutritional assessment parameters available,[46] these may be unreliable in the burned patient. Weekly monitoring of visceral protein status and weight change can be used to test efficacy in terms of outcome of nutritional support, however.[47] Moreover, Morath and others[48] have determined systematically that commonly used nutritional markers such as albumin, total lymphocyte count, energy, and serum transferrin can be used to predict which patient will develop sepsis.

### Compliance with Caloric Goals

Although actual biochemical indices may be utilized for assessment, it is advisable to measure compliance of caloric counts from diet records with nutrient goals. Bell and co-investigators[49] suggest that consumption by the patient of at least 80 per cent of his estimated needs is adequate. Methods to improve compliance include the use of modular parenteral and enteral formulas and daily recording of nutrient intakes.

### Anthropometric Measurements

Body composition measurements of fat and body cell mass may be obtained by means of upper-arm anthropometry.[46] Unfortunately, the patients who would most benefit from these measurements, those with burns greater than 50 per cent TBSA, are likely to have been injured on their upper body, thus rendering the data invalid and often unobtainable.

The serial weekly monitoring of weight should provide an appropriate index for assessing a nutritional prescription. The presence of bulky dressings, splinting apparatus, multiple escharectomies, and postoperative edema is likely to limit validity of these measurements.[10, 50] Hence, it may be prudent simply to evaluate weight change over the entire hospital course, thereby comparing premorbid weight with discharge weight. Since escharectomy weight may prove significant, adding this value to the discharge weight provides a truer picture of actual weight change incurred as a result of feeding. Bell and others[51] have demonstrated that weight loss can be limited to 10 per cent of premorbid weight after correcting for escharectomy when patients are fed twice their predicted BEE for calories.

### Biochemical Indices and Nitrogen Balance

Serum proteins, particularly albumin concentrations, have been treated as reliable indices of nutritional status of burned and nonburned hospitalized patients.[46-48] We advise caution when using these for burned patients undergoing aggressive excisions and grafting that involve frequent and lengthy operations. Whole blood volume may typically be replaced, thus yielding questionable results. Values below 2.4 gm/dl are of concern, however, and colloid replacement is needed when values are below 2.0 gm/dl. Moreover, the excess fluid administered during surgery would again weaken the validity of serum protein measurements.[10]

Perhaps the best way to assess protein status is by determining nitrogen balance. Classic studies[46, 52] suggest using the equation:

Nitrogen intake (gm) − [Urinary urea nitrogen (gm)
+ (2 gm nonurea nitrogen) + (2 gm fecal and integumental losses)]

This formula assumes that the ratio between urinary urea nitrogen (UUN) and total urinary nitrogen (TUN) is constant and that integumental nitrogen losses are small (less than 0.5 gm). Burned patients have been shown to have variable ratios of UUN to TUN, depending upon burn size and patient age.[53] Kien and colleagues[54] meticulously measured nitrogen lost through the burn wound and found that amounts fluctuated greatly depending on the percentage of open burn wounds. Therefore, a new equation to determine nitrogen balance incorporating these aspects was developed as follows:

Nitrogen balance = Total dietary nitrogen (gm) −
[TUN + fecal loss + wound nitrogen loss]

Fecal loss is estimated to be 1 gm/24 hr.[18] TUN is predicted by:

log TUN = 0.284 + 0.9084 log UUN
+ 0.002319% initial burn + 0.002146 age

Wound nitrogen loss estimated by[54]:

| Percentage Open Wound | Wound Nitrogen Loss (gm/kg/day) |
| --- | --- |
| 10% | 0.02 |
| 11–30% | 0.05 |
| ≥31% | 0.12 |

Nutritional assessment is important after the first five to seven days in order to determine response to feeding and assist in evaluating the metabolic response to burn therapy. If the patient has a high blood sugar (carbohydrate intolerance) and elevated BUN, then the serial 24-hour UUN will provide a dynamic assessment of protein metabolism in the face of 1.5 to 2.5 gm protein/kg intake and 25 to 30 kcal/day. If estimated nitrogen balance (see above equation) is greater than −2 gm daily, risks, such as a high probability of sepsis and/or organ failure, are possible. The patient would remain in the acute phase of injury. Careful monitoring for sources of infection, measurement of oxygen consumption, lactic acidemia, and fluid and electrolytes would be prudent. If adequate compliance with caloric goals and positive nitrogen balance is present, then the patient is likely to convalesce.

## FUTURE DIRECTIONS

The advances in the treatment of burned patients are remarkable. Twenty years ago, it was not uncommon for death to occur during the early resuscitative period. If the patient lived for more than a few days, he usually succumbed to invasive sepsis.[55] Today, the revolution in wound coverage in terms of artificial skin and "growing" of the patient's own epithelial cells in the laboratory is truly extraordinary.[25] In order to maintain life during the somewhat lengthy period of skin grafting, nutritional support is essential. The correct nutritional prescription should enhance the wound healing process and not produce iatrogenic complications of its own. It may even reduce the length of hospitalization required for burned patients, thus reducing treatment costs. It certainly contributes greatly to a better quality of life and minimizes long-term rehabilitation resulting from the unnecessary and excessive tissue wasting associated with semistarvation, burn injury, and stress metabolism.

## REFERENCES

1. Blocker TC, Levin WC, Nowinski WW, et al: Nutrition studies in the severely burned. Ann Surg 141:589–597, 1955.
2. Artz CP, Soroff HS, Pearson E, Hummel RP: Some recent developments in oral feedings for optimal nutrition in burns. Am J Clin Nutr 4:642–646, 1956.
3. Recommended Dietary Allowances. 9th ed. Washington, DC, National Research Council, National Academy of Sciences, 1980.
4. Levenson SM, Davidson CS, Lund CC, Taylor FHL: The nutrition of patients with thermal burns. Surg Gynecol Obstet 80:449–469, 1945.
5. Cuthbertson DP, Zagreb HC: The metabolic response to injury and and its nutritional implications: Restrospect and prospect. JPEN 3:108–129, 1979.
6. Caldwell FT, Casali RE, Flanigan WJ, Bowser B: What constitutes the proper solution for resuscitation of the severely burned patient? Am J Surg 122:655–661, 1971.
7. Baue AE, Gunther B, Hartl W, et al: Altered hormonal activity in severely ill patients after injury or sepsis. Arch Surg 119:1125–1132, 1984.
8. Blackburn BL, Miller JDB, Bistrian BR, et al: Amino acids—key nutrient in response to injury. *In* Richards JR, Kinney JM (eds): Nutritional Aspects of Care in the Critically Ill. New York, Churchill Livingstone, 1977.
9. Askart A, Long CL, Blakemore WS: Urinary zinc, nitrogen and potassium losses in response to trauma. JPEN 3:151–156, 1979.
10. Molnar JA, Wolfe RR, Burke JF: Metabolism and nutrition therapy in thermal injury. *In* Schneider HA, Anderson CE, Coursin DB (eds): Nutritional Support in Medical Practice. 2nd ed. Hagerstown, MD, Harper and Row, 1983.
11. Gooodwin CW: Parenteral nutrition in thermal injuries. *In* Rombeau JL, Caldwell MD (eds): Parenteral Nutrition. Philadelphia, WB Saunders Company, 1986.
12. Zawacki BE, Spitzer KW, Mason AD Jr, Johns LA: Does increased evaporative water loss cause hypermetabolism in burned patients? Ann Surg 171:236–240, 1970.
13. Wilmore DW, Long CL, Mason AD, et al: Catecholamines: Mediator of the hypermetabolic response to thermal injury. Ann Surg 180:653–669, 1974.

14. Wolfe RR: Caloric requirements of the burned patient. J Trauma 21:712–714, 1981.
15. Saffle JR, Medina E, Raymond J, et al: Use of indirect calorimetry in the nutritional management of burned patients. J Trauma 25:32–39, 1985.
16. Turner WW, Ireton CS, Hunt JL, Baxter CR: Predicting energy expenditures in burned patients. J Trauma 25:11–15, 1985.
17. Wolfe RR, Molnar JA: Meeting the special nutritional requirements of the burn patient. Nutr Ther News 3:1–6, 1981.
18. Serog P, Baigts F, Apfelbaum M, et al: Energy and nitrogen balances in 24 severely burned patients receiving 4 isocaloric diets of about 10MJ/M²/day (2392 kcalories/M²/day). Burns 9:422–427, 1983.
19. Cunningham JJ, Hegarty MT, Meara PA, et al: Measured and predicted calorie requirements of adults during recovery from severe burn trauma. Am J Clin Nutr 49:404–408, 1989.
20. Harris JG, Benedict FG: Biometric study of basal metabolism in man. Washington, DC, Carnegie Institute, 1919.
21. Ideal Weight Tables. Metropolitan Life Insurance Company Statistics Bulletin, November-December, 1979 (based on data from 1959).
22. Master AM, Laser RP, Beckman G: Tables of average weight and height of Americans aged 65–94 years. JAMA 172:658–662, 1960.
23. Pediatric Growth Chart. Fels Research Institute and Mead Johnson, 1978.
24. Mochizuki H, Trocki O, Dominoni L, et al: Mechanism of prevention of postburn hypermetabolism and catabolism by early enteral feeding. Ann Surg 200:297–307, 1984.
25. Burke JF, Yannas IV, Quinby WC, et al: Successful use of a physiologically acceptable artificial skin in the treatment of extensive burn injury. Ann Surg 194:413–428, 1981.
26. Rutan TC, Herdon DN, Osten TV, Abston S: Metabolic rate alterations in early excision and grafting versus conservative treatment. J Trauma 26:140–142, 1986.
27. Shelton, GF, Petersen SR, Sanders R: Hepatic dysfunction during hyperalimentation. Arch Surg 113:504–508, 1979.
28. Burke JF, Wolfe RR, Mullany CJ, et al: Glucose requirements following burn injury. Ann Surg 190:274–285, 1979.
29. Wolfe RR, O'Donnell TF Jr, Stone MD, et al: Investigation of factors determining the optimal glucose infusion rate in total parenteral nutrition. Metabolism 29:892–900, 1980.
30. Hegsted DM: Assessment of nitrogen requirements. Am J Clin Nutr 31:1669–1677, 1978.
31. Wolfe RR, Goodenough RD, Burke JF, Wolfe MH: Response of protein and urea kinetics in burn patients to different levels of protein intake. Ann Surg 197:163–171, 1983.
32. Alexander JW, MacMillam BGH, Stinnett JD, et al: Beneficial effect of aggressive protein feeding in severely burned children. Ann Surg 192:505–517, 1980.
33. Molnar JA, Burke JF: Metabolic and nutritional management. Drug Ther Oct 1984, pp 45–55.
34. Goodenough RD, Wolfe RR: Effect of total parenteral nutrition on free fatty acid metabolism in burned patients. JPEN 8:357–360, 1984.
35. Hamawy KJ, Moldwer LL, Georgieff M, et al: The effect of lipid emulsions on reticuloendothelial system function in the injured animal. JPEN 9:559–565, 1985.
36. Heymsfield SB, Horowitz J, Lawson DH: Enteral hyperalimentation. In Berk JE (ed): Developments in Digestive Diseases. Philadelphia, Lea and Febiger, 1980, pp 59–83.
37. Mochizuki H, Trocki D, Dominoni L, et al: Optimal lipid content for enteral diets following thermal injury. JPEN 8: 638–646, 1984.
38. Bell SJ, Molnar JA, Mangino JE, Burke JF: Manual of Nutritional Support for Adult and Pediatric Burn Patients, 1982 (unpublished). Copy may be obtained through Shriners Burns Institute, Boston Unit.
39. Bell SJ, Molnar JA, Burke JFG: Guidelines for the nutritional support of the burned patient. Pharm Pract News 13:1–21, 1986.
40. Multivitamin preparation for parenteral use: A statement by the Nutrition Advisory Group. JPEN 3:258–262, 1979.
41. Guidelines for essential trace element preparations for parenteral use: A statement by the Nutrition Advisory Group. JAMA 214:2051–2054, 1979.
42. Lund CC, Levenson SM, Green RW: Ascorbic acid, thiamine, riboflavin, and nicotinic acid in relation to acute burns in man. Arch Surg 55:557–583, 1947.
43. Pories WJ, Henzel JH, Rob CG, Strain WH: Acceleration of wound healing in man with zinc sulfate given by mouth. Lancet 1:121–124, 1967.

44. Condella F, Baptista RJ, Griffin RE: More efficient system for preparing total parenteral nutrient solutions. Am J Hosp Pharm 40:2146–2149, 1983.
45. Bell SJ, Molnar JA, Carey M, Burke JF: Adequacy of a modular tube feeding diet for burned patients. J Am Diet Assoc 86:1386–1391, 1986.
46. Blackburn GL, Bistrian BR, Maini BS, et al: Nutritional and metabolic assessment of the hospitalized patient. JPEN 1:11–22, 1977.
47. Delsavio N: Nutritional support for thermally injured patients: The role of the dietitian. Nutr Supp Serv 4:1014, 1984.
48. Morath MA, Miller SF, Finley RK: Nutritional indications of postburn bacteremic sepsis. JPEN 3:488–491, 1981.
49. Bell SJ, Molnar JA, Krasker WS, Burke JF: Dietary compliance in pediatric burned patients. J Am Diet Assoc 84:1329–1333, 1984.
50. Bell SJ, Wyatt J: Nutrition guidelines for burned patients. J Am Diet Assoc 86:648–653, 1985.
51. Bell SJ, Molnar JA, Krasker WS, Burke JF: Weight maintenance in pediatric burned patients. J Am Diet Assoc 86:207–211, 1986.
52. Morath MA, Miller SF, Finley RK, Jones LM: Interpretation of nutritional parameters in burn patients. J Burn Care Rehab 4:361–366 1983.
53. Bell SJ, Molnar JA, Krasker WS, Burke JF: Prediction of total urinary nitrogen from urinary urea for burned patients. J Am Diet Assoc 85:1100–1104, 1985.
54. Kien CL, Young VR, Rohrbaugh DK, Burke JF: Increased rates of whole body protein synthesis and breakdown in children recovering from burns. Ann Surg 187:383–391, 1978.
55. Mason AD, McManus AT, Pruitt BA: Association of burn mortality and bacteremia. Arch Surg 121:1027–1031, 1986.

# 11

# Complications of Burn Injury

## YOTARO SHINOZAWA and NAOKI AIKAWA

Major burn is more than a skin injury; it is a serious overall disease usually accompanied by a variety of complications. Circulatory derangement in the resuscitation phase and in the later septic phase is a major catastrophe that influences the pathophysiology of burn patients. The neuroendocrine system, metabolic function, immune system, complement system, coagulation-fibrinolysis complex, and kallikrein system are all involved to varying extents. Catecholamine, renin-angiotensin, serotonin, histamine, interleukins, and eicosanoids released at different sites, including burn wounds, increase in concentrations of these humoral mediators, affecting the vital systems, organ functions, membrane permeability, and vascular responses. Some of these responses have been called "alarm reaction" and are recognized as necessary for circulatory homeostasis, host defense against infection, or wound healing. These mediators have unfavorable aspects, however, since they contribute to the development of organ dysfunction. When these host responses are uncontrolled and severe, patients develop multiple organ failure,[1] where more than two systems or organs are affected simultaneously or sequentially. The extent and the duration of these complications depend on the severity of the thermal injury. The potential risk from complications usually exists until the surface burn is epithelialized or grafted. Pre-existing systemic diseases are exacerbated by the burn stress, especially in elderly patients. Such important masked or unrecognized diseases as hyperthyroidism require careful observation in the post-burn course. Iatrogenic complications may also occur from adverse reactions to medication and from intensive treatments that create additional stress to the patient. In this chapter, the pathophysiology and management of the complications primarily seen in the acute phase of thermal injury are discussed. Septic, neuropsychiatric, renal, and pulmonary complications are described in other chapters.

## CARDIAC COMPLICATIONS

Hypovolemia due to fluid loss from the burn wound and the fluid shift from circulation into the interstitial and intracellular spaces is primarily responsible for the decreased cardiac output seen in the early post-burn phase. Optimal fluid resuscitation will improve the cardiac dysfunction; however, volume replacement alone is often inadequate to return cardiac output to normal in the first post-burn hours. In the patients with burns of more than 70 per cent of total body surface area (TBSA), acute left ventricular failure occasionally occurs in the absence of pulmonary edema and it is usually fatal.

Congestive heart failure may occur in the course of acute resuscitation during the first 24 hours, but more commonly in the fluid mobilization phase three to seven days post burn. Pulmonary edema may follow the latter. In patients with ischemic heart disease these can occur throughout the hospital course.

There are many reports, mostly experimental, demonstrating that myocardial depressant factor (MDF) is responsible for the cardiac dysfunction in the early shock and in later septic shock phases. One experimental study[2] demonstrated ultrastructural alterations of the mitochondria of cardiac septal preparations perfused with burn shock plasma. Another experimental study[3] showed that MDF activities, determined by cat papillary muscle bioassay technique, were 28 ± 3 units in patients with 61.9 per cent of mean burn surface area on day one and 56 ± 4 units on days four and five, while in control patients MDF activities were 23 ± 3 units. At the time when MDF was high, cardiac output was well maintained. Although cardiac output is affected by many factors, this suggests that the effects of MDF on the cardiac function are still controversial. The fact that significant elevations in MDF activity were followed by circulatory shock may give credence to the potential usefulness of plasma MDF activity as a predictor of risk of myocardial dysfunction in patients with severe burns.

MDF has been reported as a toxic glycoprotein that is produced in the inadequately perfused pancreas[4] or by splanchnic vasoconstriction.[5] It is also suspected that burned skin produces toxic glycoprotein,[6] which reduces cardiac contractility. It is reported that endogenous nickel, which is increased fivefold in the first two days after burn, may induce coronary vasoconstriction and myocardial ischemic injury in rats with third-degree burns of 20 to 25 per cent TBSA.[7]

In extensively burned patients, decreased cardiac output in the presence of adequate filling pressure suggests direct myocardial depression in the early post-burn period. Dopamine therapy in certain individual patients may be useful, the dose titrated according to the patient's hemodynamic response.[8, 9] It is crucial to administer sufficient fluids before the commencement of dopamine drip, and this is ensured by observing filling pressures and urine output. During the early phase of fluid resuscitation, administration of fresh frozen plasma induces a marked increase in cardiac output in most cases (Fig. 11–1). This is not necessarily accompanied by an increase in preload, suggesting that fresh frozen plasma has the ability to improve cardiac function.[9] It is important to remember, however, that this form of therapy has limited application in the present day because of blood transfusion–related infections. Hypoxia or carboxyhemoglobin can aggravate the cardiac muscle dysfunction. With the advent of the Swan-Ganz catheter (SGC) in 1970, bedside monitoring of cardiac function and assessment of the effectiveness of the therapy became available for the management of critically

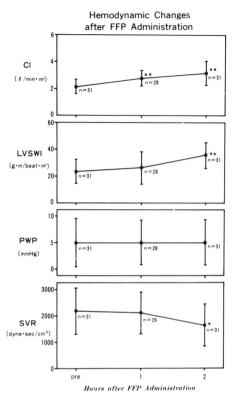

Hemodynamic Changes
after FFP Administration

**FIGURE 11–1.** Effects of fresh frozen plasma (FFP) on hemodynamics in 31 burned patients with burn size of 63.3 ± 20.1 per cent TBSA. FFP was infused for an average of 0.065 ml/kg per cent burn, but total fluid load per hour was not increased as crystalloid infusion was decreased. The FFP infusion resulted in a significant increase in cardiac index (CI) after one hour. Left ventricular stroke work index (LVSWI) was also increased and systemic vascular resistance (SVR) was decreased after two hours of plasma infusion, while pulmonary wedge pressure did not change. Values = mean ± SD, $*P<0.05$, $**P<0.01$ (vs pre-value).

burned patients. The management of the functional cardiac complications can be guided by SGC monitoring; the amounts of intravenous fluids and inotropic agents being adjusted with the data derived.[9]

Arrhythmia in the form of premature atrial or ventricular beats, supraventricular tachycardias, or life-threatening ventricular arrhythmia is rare in the first 24 hours, except in the case of electrical injuries. Arrhythmias are more likely to be present in the first 72 hours in those patients with hypokalemia. The use of diuretics and digitalis can precipitate the arrhythmias. The late onset of arrhythmias may signal a silent myocardial infarction or, in septic patients, hematogenous seeding of the myocardium. As a relatively later cardiac complication, endocarditis is often noted with symptoms of fever of unknown origin, tachycardia, heart murmur, or hypertension. An increased risk of endocardial vegetation is reported when an SGC has been indwelling for a long period (Fig. 11–2); this may result in endocarditis particularly when a catheter is used in extensive burns for more than five days (Fig. 11–3).[8] Myocardial infarction and the possible appearance of angina after injury should also be kept in mind.

At postmortem examination, heart muscle degradation, extra- and intracellular edema, rupture of sarcoplasmic reticulum, swelling and vacuolization of

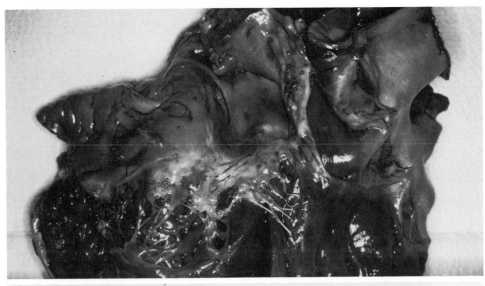

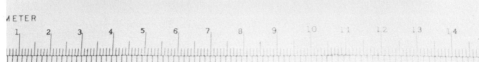

**FIGURE 11–2.** Endocardial vegetations on the tricuspid and pulmonary valves found at autopsy of a 41-year-old male with 84 per cent TBSA and inhalation injury. A Swan-Ganz catheter had been indwelling for 206 hours during the initial resuscitation. The patient died of septicemia on the sixteenth post-burn day.

mitochondria with unfolded and ruptured cristae, and rupture of the myofilaments are seen.

## HEMOGLOBINURIA

Hemoglobinuria is a contributing factor to the development of renal dysfunction in the early phase. In extensive third-degree burns, acute massive hemolysis occurs, releasing free hemoglobin into the plasma. The free hemoglobin is usually conjugated with haptoglobin and metabolized in the liver. However, when a large amount of free hemoglobin is released in a short period of time, plasma haptoglobin is depleted and free hemoglobin passes through the glomeruli and is excreted in the urine, causing a degenerative necrosis of the tubular cell or the occlusion of the renal tubules with hemoglobin casts. Free hemoglobin alone does not necessarily cause acute renal failure; however, the combination of hemoglobinemia and other factors such as dehydration, hypovolemic shock, and endotoxemia promotes initiation of the renal failure. Haptoglobin adminis-

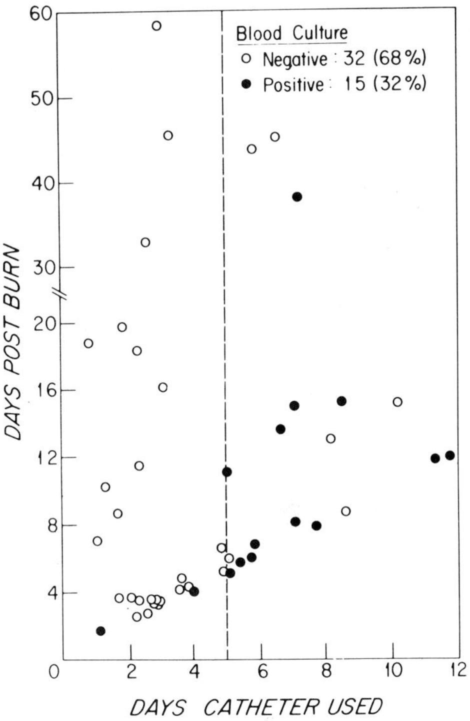

**FIGURE 11–3.** The relationship of positive arterial blood culture to days after burn (ordinate) and days of Swan-Ganz catheter use (abscissa). The rate of positive blood cultures (closed circles) is high among patients who had been monitored for more than five days (dashed line). (Adapted from Aikawa N, Martyn JAJ, Burke JF: Pulmonary artery catheterization and thermodilution cardiac output determination in the management of critically burned patients. Am J Surg 135:811–817, 1978, with permission.)

tration has been proposed for prevention of renal failure in the early phase.[10] The duration of macroscopic hemoglobinuria is reduced by haptoglobin administration, which increases serum free haptoglobin levels (Fig. 11–4). Hemoglobin precipitation in the tubules is also prevented by other measures such as alkalization of urine by sodium bicarbonate administration.

## HEPATIC COMPLICATIONS

Clinical characteristics and the natural course of acute liver complication in thermal injury are not fully understood. Elevated transaminase levels, increased alkaline phosphatase, bilirubinemia, hypoalbuminemia, and prolonged prothrombin time usually indicate liver dysfunction in a clinical setting. Czaja et al[11] reported that the incidence of liver complications occurring within the first week after burn was 58 per cent and that the liver damage could occur as early as 24 hours after burn. In their series, the mean size of burns in patients with liver complication was 57.9 per cent of TBSA (ranging from 14 to 96 per cent), and the mortality of this group was 74.5 per cent. The occurrence of liver dysfunction

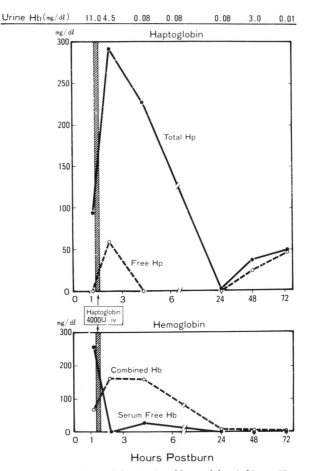

KM  60yrs. male 58% (44% 3rd) BSA Burn

**FIGURE 11–4.** Changes in serum haptoglobin (Hp) and hemoglobin (Hb) in a 60-year-old patient with 14 per cent TBSA second-degree and 44 per cent TBSA third-degree burns. Hemoglobinuria was noted at 60 minutes post burn, and 4000 units of Hp preparation was administered 15 minutes later. The serum free Hb level was 254 mg/dl, and there was no free Hp in the serum before the Hp administration. Hp infusion resulted in a decrease in urine Hb from the pretreatment level of 11 mg/dl to 0.08 mg/dl three hours after Hp infusion. (Adapted from Aikawa N, Ishibiki K, Okusawa S, et al: Use of haptoglobin to prevent renal damage due to hemolysis in extensive third-degree burns. J Burn Care Rehabil 5:20–24, 1984, with permission.)

in the early phase is related to the severity of hemodynamic alterations. Acute reduction of cardiac output, increased viscosity of blood, and splanchnic vasoconstriction can cause hepatic hypoperfusion and ischemia, although liver dysfunction is not always concomitant with underlying shock and hypoxemia. Centrilobular hepatic congestion due to a decreased cardiac output or overzealous administration of fluid in the resuscitation phase cause early hepatomegaly and are responsible for liver dysfunction as well as hepatocellular injury. Caloric deficiency or a catabolic process predominating in the first few days may also be attributable to the parenchymal liver damage. Transaminase levels increase as early as 24 hours after burn, and the peak levels of bilirubin are seen in severely burned patients around the fifth post-burn day or later. Large numbers of damaged red blood cells may cause a disproportionate load on the liver cells to conjugate the indirect bilirubin, causing hyperbilirubinemia. This appears around the second day and subsides within five days. In the Czaja series, severely burned patients had a prolonged hyperbilirubinemia (2.6 to 28.5 mg/dl) in the second week after burn associated with increased alkaline phosphatase and subsiding transaminases. It was composed mainly (75 per cent) of conjugated bilirubin. Other possible causes of acute liver dysfunction in the early phase are cholestatic drugs such as triacetyl oleandomycin, erythromycin esterate, anabolic hormones, chlorpromazine, blood transfusion, anesthetic agents, and burn toxin.

Liver dysfunction in the later phase of burn injury resembles hepatitis, but its cause is not clearly understood. Possible causes include non-A, non-B hepatitis induced by blood products, fatty change, and infection-related mechanisms.[11] Conjugated hyperbilirubinemia and increased alkaline phosphatase are usually the signs of nonspecific reactive hepatitis, or benign intrahepatic cholestasis. Late hyperbilirubinemia that develops in tandem with sepsis is closely associated with poor prognosis. Compromised reticuloendothelial function of the liver is also seen in septic burn patients. As the excretion of conjugated bilirubin by the Golgi apparatus of the hepatocyte is energy-dependent, the increased oxygen demand in sepsis and depleted caloric intake impair the excretory function of the hepatocytes, resulting in intrahepatic cholestasis. These enzyme abnormalities resolve with the improvement in the patient's general condition, but the level of alkaline phosphatase remains twice as high as normal even after other enzymes normalize. This late rise of alkaline phosphatase could be a reflection of hepatic regeneration similar to that described in patients recovering from acute viral or alcoholic hepatitis.[13]

Microscopic abnormalities of the liver are usually diffuse and nonspecific, with the degree of histological change not always consistent with the degree of clinical findings. Congestion of the sinusoids and central veins, cellular swelling, separation of Disse's spaces, anoxic cytoplasmic vacuolation of centrilobular hepatocytes, and centrilobular hepatocyte necrosis are dominant in the acute phase. Mild to moderate fatty degeneration in a centrilobular location is also seen as an early pathological change in severely burned patients. Patients with hyperbilirubinemia sometimes demonstrate canalicular cholestasis, acute and chronic inflammation of the portal tracts, inflammatory foci within the hepatic parenchyma, Kupffer cell hyperplasia, and depositions of centrilobular fat.

The liver dysfunction seen in the post-burn period usually improves as long as the clinical status is normalized. In the presence of sepsis, liver dysfunction continues. The prophylaxis and/or therapy of the post-burn liver dysfunction include the maintenance of sufficient hepatic blood supply, management of sepsis, and conservative hepatoprotective therapy. Early removal of necrotic skin tissue and covering of the wound surface are also recommended. In severe cases, steroids may be effective. Adenosine triphosphate,[14] ATP-MgCl$_2$, growth hormone, and glucose are used to re-establish the reticuloendothelial function of the liver. Plasma exchange or glucagon-insulin therapy[15] is advocated for liver failure. Although the incidence of hepatitis is low, the prophylactic use of hyperimmune gamma globulin should be considered.[16]

## MULTIPLE ORGAN FAILURE

Multiple organ failure (MOF) is a clinical syndrome in which two or more vital organs, including the lung, kidney, liver, heart, and coagulation system, are affected simultaneously or sequentially. The incidence is variable depending on the severity of injury. Among patients with more than 30 per cent TBSA burn and/or inhalation injury, the incidence of MOF was 48.1 per cent (Table 11–1), and the mortality rate was as high as 76.9 per cent (Fig. 11–5).[1] Bacteremia or toxemia resulting from severe shock, inhalation injury, or wound sepsis is closely related to the development of MOF. Endotoxemia resulting from the patient's own intestinal flora may be responsible for early multiple organ failure seen in the first few days after injury. Organ dysfunction is caused by the activation or release of various mediators such as interleukin-1, tumor necrosis factor (TNF), eicosanoids, complements, kallikrein-kinin systems, or interleukins. Therapy includes treatment of the underlying sepsis and shock, blocking of the activation of mediators, and artificial support of function of the organs affected.

## GASTROINTESTINAL COMPLICATIONS

Curling's ulcer is known as the major gastrointestinal complication. Its incidence varies widely, depending mostly on the method of survey. In post-

**TABLE 11–1. Incidences of Organ Failure and Multiple Organ Failure in Burned Patients**

| Severity | Organ | | | | | |
|---|---|---|---|---|---|---|
| | *Lung* | *Kidney* | *Liver* | *Heart* | *DIC* | *MOF* |
| Severe (54 pts) | 30 pts 55.6% | 17 pts 31.5% | 15 pts 27.8% | 21 pts 38.9% | 7 pts 13.0% | 26 pts 48.1% |
| Not severe (104 pts) | 0 | 0 | 1 pt 1.0% | 0 | 0 | 0 |
| Total (158 pts) | 30 pts 19.0% | 17 pts 10.8% | 16 pts 10.1% | 21 pts 13.3% | 7 pts 4.4% | 26 pts 16.5% |

91 organ failures were observed in 34 patients; 8 patients had a failure in one organ, 7 patients in two organs, 10 patients in three organs, 6 patients in four organs, and 3 patients in five organs. pts = Patients; DIC = disseminated intravascular coagulation; MOF = multiple organ failure.

Adapted from Aikawa N, Shinozawa Y, Ishibiki K, et al: Clinical analysis of multiple organ failure in burned patients. Burns 13:103–109, 1987, with permission.

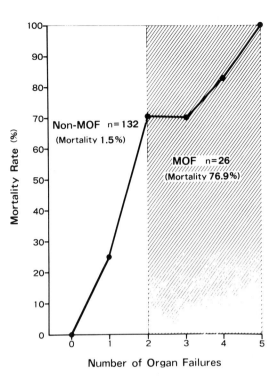

**FIGURE 11-5.** Relationship between the mortality rate and number of organ failures. The mortality rate of burned patients increases as the number of organ failures in a patient increases. The mortality rate of 132 patients without multiple organ failure (MOF) was 1.5 per cent whereas the patients with MOF had a 76.9 per cent mortality rate (*P*<0.05 by chi square test). (Adapted from Aikawa N, Shinozawa Y, Ishibiki K, et al: Clinical analysis of multiple organ failure in burned patients. Burns 13:103–109, 1987, with permission.)

mortem studies, the incidence of Curling's ulcer is approximately 25 per cent,[17, 18] whereas clinical studies indicate the incidence to be around 10 per cent.[19, 20] In a more recent clinical survey of 2700 patients, the incidence is reported to be as low as 0.3 per cent.[21] With the advent of histamine $H_2$ receptor antagonists and improved management of the early shock period, including early enteral feedings, the incidence of Curling's ulcer has been decreasing for the last decade. The ulcer is more frequently localized in the stomach than in the duodenum. Serial endoscopy has been used to demonstrate acute, superficial gastric and duodenal lesions as early as five hours after burn, but progression to life-threatening ulceration such as perforation or hemorrhage occurs later.[22]

As for the signs and symptoms, Pruitt and Goodwin[23] reported that hematemesis and melena were seen in 64 per cent of patients with Curling's ulcers, 43 per cent of whom had massive hemorrhage or accompanying shock. Perforation occurred in 12 per cent. Pain is an uncommon sign, occurring in only 4 per cent of patients. Serial endoscopic examination revealed that many burn patients with acute ulcers remain asymptomatic,[24] although gastric changes, such as erythematous macular lesions superimposed on a usually pale mucosa, focal mucosal hemorrhage, and superficial lesions were observed as early as five hours post burn.

Post-burn upper gastrointestinal stress ulcers are commonly superficial and only infrequently penetrate below the muscularis layer. Gastric ulcers are predominantly multiple and round in configuration, and their greatest diameter is usually less than 2 cm, although they can be solitary, irregular, and large (Fig. 11–6). Duodenal ulcers are usually solitary, but they too can be multiple.[23] The frequency of mucosal changes is related to burn size. Stress ulcers in patients with more than 50 per cent TBSA are caused by the stress of burn itself, but those in patients with less than 50 per cent TBSA are caused predominantly by sepsis. Shock and hypoxemia are also contributing factors to the development of gastrointestinal lesions. In the pathogenesis of Curling's ulcer, gastrin secretion itself does not correlate with ulcer formation. In extensively burned patients without gastroduodenal disease, fasting serum gastrin levels were $139.0 \pm 24.6$ pg/ml (normal range 50 to 250 pg/ml), whereas in patients with superficial gastroduodenal disease the levels were $113.2 \pm 16.7$ pg/ml. On days three through five when hemodynamics were stable, the gastrin levels were $83.8 \pm 11.5$ pg/ml.[22] The total titratable acidity of unstimulated gastric secretion did correlate with the degree of gastroduodenal disease, however. It is reported that the acid output was lowest ($1.19 \pm .038$ mEq/hr) in those with normal gastro-duodenal mucosa, higher ($2.80 \pm 0.66$ mEq/hr) in those with superficial erosion, and highest ($8.53 \pm 4.96$ mEq/hr) in those with ulcerative disease.[22] There was no correlation between gastrin levels and acidity; in other words, some patients with low acid secretion had ulcerative disease. Thus, high acid secretion alone is not primarily pathogenetic. A possible implication is that acute mucosal injury because of ischemia and acidosis immediately after the burn precedes Curling's ulcer. General hemodynamic alterations, hemoconcentration, local vasoconstric-

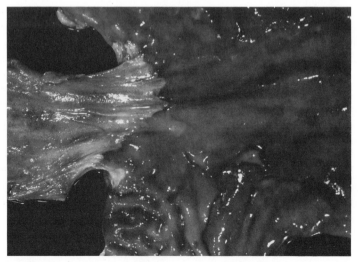

**FIGURE 11–6.** Curling's ulcers seen at autopsy of a two-year-old boy with 64 per cent TBSA burn who died on the eighth post-burn day. There are multiple small superficial ulcers in the stomach.

tion, and submucosal arteriovenous shunts[25] can influence the gastric mucosal ischemic process and make the mucosa susceptible to erosion even in the presence of a normal amount of the intraluminal acid.[22]

Superficial duodenal injury usually occurs immediately after burn injury. The secretion of enterogastrone from the acutely injured duodenum may be impaired, and the normal feedback mechanism for controlling gastric acid secretion and for neutralizing hydrochloric acid may be disturbed.[26] Bile salts and lysolecithin reflux, whether or not associated with ileus in the early post-burn period, and digestive enzymes[27] also contribute to the deterioration of the mucosa. The role of gastric mucus in protecting the gastric mucosa is controversial. It is reported that the content and secretion rates of gastric mucus decrease following burn injury[28]; however, another report shows that gastric mucous content is normal even in the patients with acute mucosal disease.[29] Acid secretion is also diminished by altered gastric mucosal blood flow because of the elevated levels of circulating catecholamines[30] or glucagon.[31] The high concentration of carbonic anhydrase in the surface cells may have a protective effect by increasing the secretion of bicarbonate to neutralize acid. Judging from the pepsinogen levels, the participation of pepsin does not seem important.

Prophylactic measures against the development of gastroduodenal ulcers include the maintenance of hemodynamics to assure sufficient splanchnic circulation, early diagnosis and effective treatment of sepsis, ventilatory support to prevent anoxia or respiratory acidosis, and provision of adequate calories to meet the accentuated metabolic needs. As ulceration can occur as early as 96 hours post burn, attempts to reduce the acidity of gastric contents should be instituted during the resuscitation period. The placement of a nasogastric tube is required. To maintain the pH of gastric aspirate above 4.0, antacids such as magnesium and aluminum hydroxides (Maalox) are administered every two to six hours, and the rate of administration can be increased if the pH level is not maintained. An excessive amount of Maalox may form a bezoar and cause obstruction. In unintubated patients who can eat, the gastric tube should be removed as soon as bowel function is regained in order to avoid nasal bleeding and esophagitis. Recently, histamine $H_2$-receptor antagonists (cimetidine, ranitidine hydrochloride, famotidine, roxatidine acetate hydrochloride) have come into use to reduce the production of gastric acid. Cimetidine has been proven beneficial in preventing post-burn gastrointestinal bleeding.[32, 33] As the biological half-life of cimetidine is reduced by rapid clearance, the dosage and schedule need to be altered in burned patients.[34] Enteral tube feeding is effective in maintaining gastric pH above 5.0 in addition to supporting the nutritional state.[33, 35] With an appropriate combination of antacid therapy, enteral feedings, and cimetidine, the incidence of Curling's ulcer has become less than 1 per cent in the burn patient population.[36]

When surgical intervention is required for Curling's ulcer, vagotomy and antrectomy are the procedures of choice for reducing acid secretion. The indications for surgery for gastrointestinal bleeding in burn patients are somewhat more conservative than in nonburn patients, since the risk of wound dehiscence, wound infection, anastomotic leakage, and peritonitis are greater in burn patients. Free perforation is the absolute indication for surgery; allowing for spontaneous omental plugging of the perforation is not an effective method of treatment in burn patients.[37]

In spite of reduction in the incidence of gastroduodenal ulcer by prophylactic management, acute ulcers of the colon have been identified clinically or at autopsy in burn patients with severe sepsis. This is related to the changes in gastrointestinal flora by the antibiotics administered for the prevention and treatment of infection. Antibiotic-associated diarrhea has been observed with almost all antibiotics and particularly with lincomycin and clindamycin. Ampicillin, amoxicillin, and several third-generation cephalosporins may also cause enterocolitis. The pseudomembranous colitis, which manifests as severe diarrhea and melena with subsequent hypovolemia, is sometimes a catastrophic complication. Diagnosis is made from the symptoms and is confirmed by fiberoptic colonoscopy. The stool should be sent for anaerobic culture of *Clostridium difficule* and exotoxin determination. Treatment includes prompt cessation of the antibiotic and oral vancomycin, 250 mg qid, should be administered together with adequate intravenous fluids. Precautions against infectious hazard should be instituted because contamination of the burn unit by stools containing spores will cause an endemic infection.

Paralytic ileus occurs two to three days after thermal injury in patients with burns exceeding 20 per cent TBSA. Lescher et al[38] described five cases of acute obstruction of the colon in the absence of any organic cause of obstruction in 529 thermally injured patients. After the first few post-burn days, abdominal distention can be the initial clinical sign of wound sepsis or silent perforated peptic ulcer in the critically ill or the aged. Hypokalemia, anemia, and hypoalbuminemia also cause adynamic ileus. Nausea, vomiting, and abdominal distention are diagnostic. High-pitched, hypoactive bowel sounds are heard in pseudo-obstruction of the colon. Radiographic studies of the abdomen are helpful in diagnosis, and a contrast enema is necessary to rule out distal mechanical obstruction. The ileus sometimes causes pulmonary dysfunction by abdominal dilatation, and tracheal aspiration of the gastric contents is sometimes fatal. For decompression of the stomach, a nasogastric tube should be used instead of Muller-Abott or Dennis-type long intestinal tubes, which are not indicated in paralytic ileus. Colonoscopic decompression is effective in cases of colon dilatation. Medical treatment of the underlying pathological conditions is also required. The indications for operative intervention include signs of perforation and peritonitis, failure of conservative treatment, severe respiratory embarrassment, and cecal diameter greater than 12 cm, which suggests there is pseudo-obstruction of the colon.

## SUPERIOR MESENTERIC ARTERY SYNDROME (SMAS)

Lescher et al[39] reported that 37 (1 per cent) of 3536 burn patients with average burns of 34 per cent TBSA developed SMAS. The average burn surface in the 37 cases of SMAS was 52 per cent TBSA. The mesenteric artery compresses and wedges the third duodenal portion between the SMA and the abdominal aorta, causing obstruction and massive duodenal dilatation. The loss of mesenteric and retroperitoneal fat associated with general weight loss and anatomical variation is responsible for this complication. In their series, mean weight loss was 24 per cent, ranging from 6 to 53 per cent. Bilious vomiting is the initial symptom in the majority of patients. Postcubital abdominal fullness, eructation, and early satiety are other early complaints commonly occurring after an average of 30 days of hospitalization. Prolonged bed rest in the supine position induces this complication. Acute gastroduodenal ulceration is a factor in 25 to 30 per cent of the patients with this syndrome. Roentgenographic studies using fluoroscopy of the gastrointestinal tract confirm the syndrome. Roentgenographic findings of barium contrast include dilatation of the proximal duodenum, apparent antiperistalsis of the duodenum, abrupt oblique obstruction of the distal duodenum, duodenal elongation or redundancy, and positional relief of the obstruction, which is usually seen by placing the patient in the left lateral decubitus position.

The treatment is as follows: place the patient in an appropriate position to avoid a prolonged supine position; maintain nasogastric suction; institute intravenous hyperalimentation; and administer antacids for gastroduodenal erosion and ulceration. The obstruction is usually relieved in one to two weeks, except when intestinal motility is impaired by sepsis. If surgical intervention is necessary, the most popular operation is the side-to-side duodenojejunostomy with anastomosis of the second part of the duodenum to the proximal loop of the jejunum.[37] If peptic ulcer is a factor, truncal vagotomy with either a pyloroplasty or gastroenterostomy should be performed.

## ACALCULOUS CHOLECYSTITIS

Acute acalculous cholecystitis is observed in a variety of clinical settings, including bacterial sepsis, severe trauma such as surgical trauma and burns, and multiple transfusions.[40] One report showed that out of 1560 burn admissions, seven developed acalculous cholecystitis in the period between 10 and 37 days post burn.[41] There is a report of a 10-year-old boy who suffered gallbladder perforation eight days after thermal injury.[42] The causes of this complication are thought to be dehydration, bacteremia, transient state of shock, obstruction of the superior mesenteric artery, and fat embolism. These affect microcirculation in the gallbladder and cause subsequent gallbladder ischemia. Other possible causes include stagnation of the bile and precipitation of irritative bile salts, prolonged ileus, Shwartzman's reaction, vascular manifestations of allergy, autolytic effects of trypsin associated with biliary stasis, and drugs to alleviate pain, among others. Factor XII is also thought to induce this complication. Severe injury activates Factor XII, which stimulates the release of bradykinin and may injure the vessels in the muscularis and serosal layers of the gallbladder. Burned skin is known to have a Factor XII–like substance, and albumin infused in the post-burn phase contains Factor XII fragments. Collagen in the plasma, the products of necrotic tissue, and endotoxin also activate Factor XII.

Pathologically, the common features are an intense injury of blood vessels in the muscularis and serosa, acute inflammation throughout the entire wall, fibrin patches on the serosa, degenerative changes in the muscle, and septic necrosis of the muscle. Because of the intensity of the vascular injury, acute acalculous cholecystitis with minimal clinical manifestations may rapidly progress to gangrene and perforation.

Interestingly, the lung and gallbladder are likely targets of these kinds of events induced by Factor XII. Diagnosis is made by a progressive elevation of serum bilirubin and right quadrant pain with rebound tenderness. Peritonitis, pancreatitis, and thrombophlebitis are sometimes associated findings. Since the perforation of the infectious gallbladder is usually fatal, early recognition and undelayed surgical treatment including cholecystectomy and drainage are vital.

## PANCREATITIS

The symptoms are the same as those of pancreatitis occurring in nonburn patients. Clinically, elevated serum amylase is noticed first; elastase and trypsin are also released from the inflamed pancreas. Abdominal pain, rebound tenderness, and paralytic ileus with elevated pancreatic amylase in the serum and urine are diagnostic. Pathological changes are edema, hemorrhage, necrosis, and abscess formation, depending on the severity and stage of the disease. The association of the thermal injury with this complication is based on hypoperfusion, hemolysis, Shwartzman's reaction, a part of the generalized septic process, or impaired gastrointestinal motility. In severe cases, formidable complications such as ARDS, renal failure, liver failure, DIC, gastrointestinal hemorrhage, metabolic disorders are involved.

## ANEMIA AND LEUKOPENIA

Anemia is invariably seen in severely burned patients, and if it is prominent enough to impair oxygen delivery, it may contribute to the various organ dysfunctions described in this chapter. Many factors contributre to the anemia. In the early post-burn phase, anemia is induced by the direct destruction of red blood cells (RBCs) by heat. This anemia appears even within hours after the burn, and it is accompanied by hemoglobinemia and hemoglobinuria. In spite of a decreased total RBC mass, the hematocrit is sometimes elevated because of massive plasma loss through the capillary walls. The damaged erythrocytes are removed from the circulation during the first two days after injury.[43] Younger cells are primarily affected by the heat and are lost, which contributes to the reduced average life span of RBCs.[44] Cell surface abnormality observed in transfused cells suggests that heat is not the sole cause of the shortened RBC survival.[45] The abnormality of red cell membrane metabolism, such as lysolecithin-induced lipid molecule alteration, and decreased deformability contribute to hemolysis. The damaged RBCs are eliminated in the spleen and liver. A burn of 15 to 40 per cent TBSA reduces the circulating RBC mass by 20 to 30 per cent.[46] Fluid loss from the circulation causes an intravascular increase of high molecular weight protein such as fibrinogen and its degradation products, which favor thrombus formation, and results in RBC loss. In the first two days, RBCs are also lost by surface bleeding and sequestration. Hemorrhage from the gastrointestinal tract occurs in the later period.

There is a report showing that the plasma taken from burn patients three to four weeks after burn injury inhibits RBC colony growth.[47] This serum substance is not present in the immediate post-burn period but develops gradually, with maximum intensity between post-burn days 20 and 30. Erythropoietin production is variable, and even when it increases in response to the reduced oxygen delivery to the tissues, levels are insufficient to promote erythropoiesis and correct RBC deficit.[48] This anemia is normocytic and normochromic and is accompanied by low serum iron and low iron-binding capacity. A bone marrow specimen shows a decrease in sideroblasts and an increase in stored iron. These features therefore suggest that bone marrow function is suppressed and inhibition of erythropoiesis plays a role in the pathogenesis of the anemia after thermal injury. Thus, despite anemia, reticulocytopenia rather than reticulocytosis occurs.

Anemia also occurs in the later phase, usually accompanying treatment such as graft operation, dressing change, or frequent blood sampling for diagnostic purposes. Topical medications or bacterial sepsis alone does not inhibit in vitro RBC colony growth,[47] although mafenide acetate (Sulfamylon) induces the echinocytosis. Other topical chemotherapeutics such as silver nitrate, silver sulfadiazine, and chlorhexidine are implicated in the sudden onset of often severe hemolytic anemia. Acquired autoimmune hemolytic anemia is rarely reported when plasma is used as fluid volume replacement.

Granulocytopenia often accompanies severe infection in burn patients. It is attributed to the acute deposition of granulocytes in the microcirculation at the site of thermal injury and in the lung. Granulocytopenia might be due to the regulatory defect in white blood cell production. Peterson et al[49] have suggested that the colony-stimulating factor (CSF) is reduced in the burn patients, especially when sepsis is complicated. Changes in polymorphonuclear neutrophil count after burn are similar in survivor and nonsurvivor groups of burned patients, but lymphocyte and monocyte counts are lower in the nonsurvivor group between days 5 and 18. Lymphocytes and monocytes regulate the production of CSF, a glycoprotein with an approximate molecular weight of 45,000.[50] An inappropriately low level of CSF in serum is associated with neutropenia and, consequently, with infection in burned animals.[51] Topical silver sulfadiazine cream and antibiotics or histamine $H_2$ blockers are known to cause leukopenia.

## HYPERTENSION IN CHILDREN

Arterial hypertension is commonly complicated in thermally injured children. Popp et al[52] reviewed 987 burned children and documented 195 patients (19.8 per cent) who developed hypertension in which a diastolic blood pressure above 90 mm Hg was sustained for at least 24 hours and treatment with antihypertensive agents was required. The problem occurred more frequently in males (23.3 per cent) than in females (14 per cent) and in the 7- to 10-year age group (30.2 to 32.3 per cent). The incidence increased with burn severity up to 40 per cent TBSA. Patients with burns of 40 per cent TBSA or larger had approximately a 40 per cent incidence of hypertension. A lesser incidence seen in the patients with more than 70 per cent TBSA can be attributed to the number of patients who were extremely ill and died early of burn shock. Fifteen of the 195 patients had hypertensive encephalopathy such as lethargy, irritability, headache, or somnolence and seizure. The problem could not be related to the location of burn wound, drug treatment, or differences in blood transfusion and fluid therapy, but all patients were in the acute phase of wound treatment. A matched study[52] consisting of 21 normotensive patients (mean burn index 39.5) and 21 hypertensive patients (mean burn index 40.7) showed that the mean of the highest daily blood pressure was 123/78 mm Hg in the former group and 145/100 mm Hg in the latter. The mean blood pressures during convalescence were 114/75 mm Hg in the normotensive group and 118/76 mm Hg in the hypertensive group. The hypertension subsided after complete autograft.

Akrami et al[53] described markedly elevated plasma renin activity in hypertensive burned children in the early phase of burn. Hypovolemia in the early phase reduces the renal flow; intrarenal redistribution of the renal flow from the outer cortex to the inner cortex and juxtamedullary region stimulates the renin-angiotensin-aldosterone (RAA) system. Angiotensin-induced vasoconstriction may be most important as a cause of burn-related hypertension in the initial phase. Increased catecholamine, chronic hypoxia due to anemia, stimulation of the sympathetic nervous system, and release of renin may contribute to hypertension in the later phase.

The onset of hypertension generally occurred within the first few days following thermal injury, and in the cases of sustained hypertension, the onset was within the first nine days.[54] It is also known that the hypertension is accompanied by tachycardia.[54] The cardiovascular system of the younger child may be more vulnerable to the effects of the various alterations in physiological and metabolic function generated by burn injury, whereas the more mature cardiovascular system of adolescent patients may render them more resistant to the mechanisms that generate the hypertensive response. Hypertension itself does not worsen the prognosis, but the problems of encephalopathy and seizure indicate the need for careful blood pressure monitoring and effective antihypertensive therapy in the treatment of burned children.

## ADRENAL INSUFFICIENCY

Acute adrenal insufficiency with massive hemorrhage and necrosis of the adrenal gland may occur after severe shock because of hypovolemia or sepsis. Cardiovascular collapse and cyanotic mottling of the skin, often accompanied by upper abdominal pain and tenderness, are the most frequent clinical features. Eosinocytosis, hyperkalemia, hyponatremia, and glucose metabolic derangement usually occur. Therapeutic doses of appropriate steroids should be administered.

## ELECTROLYTE IMBALANCES

SODIUM. In the early phase of severe burn, sodium and water are shifted from the extracellular into the intracellular or interstitial spaces. They are absorbed or bound to the injured or destroyed collagen macromolecules depending on the gel-sol physical state of the surrounding medium. As a result, large amounts of sodium are lost from the extracellular space or plasma. If excess hypotonic solution is used for resuscitation in this situation, hyponatremia is induced. It has been reported that the syndrome of inappropriate antidiuretic hormone contributes to post-burn hyponatremia with hypertonic urine in post-burn days 4 to 58, and volume depletion or adrenal insufficiency does not play a role in the pathogenesis.[55] It has been suggested that burn injury resets the osmoregulatory mechanism to link plasmatonicity and vasopressin secretion to a lower level of tonicity.

Topically applied 0.5 per cent silver nitrate solution is a hypotonic (29.4 mEq/L) solution that forms $AgCl_2$ on the burn wound with a subsequent decrease in plasma chloride and sodium. When silver nitrate is used on a large surface area, a careful monitoring of serum and urine electrolytes and salt supplementation is required. The estimated amount of sodium chloride lost through the burn surface is approximately 350 mEq/m$^2$/day.[56]

When a patient is on hypertonic lactate saline resuscitation, hypernatremia is encountered. In addition, hypernatremia is often associated with dehydration in patients given inadequate fluid resuscitation in the early phase. Half-normal saline is the treatment of choice in patients whose serum sodium levels exceed 150 mEq/L.

POTASSIUM. Hyperkalemia is often observed in burn patients as thermally injured cells, including erythrocytes, release intracellular potassium into circulation. Unless acute tubular necrosis supervenes, however, hyperkalemia is transient and cardiac arrhythmia because of it is no problem in uncomplicated cases. Hypokalemia may be seen when hyperventilation occurs because of respiratory distress, usually during post-burn days three to ten.

**CALCIUM.** In severely burned patients, hypocalcemia may present at 12 to 24 hours after the burn, presumably owing to saponification of fat in the thermally injured subcutaneous adipose tissue. The onset of hypocalcemia can be profound and early in children.[57]

**PHOSPHORUS.** Nordstrom et al[57] described the lowering of serum phosphate levels (0.8 to 1.5 mMol/L) in patients having burns of 20 to 85 per cent TBSA in post-burn days three to nine. The serum phosphate level is lowest at the fifth day and then returns to normal except in patients who die. The increased secretion of parathyroid hormone (PTH) mediated through the adrenergic nervous system may participate in the lowering of the serum phosphate level. As urinary loss of phosphate does not occur, phosphate depletion from burned skin is speculated. Aluminum hydroxide, antacid agents, phosphate-poor hyperalimentation, and starvation are also positive factors causing hypophosphatemia. The acute physiological consequences of hypophosphatemia have not been clarified. Dysfunction of RBCs, platelets, and brain cells and the lowered phagocytic activity of leukocytes and respiratory failure may be associated with hypophosphatemia. The cells in the hypophosphate media are deficient in ATP derived from glycolysis. The oxygen delivery of hemoglobin is diminished via the 2,3-DPG mechanism in hypophosphatemic states, and glycolysis is depressed in the erythrocytes. These indicate that hypophosphatemia has a deleterious influence on oxygenation and other important metabolic mechanisms and thus potentially contributes to increased morbidity. In the series of Nordstrom et al,[58] patients died if their serum phosphate levels did not recover.

## HYPEROSMOLAR HYPERGLYCEMIC NONKETOTIC COMA (HHNKC)

Diabetic patients are prone to suffer from HHNKC when dehydration combines with other stressful events such as extensive burn and infection. As a therapy, infusion of half-normal saline (0.45 per cent) as well as the administration of adequate insulin and adjustment of electrolyte imbalances is recommended if the patient is not hypotensive.

## VASCULAR, SKELETAL, AND MUSCLE COMPLICATIONS

Vascular complications of hand and foot occur from a circumferential third-degree burn with a decreased arterial flow because of arterial compression. Diagnosis is made from loss of pulsation, pain, and the inability to move the fingers and toes. These usually occur 12 hours after burn as tissue edema progresses. Peripheral neuropathies have been observed, usually under the area of the burn. Escharotomy or escharectomy is effective for treating peripheral impairment by relieving compression. As for skeletal complications, asymptomatic effusion into the joint underlying a major burn is quite common and causes swelling and limitation of motion. This may last for several weeks. Needle aspiration should be withheld, since that procedure introduces infection. Sometimes bone is involved in burn. The common site is the subcutaneous surface of the tibia and extensor surface of the phalanges. Splinting to maintain the position of function followed by early skin grafting will improve function.

Deep vein thrombosis can occur in burn patients. High viscosity of the blood in the early phase and hypercoagulability by activation of tissue thromboplastin or Factor XII in the stress state are the main causative factors. Prolonged bed rest and immobilization of the lower legs should be avoided.

## REFERENCES

1. Aikawa N, Shinozawa Y, Ishibiki K, et al: Clinical analysis of multiple organ failure in burned patients. Burns 13:103–109, 1987.
2. Raffa J, Trunkey DD: Myocardial depression in acute thermal injury. J Trauma 18:90–93, 1978.
3. DeSantis D, Phillips P, Spath MA, et al: Delayed appearance of a circulating myocardial depressant factor in burn patients. Ann Emerg Med 10:22–24, 1981.
4. Lefer AM, Martin J: Origin of myocardial depressant factor in shock. Am J Physiol 218:1423–1427, 1970.
5. Baxter CR, Cook WA, Shires GT: Serum myocardial depressant factor of burn shock. Surg Forum 17:1–2, 1966.
6. Rosenthal SR, Hakim AA, Hawley PL: Purified burn toxic factor and its competition. In Matter P et al. (eds): Research in Burns, Transactions of the 3rd International Congress on Research in Burns, Prague, 1970. Bern, Huber, 1971.
7. Rubanyi G, Szabo K, Balogh I, et al: Endogenous nickel release as a possible cause of coronary vasoconstriction and myocardial injury in acute burn of rats. Circ Shock 10:361–370, 1983.
8. Aikawa N, Martyn JAJ, Burke JF: Pulmonary artery catheterization and thermodilution cardiac output determination in the management of critically burned patients. Am J Surg 135:811–817, 1978.
9. Aikawa N, Ishibiki K, Naito C, et al: Individualized fluid resuscitation based on haemodynamic monitoring in the management of extensive burns. Burns 8:249–255, 1982.
10. Aikawa N, Ishibiki K, Okusawa S, et al: Use of haptoglobin to prevent renal damage due to hemolysis in extensive third-degree burns. J Burn Care Rehabil 5:20–24, 1984.
11. Czaja AJ, Rizzo TA, Smith WR, Pruitt BA: Acute liver disease after cutaneous thermal injury. J Trauma 15:887–894, 1975.
12. Aldrich RH: Role of infection in burns. N Engl J Med 208:229–309, 1933.
13. Ross RS, Iber FL, Harvey AM: The serum alkaline phosphatase in chronic infiltrative disease of the liver. Am J Med 21:850–856, 1956.
14. Zaki MS, Burke JF, Trelstad RL: Protective effects of adenosine triphosphate administration in burns. Arch Surg 113:605–610, 1978.
15. Wilmore DW, Moylan JA Jr, Bristow BF et al.: Anabolic effects of human growth hormone and high caloric feedings following thermal injury. Surg Gynecol Obstet 138:875–884, 1974.
16. Chlumsky J, Chlumska A, Vrabec R, et al: Liver changes after burn illness. Acta Chir Plast 21:120–124, 1979.
17. Law EJ, Day SB, MacMillan BG: Autopsy findings in the upper gastrointestinal tract of 81 burn patients. Arch Surg 102:412–416, 1971.
18. Linares HA: A report of 115 consecutive autopsies in burned children: 1966–80. Burns 8:263–270, 1981.
19. Bruce HM, Pruitt BA Jr: Curling's ulcer in children: A 12 year review of 63 cases. J Trauma 12:490–496, 1972.

20. Pruitt BA Jr, Foley FD, Moncrief JA: Curling's ulcer: A clinical pathology study of 323 cases. Ann Surg 172:523–539, 1970.
21. Mc Connell CM, Hummel RP: Perforating Curling's ulcer: A rare but lethal complication. Burns 7:203–207, 1980.
22. Rosenthal A, Czaja AJ, Pruitt BA: Gastrin level and gastric acidity in the pathogenesis of acute gastroduodenal disease after burns. Surg Gynceol Obstet 144:232–234, 1977.
23. Pruitt BA Jr, Goodwin CW: Stress ulcer disease in the burned patients. World J Surg 5:209–222, 1981.
24. Czaja AJ, McAlhany JC, Pruitt BA Jr: Acute gastroduodenal disease after thermal injury: An endoscopic evaluation of incidence and natural history. N Engl J Med 291:925–929, 1974.
25. Kitajima M, Wolfe RR, Trelstad RL, et al: Gastric mucosal lesions after burn injury: Relationship to H$^+$ back-diffusion and the microcirculation. J Trauma 18:644–650, 1978.
26. Czaja AJ, McAlhany JC, Pruitt BA Jr: Acute duodenitis and duodenal ulceration after burn. JAMA 232:621–624, 1975.
27. Czaja AJ, McAlhany JC Jr, Andes WA, et al: Acute gastric disease after cutaneous thermal injury. Arch Surg 110:600–606, 1975.
28. O'Neill JA Jr, Ritchey CR, Mason AD Jr, et al: Effect of thermal burns on gastric mucous production. Surg Gynecol Obstet 131:29–33, 1970.
29. McAlhany JC Jr, Czaja AJ, Cathcart RS III, et al: Histochemical study of gastric mucosubstances after thermal injury: Correlation with endoscopic evidence of acute gastroduodenal disease. J Trauma 15:609–612, 1975.
30. Wilmore DW, Long JM, Mason AD Jr, et al: Catecholamines: Mediator of the hypermetabolic response to thermal injury. Ann Surg 180:653–669, 1974.
31. Wilmore DW, Lindsey CA, Moylan JA, et al: Hyperglucagonaemia after burns. Lancet 1:73–75, 1974.
32. Liu YL, Yuan KJ: Prevention of stress ulcer bleeding with cimetidine in severe burns. Burns 9:327–329, 1983.
33. Moscona R, Kaufman T, Jacobs R, et al: Prevention of gastrointestinal bleeding in burns: The effects of cimetidine or antacids combined with early enteral feeding. Burns 12:65–67, 1985.
34. Martyn JA, Greenblatt DJ, Abernethy DR: Increased cimetidine clearance in burn patients. JAMA 253:1288–1291, 1985.
35. Choctaw WT, Fujita C, Zawacki BE: Prevention of upper gastrointestinal bleeding in burn patients. A role for "elemental" diet. Arch Surg 115:1073–1076, 1980.
36. Curreri PW: Invited commentary for stress ulcer disease in the burned patient. World J Surg 5:221–222, 1981.
37. Munster AM: Burn Care for the House Officer. Baltimore, Williams & Wilkins, 1980.
38. Lescher TJ, Teegarden DK, Pruitt BA Jr: Acute pseudo-obstruction of the colon in thermally injured patients. Dis Colon Rectum 21:618–622, 1978.
39. Lescher TJ, Sirinek KR, Pruitt BA Jr: Superior mesenteric artery syndrome in thermally injured patients. J Trauma 19:567–571, 1979.
40. Glenn F, Becker CG: Acute acalculous cholecystitis. Ann Surg 195:131–136, 1982.
41. Alawneh I: Acute non-calculous cholecystitis in burns. Br J Surg 65:243–245, 1978.
42. TeWater WF: Spontaneous gallbladder perforation. S Afr Med J 56:423, 1979.
43. Baar S: Anemia of burns. Burns 6:1–8, 1979.
44. Loebl EC, Marvin JA, Curreri PW, et al: Erythrocyte survival following thermal injury. J Surg Res 16:96–101, 1974.
45. Baar S, Arrowsmith DJ: Thermal damage to red cells. J Clin Pathol 23:572–576, 1970.
46. Topley E, Jackson DMG, Cason JS, et al: Assessment of red cell loss in the first two days after severe burns. Ann Surg 155:581–590, 1962.
47. Wallner SF, Vautrin RM, Buerk C, et al: The anemia of thermal injury: Studies of erythropoiesis in vitro. J Trauma 22:774–780, 1982.
48. Andes WA, Rogers PW, Beason JW, et al: The erythropoietin response to the anemia of thermal injury. J Lab Clin Med 88:584–592, 1976.
49. Peterson VP, Hansbrough J, Buerk C, et al: Regulation of granulopoiesis following severe thermal injury. J Trauma 23:19–24, 1983.
50. Golde DW, Cline MJ: Identification of the colony stimulating cells in human blood. J Clin Invest 51:2981–2983, 1972.
51. McEuen DD, Ogawa M, Eurenius K: Myelopoiesis in the infected burn. J Lab Med 89:540–543, 1977.

52. Popp MB, Friedberg DL, MacMillan BG: Clinical characteristics of hypertension in burned children. Ann Surg 191:473–478, 1980.
53. Akrami C, Falkner B, Gould AE, et al: Plasma renin and occurrence of hypertension in children with burn injuries. J Trauma 20:130–134, 1980.
54. Falkner B, Roven S, DeClement FA, et al: Hypertension in children with burns. J Trauma 18:213–217, 1978.
55. Shirani KZ, Vaughan GM, Robertson GL, et al: Inappropriate vasopressin secretion (SIADH) in burned patients. J Trauma 23:217–224, 1983.
56. Bondoc CC, Morris PJ, Wee T, et al: Metabolic effects of 0.5% silver nitrate therapy for extensive burns in children. Surg Forum 17:475–477, 1966.
57. Szyfelbein SK, Drop LJ, Martyn JAJ: Persistent ionized hypocalcemia in patients during resuscitation and recovery phase of body burns. Crit Care Med 9:454–458, 1981.
58. Nordstrom H, Lennquist S, Lindell B, et al: Hypophosphataemia in severe burns. Acta Chir Scand 143:395–399, 1977.

# 12

# Clinical Pharmacology and Therapeutics in Burns

## J. A. JEEVENDRA MARTYN

Irrespective of the type—electrical, chemical, scald, or flame—burns involving significant body surface area induce a cascade of systemic and physiological responses.[1, 2] A burn injury that exceeds 10 to 15 per cent of the total body surface area (TBSA) causes pathophysiological alterations in the cardiovascular, pulmonary, renal, and hepatic systems as well as fluctuations in plasma protein concentrations. These changes may be the result either of direct damage to the skin itself or of the body's pathophysiological response to injury. Significant changes in the pharmacokinetics and pharmacodynamics of many drugs are induced by metabolic derangements, neurohumoral responses, massive fluid shifts, sepsis, and systemic effects of massive tissue destruction. This chapter gives an overview of the altered pathophysiology and its influence on pharmacology.

## PATHOPHYSIOLOGICAL CHANGES AFFECTING DRUG PHARMACOLOGY

### Cardiovascular Effects

The clinical course of the burned patient is marked by two distinct metabolic phases. In the immediate post-burn period (up to 24 to 36 hours after injury), blood flow to organs and tissues decreases,[2, 3] often owing to the rapid reduction in circulating blood volume or to the severe compressive effects of circumferential burns.[4] Despite adequate cardiac filling pressures, some patients continue to have reduced cardiac output, which suggests other contributing factors, such as the direct myocardial depressant effect of burn injury; the presence of myocardial depressant factor has been shown in both laboratory animals and humans, particularly in subjects with extensive third-degree burns.[2, 5] The release of vasoconstricting substances that increase peripheral resistance and the increase in blood viscosity also contribute to this decreased blood flow.[2, 6, 7]

Decreased blood flow to organs and tissue can cause altered drug kinetics, especially for high-extraction drugs, the clearance rates for which are almost exclusively dependent on blood flow through the organ.[8] Moreover, hypovolemia may result in higher-than-normal plasma concentrations for a given dose because of the decrease in central volume of distribution. Patients can be extremely sensitive to the effects of any drug during this stage.[9] This sensitivity can be confounded by the increased loss of a drug through a burn wound,[10, 11] which can effectively decrease the plasma concentration and consequently the effect of a drug.[10] During the hypovolemic (resuscitation) phase, as indicated previously, blood flow to organs and tissues (e.g., stomach, muscle) is decreased, which results in decreased absorption, decreased bioavailability, and nonlinearity of drug absorption from these sites. If higher doses are administered to overcome poor absorption through the peripheral tissues, later restoration of perfusion may lead to unexpectedly rapid uptake of medication from these sites, with toxic effects. Thus, small, repetitive doses of intravenous drugs generally are more effective during this initial phase than the administration of drugs via gastrointestinal, intramuscular, or subcutaneous routes.

Following the resuscitation period, the second phase of burn injury begins (after 24 to 36 hours post burn): the hypermetabolic or recovery phase. Blood flow to the organs and tissues increases,[2, 12, 13] although in the geriatric patient this response is usually either delayed or absent. Cardiac output rises to one and one-half to three times normal; the elevated basal metabolic rate invariably present following thermal injury only partially accounts for this increase in cardiac output.[14] Even during general anesthesia cardiac output continues to be higher than normal in burned patients,[15] although there is some lessening of flow. The increased cardiac output is associated with increased splanchnic and skin blood flow,[13, 16] which can have an effect on both total and individual organ clearance of drugs. Drugs administered via the intramuscular route may be rapidly absorbed because of the enhanced blood flow. The efficiency and rate of drug absorption via the gastrointestinal tract have not been determined, but clinical impression suggests that absorption is not impaired during the hypermetabolic phase.

## Protein-Binding Changes

Plasma protein concentrations are altered in both the resuscitative and recovery phases of burn injury.[17] Although total plasma protein concentrations decrease, the concentrations of individual proteins may decrease or increase, depending on the protein, the amount of time post burn, and the magnitude of the burn. Alterations are attributable to various factors, including the loss of proteins, altered protein synthesis rates, and catabolism by the liver.[1]

Two pharmacologically important drug-binding proteins have been identified: albumin and alpha$_1$-acid glycoprotein, a component of alpha$_1$-globulin.[18] Bloedow et al, studying burned patients with mean TBSA burns of 20 per cent or more, divided subjects into two groups: those in the acute stage, the period up to eight days post burn, and those in the convalescent stage, about one month post burn.[19] In the first group, total protein concentrations were about 30 per cent lower than normal and returned to control levels during the convalescent phase of burn injury. Albumin levels, however, remained at approximately 50 per cent of control throughout the observation period. Levels of alpha$_1$-globulin in both groups were increased two- to threefold over controls, as were the concentrations of alpha$_1$-acid glycoprotein.

The effects of these concentration variances, particularly those of albumin and alpha$_1$-acid glycoprotein, on the plasma binding properties of drugs have also been studied. Drugs that bind predominantly to albumin, including diazepam, phenytoin, and salicylic acid, showed an increase in the free fraction in plasma.[18–20] In contrast, the free fractions of imipramine, lidocaine, meperidine, and propranolol were decreased in plasma, primarily owing to increased binding to alpha$_1$-acid glycoprotein.[18–20] Changes in drug binding due to burn-induced alterations in plasma protein concentrations can also affect kinetics and may result in alterations in the distribution and clearance volumes.[20, 21] Increased binding generally leads to a decreased volume of distribution, whereas decreased binding has the opposite effect. Changes in protein binding affect only the clearance of low-extraction drugs; in the kidney, for example, increased binding results in decreased elimination of glomerulus-filtered drugs, since only the free fraction is filtered. Decreased binding, therefore, may lead to enhanced elimination by glomerular filtration.

Similar directional changes can occur in the liver with respect to low-extraction drugs,[22] and the decrease in binding (increased free fraction) seen following burn injury may partly account for the rapid clearance of phenytoin and lorazepam in burned patients.[20, 23] Recent documentation suggests that lidocaine and meperidine, drugs that are dependent on blood flow for clearance, may have an impaired clearance, either because of drug interaction (e.g., cimetidine) or because of the burn itself,[24, 25] despite the known increases in hepatic blood flow following burns.[13, 14] The mechanisms for this impaired clearance are unclear, although the increased protein binding of drugs may play a role. Finally, changes in the plasma binding of drugs complicate the interpretation of concentrations of drugs reported by laboratories. Since plasma levels reported by various laboratories include both free and bound (total) concentrations when changes in binding are present, it is difficult to know whether the reported concentrations are therapeutic, subtherapeutic, or toxic.

## Hepatic Changes

The liver may be damaged by hypoperfusion during the early post-burn phase as a result of hypovolemia, hypotension, hypoxemia, or inhaled or absorbed chemicals. Later hepatic dysfunction may result from drug toxicity, sepsis, or blood transfusions. Hepatic blood flow is increased and protein synthesis and breakdown are enhanced, as is hepatic gluconeogenesis.[1] Conversely, hepatic enzyme levels such as SGOT and SGPT are elevated, suggesting hepatotoxicity.[26] Thus, depending on the test performed, the function of the liver may indicate impaired or enhanced function. As a result of the paucity of pharmacological studies in burned patients, whether or not the drug-metabolizing capacity of the body is altered following burn injury is unclear. Based on pharmacological studies in other disease states, phase I reactions are expected to be impaired and phase II reactions unaltered following burn injury.[8, 27] Phase I reactions include oxidation, reduction, hydroxylation, and demethylation reactions, while phase II reactions are conjugation reactions and include acetyl, sulfate, glucuronide, and methyl conjugations.

## Renal Effects

Renal function may be adversely affected soon after injury owing to myoglobinuria and hemoglobinuria; the former is most common in electrical injury, while the latter is seen following severe cutaneous burns. Hypovolemia and hypotension may further aggravate renal dysfunction and result in acute tubular necrosis. In adequately resuscitated patients the glomerular filtration rate increases three to seven days post burn, along with similar directional changes in cardiac output and metabolic rate.[28, 29] Renal blood flow in burned patients is approximately 80 per cent higher than normal as a result of cellular hypertrophy and hyperplasia, and the kidney appears approximately 60 per cent heavier.[30] The increased glomerular filtration rate may be due to elevated prostaglandin and glucagon release.[31] Patients with burns of more than 40 per cent TBSA demonstrate renal tubular dysfunction, evidenced primarily by an inability to concentrate the urine.[6, 32] During hyperosmolar states antidiuresis is not seen, which suggests an inadequate renal response to antidiuretic hormone and aldosterone. Thus it is possible to observe good urine output in the presence of hypovolemia. From these observations it is evident that drugs filtered by the glomerulus may exhibit enhanced elimination, whereas tubularly secreted drugs may or may not have altered kinetics.

## Pulmonary Effects

Pulmonary function may be adversely affected by burn injury because of direct inhalation injury or the secondary effects of cutaneous burns. The lung plays an increasingly significant role in the uptake, distribution, and elimination of endogenous and exogenous substances.[33, 34] However, it has yet to be determined how burns and concomitant pulmonary changes alter drug kinetics and dynamics. Drug disposition and response may be further complicated by the presence of sepsis, drugs that induce[35] or inhibit[36] drug metabolism, hepatotoxic or nephrotoxic drugs, malnutrition, parenteral nutrition, pre-existing systemic disease, and endogenously released burn-induced substances.

## PHARMACOLOGICAL STUDIES IN BURNED PATIENTS

## Antibiotics

Antibiotics are key therapeutic agents because of the common complication of sepsis after burn trauma. The antibiotic (tobramycin, gentamycin, amikacin) dosage requirement in burned patients is usually higher than normal,[29, 37] as normal doses do not result in adequate therapeutic concentrations because of the increased clearance. The two major reasons for this clearance are (1) enhanced drug elimination by the kidney due to the burn-induced increase in the glomerular filtration rate[28–30] and (2) the escape of drugs through the burn wound.[11] For drugs with minimal protein-binding capacity, creatinine clearance may provide an accurate estimate of the capacity of the burned patient to excrete antibiotic drugs via glomerular filtration. The elimination half-life or clearance of drugs such as tobramycin, vancomycin, and gentamycin directly correlates with changes in creatinine clearance.[29, 38]

Drug loss through the burn wound may be more significant in the infant and child than in the adolescent or adult because of the relatively high ratio of body surface area to body weight. However, antibiotic therapy must be monitored carefully and modified in the presence of renal failure, since the predominant route of elimination is renal excretion. Since little binding of most antibiotic agents to plasma proteins occurs (less than 10 per cent),[39] measured plasma concentrations reflect true (free) concentrations.

Just as systemically administered antibiotics can leach out through a burn wound, topical antibiotic agents applied to a burn wound can be absorbed into the blood stream and cause toxic reactions.[2, 31] This subject is discussed in Chapter 19 on Infection and Antibiotics.

## H₂-Receptor Antagonists

Acute stress ulceration of the stomach and duodenum is the most common life-threatening gastrointestinal complication of burn injury. Czaja et al[40] found gastric erosions in 86 per cent of adults who suffered burns covering more than 40 per cent of TBSA within 72 hours of injury; 28 per cent of these patients progressed to gastric or duodenal ulceration. The incidence of life-threatening hemorrhage was 5 per cent. In Curling's report[41] on acute stress ulceration, all 12 patients were children; this high incidence has been confirmed in a report by Sevitt,[42] who found a twofold increase in the incidence of acute ulceration in burned pediatric patients compared to adult patients (14 per cent versus 7.3 per cent). The exact cause of this ulceration is unknown, but its relationship to increased acidity, with and without bacteremia and sepsis, has been emphasized.

The control of increased gastric acidity and bleeding in critically ill patients includes early enteral feeding and the administration of oral antacids and/or H₂-receptor antagonists[43, 44]; however, these regimens cannot be instituted in all patients with major burns, either because of burn- or sepsis-induced gastrointestinal ileus or because of the need for perioperative fasting. Feeding or oral antacid administration during this time can result in pulmonary aspiration of gastric contents. In these instances H₂-receptor antagonists such as cimetidine and ranitidine, which can be administered parenterally, are useful chemoprophylactic agents.

The efficacy of cimetidine in patients has been evaluated in several studies in burned patients.[28, 45-48] In adults given cimetidine within the first 18 hours post burn, the number of oral antacid (Mylanta) doses required to maintain gastric pH at 6.0 or above was significantly reduced. Between 18 and 42 hours post burn, however, cimetidine was less effective.[46] Subsequent pharmacokinetic studies[10, 28] explained this phenomenon. During the early resuscitation phase of burn injury (up to 18 hours post burn), although urinary excretion was decreased, the total cimetidine clearance was comparable to that of normal patients because of the increase in nonrenal clearance.[10] In the later phase, however, the clearance of cimetidine by both renal and nonrenal routes was increased, resulting in rapid elimination of the drug.[28] The larger the burn, the faster cimetidine was eliminated. From these studies we can conclude that the usual adult dose of 5 to 6 mg/kg every six hours should suffice for the first 24 hours after burn. However, to compensate for the enhanced clearance in the period that follows, both the dosage and the frequency of administration may need to be increased. In adults doses should be at least 400 mg every four hours.[47]

The control of gastric pH and stress ulceration is more complicated in children. As indicated previously, the incidence of acute stress ulceration in children is approximately twice that in adults. Normal children tolerate and indeed require a greater daily dosage of many drugs, including cimetidine, to achieve the same serum concentration or effect.[49] In the presence of burn this increased dosage requirement is further enhanced; administration of 10 to 15 mg/kg of cimetidine was not sufficient to maintain gastric pH for longer than four to five hours.[48] In both children and adults it was noted that creatinine clearance, a reflector of the glomerular filtration rate, was increased following burns (Table 12–1), and the enhanced elimination kinetics of cimetidine was directly related to the increased glomerular filtration rate (Fig. 12–1). Previous studies in adult burn and normal patients have documented that plasma cimetidine concentrations of 0.5 μg/ml or greater effectively control gastric pH at 4.0 or above. In burned children, however, these levels proved ineffective; plasma cimetidine concentrations of 1.0 μg/ml or greater were required, suggesting that burn injury to a

**TABLE 12–1. Cimetidine Kinetics\***

|  | Pediatric Burns (n = 21) | Adult Burns (n = 8) | Controls (n = 9) |
|---|---|---|---|
| Weight (kg) | 25.6 ± 4.1 | 69.3 ± 4.9 | 72.4 ± 2.0 |
| Creatinine clearance (ml/min/70 kg) | 139.7 ± 26.2 | 171.5 ± 19.0 | ~125 |
| Distribution volume (L/kg) | 1.38 ± 0.09 | 1.59 ± 0.17 | 1.53 ± 0.12 |
| Cimetidine clearance (ml/min/kg) | 16.22 ± 1.46 | 14.04 ± 1.85‡ | 8.21 ± 0.64 |
| Half-life (hours) | 1.06 ± 0.07† | 1.52 ± 0.14‡ | 2.21 ± 0.17 |
| Urinary excretion (% dose)§ | 40.7 ± 3.8 | 63.4 ± 9.2 | 44.8 ± 8.2 |
| Cimetidine therapeutic level (μg/ml) | ≥1.0 | ≥0.5 | ≥0.5 |

\*Mean ± SE.
†Pediatric burns vs. adult burns ($p < 0.025$).
‡Adult burns vs. adult controls ($p < 0.01$).
§Urinary excretion at 8 hours for burn groups and at 24 hours for controls.
Data from Martyn et al[28, 48]

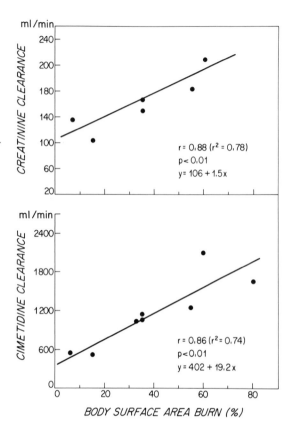

**FIGURE 12–1.** Relation of clearance of creatinine (*above*), a reflector of glomerular filtration rate, and of cimetidine (*below*) to extent of burn injury. As burn size increases, glomerular filtration increases. The clearance of cimetidine parallels the increase in glomerular filtration. (From Martyn JAJ, Abernethy DR, Greenblatt DJ: Increased cimetidine clearance in burn patients. JAMA 258:1288–1291, 1985. Copyright 1985, American Medical Association.)

child is associated with alterations in the pharmacokinetic profile as well as the pharmacodynamic responses to cimetidine. Although a previous study[50] in critically ill intensive-care patients documented the effective control of gastric pH during continuous infusions of cimetidine, preliminary studies in burned children indicate that a bolus dose of 5 mg/kg of cimetidine, followed by a continuous infusion at a rate of 2 mg/kg/hour, are ineffective.

Studies in adult burn patients indicate that 50 mg of ranitidine effectively controls the gastric pH in most patients.[51] The additional advantage of ranitidine is its lack of side effects or interaction with drug-metabolizing enzymes. The effectiveness of sucralfate for control of gastric ulceration has not been studied in burned patients.

## Sedatives and Narcotics

**Benzodiazepines.** Benzodiazepines such as chlordiazepoxide (Librium), diazepam (Valium), and lorazepam (Ativan) are commonly used sedatives, all of which bind highly (greater than 90 per cent) to plasma proteins; they are eliminated by hepatic metabolism and have low metabolic clearances.[27] When a single dose of diazepam or chlordiazepoxide is administered, its therapeutic efficacy is short-lived owing to its rapid uptake by peripheral tissues. Diazepam and chlordiazepoxide are metabolized by phase I– or cytochrome p450–dependent pathway.[27] Thus, although the elimination half-life of these drugs is prolonged in normal and burned patients,[52] the duration of action of a single dose is usually quite short[27, 31] (Table 12–2). Repeated administration of these drugs, however, can saturate the tissue uptake sites, and the termination of effect then depends not on redistribution but on biotransformation by hepatic enzymes, which can be quite depressed in burned patients.[52] Thus, following repeated administration of drugs such as diazepam and chlordiazepoxide, recovery from sedative effects will be prolonged. The metabolites of these drugs are also pharmacologically active and can prolong and potentiate the sedative effects of the parent compound. Thus, if diazepam and chlordiazepoxide are used to sedate patients who are on respirators, weaning these patients from respirators might become a problem because of the drugs' long durations of action.

Lorazepam possesses some features that distinguish it from diazepam and chlordiazepoxide. First, lorazepam is metabolized by conjugation (phase II– or cytochrome p450–independent pathway) to a pharmacologically inactive glucuronide metabolite.[27] Second, the drug's clearance occurs at a faster rate in burned patients than in controls (Fig. 12–2) and is unaffected by concomitantly administered drugs such as cimetidine.[23, 53] Thus, even after repeated administration of the drug, the rate of metabolic clearance of lorazepam from the body is faster than that of either diazepam or chlordiazepoxide (Table 12–2). For these reasons lorazepam may be the preferred drug when repeated administrations are necessary. It should be remembered that post-burn delirium may be associated with the use of benzodiazepines, particularly in the presence of pain or other metabolic abnormalities.[54]

**PSYCHOPHARMACOLOGICAL AGENTS.** Critically ill burn patients are at risk for the development of a variety of neuropsychiatric complications. In such instances a common drug of choice has been parenteral or oral haloperidol. Although the pharmacology of haloperidol has not been studied in sufficient detail in burn

**TABLE 12–2. Comparative Pharmacokinetics of Diazepam and Lorazepam***

|  | Half-life (hr) | Distribution Volume (L/kg) | Clearance (ml/kg/min) |
|---|---|---|---|
| **Diazepam** |  |  |  |
| Controls | 36 ± 5 | 131 ± 18 | 46 ± 7 |
| Burns | 72 ± 26 | 94 ± 17 | 24 ± 6† |
| **Lorazepam** |  |  |  |
| Controls | 13.92 ± 0.8 | 1.39 ± 0.1 | 1.16 ± 0.10 |
| Burns | 9.59 ± 1.26† | 2.66 ± 0.55† | 4.28 ± 1.2† |

*Mean ± SE.
†p < 0.05, significantly different from controls.
Data from Martyn et al[23, 52].

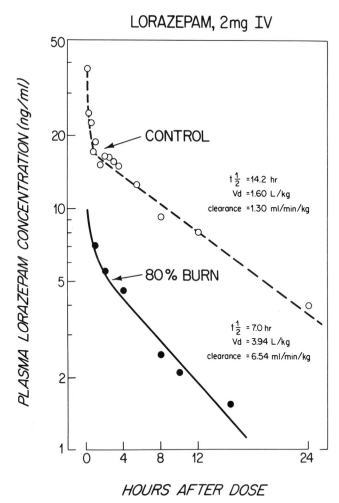

**FIGURE 12–2.** Plasma concentration of lorazepam (2 mg IV) in a 25-year-old healthy subject and an 18-year-old male burn patient with 80 per cent TBSA who was studied 25 days post burn. Despite administration of equal doses, the burned patient had a faster clearance rate. (From Martyn JAJ, Greenblatt DJ: Lorazepam conjugation unimpaired in burn trauma. Clin Pharmacol Ther 43:250–255, 1988.)

patients, severe haloperidol-induced dystonias and akathisias led one group to discourage its use in burn patients.[55] The extrapyramidal symptoms are believed to be caused by an imbalance between the central nervous system's cholinergic and dopaminergic receptors. Acute dystonic reactions are characterized by disturbances in muscle tone and abnormal posturing, with involuntary movements that are spasmodic and uncoordinated. Although more often seen with haloperidol, such reactions have also been observed following administration of the long-acting drug fluphenazine.

With these drugs the incidence of extrapyramidal symptoms seems higher in burn patients than in controls,[55] possibly as a result of the increased sensitivity of the neuromuscular junction to the effects of acetylcholine (see following discussion on neuromuscular relaxants). This could occur because of increased concentrations of nicotinic acetylcholine receptors, which become supersensitive to the acetylcholine present at the muscle membrane. The extrapyramidal symptoms observed with haloperidol are not specific to the drug itself but can also be observed with other antipsychotic drugs such as phenothiazine and its derivatives. It should be stressed that the plasma binding of tricyclic antidepressants is increased,[18] and, at least initially, doses have to be increased to achieve therapeutic free concentrations. On the other hand, once these drugs are administered, their clearance may be impaired because of altered hepatic activity and increased binding.[18, 22]

**NARCOTICS.** The pharmacology of narcotics is discussed in a separate chapter (Chapter 13). However, it should be pointed out briefly here that concern about possible addiction or the inability of burn patients to eliminate administered drugs has led to undermedication.[56] The studies of morphine and sufentanil pharmacokinetics[57, 58] in burn patients show clearances similar to those of normals or somewhat enhanced. On the other hand, the clearance of meperidine may be impaired.[24] Thus, no pharmacokinetic reason is apparent for withholding at least morphine and sufentanil from burned patients. In fact, clinical impressions suggest that the narcotic requirements of burn patients increase in proportion to the magnitude of burn injury.

Recently efforts have been made to understand the physiological significance of the hypermetabolic (stress) response trauma, and techniques to modify this response have been suggested. The afferent responses that increase metabolism can be accentuated by the brain, particularly in the presence of pain and anxiety.[1, 59] In this context, high-dose morphine and beta-blockers have been shown to decrease the hypermetabolic response to trauma.[59, 60] In a preliminary study[59] Demling reported that patients with persistently high levels of endorphins and possibly catecholamines developed sepsis; the question has been raised whether these substances will decrease oxygen delivery, alter the immune response, and open the way for sepsis.[59] Demling further demonstrated that sedatives and opiate administration decrease endogenous opioid levels, and patients receiving this treatment did quite well. Although more studies are indicated, it appears that the administration of exogenous opioids and sedatives is not harmful to burned patients.

## Anesthetic Agents

**INTRAVENOUS DRUGS.** The uptake, elimination, and distribution of anesthetic drugs have not been adequately characterized in burn patients. The most extensively used intravenous anesthetic is ketamine[61]; its advantages include cardiovascular-stimulating properties, intensive postoperative analgesia, and the ability to be administered intramuscularly. Low-dose ketamine (1.5 to 2 mg/kg intramuscularly) produces adequate amnesia and analgesia, with rapid re-estab- lishment of activity, such as eating. Intramuscularly administered ketamine (4 to 5 mg/kg) can produce good operative conditions for tangential excision.[62] When used as the sole anesthetic agent in acutely burned patients, the prolonged awakening period associated with ketamine gives the nursing staff extra time to position and provide care for the freshly grafted wound areas. Although ketamine most often produces tachycardia and hypertension, hypotension has also been known to occur, probably owing to the inability of the already stimulated sympathetic nervous system to counterbalance the direct myocardial depressant and vasodilating effects of the drug.[61] Patients develop a tolerance to ketamine with repeated use, so doses should be titrated according to the needs of the patient. Whether similar tolerance to barbiturates develops in the acute phase of thermal injury is unknown, although the repeated administration of thiobar- biturates to recovered burn patients is known to induce tolerance.[63]

**INHALATION AGENTS.** Inhalation agents continue to be the anesthetic of choice for patients in many burn units. Thus far there are no reports of any incidence of halothane-related hepatitis in burned patients[64]; our unpublished observations at the Shriners Burns Institute over the last 20 years have confirmed this impression. With the multiple complicating and compounding factors affecting the burned patient, it will always be difficult to pinpoint halothane or any other agent as the cause of hepatitis.

The effects of enflurane on oxygen supply-demand balance have been studied in the hypermetabolic-hyperdynamic state of burned patients undergoing excision and skin grafting procedures.[65] The patients studied were without any apparent cardiac, pulmonary, hepatic, or kidney dysfunction, and they were not septic. Following the induction of anesthesia and enflurane administration, cardiac output decreased, but an adequate oxygen supply-demand balance was main- tained, with no evidence of metabolic acidosis.[65] The effects of anesthesia and positive-pressure ventilation on early (1 to 12 hours) post-burn cardiopulmonary changes were assessed during halothane anesthesia.[66] Similar to enflurane, halothane and positive-pressure ventilation decreased cardiac output and oxygen demand roughly equally; thus, no metabolic acidosis was seen. These changes reverted to baseline levels with discontinuation of the anesthetics. It was noted that infusion of low molecular weight dextran prevented the increase in systemic vascular resistance and the decrease in cardiac output.[66]

Morphine, administered in an average dose of 0.38 mg/kg/hour for a mean of 3.4 hours, has also been shown to decrease oxygen consumption in burned patients.[67] At this dose, morphine exerts important depressant influence on the central nervous system and behaves very much like an inhalation anesthetic drug. Since the central nervous system plays a major role in the reflex arc that initiates and maintains the post-traumatic metabolic response,[67] it is conceivable that enflurane, halothane, and morphine decrease the hypermetabolism of burn patients because of their depressant effects on the central nervous system. The hypothermia observed during general anesthesia in burn patients may be partly related to these central nervous system effects.

Anesthetics also have an effect on the specific and nonspecific immune systems.[68] Profound depression of the bone marrow, leading to depression of white blood cells, was observed following the exposure of intensive care, nonburned patients to nitrous oxide, in some patients after an exposure of only two hours.[69] Similar exposure to clinical concentrations of halothane and the administration of barbiturates or morphine reduced phagocytic activity by about 40 to 50 per cent. Sedatives such as chlorpromazine and diazepam cause even more depression of phagocytic activity, whereas anesthetic agents in general have no depressant effect involving cellular immunity.[68] Lymphocyte reactivity to antigens is depressed after halothane or enflurane anesthesia only in combination with major surgery.[70] After neuroleptanesthesia and major surgery, depression of lymphocyte reactivity is the same as that seen after administration of inhalation agents.[70] All evidence points, therefore, to the stress of surgery rather than to the direct effect of inhalation agents as the most important factor in reducing immunocompetence.

## Adrenergic Agonists and Related Compounds

In some instances volume replacement alone is inadequate, and the use of adrenergic agents has been advocated both during resuscitation and when complications such as sepsis occur. Aikawa et al, using the left ventricular stroke work index as an indicator of myocardial function, provided preliminary evidence that this parameter could be improved with the use of low-dose dopamine in a small number of patients.[3] Subsequent studies in burn patients during the acute phase of burn injury have not confirmed these observations. For instance, Cone et al[71] studied the effects of 5 to 10 μg/kg/min of dopamine to improve cardiac output during the first 24 hours after burn injury and found no changes in hemodynamic parameters.

The usefulness of dopamine therapy has also been evaluated in the latter phase of burn injury. When the thermodilution technique was used to measure right ventricular end-diastolic volume, right ventricular ejection fraction, and cardiac output, no change in any of these parameters was observed during dopamine therapy of 3 to 9 mg/kg/min.[72] However, in the same study the authors noted significant elevation of mean pulmonary arterial pressures, particularly in patients in whom pulmonary artery pressures were elevated above 25 mm Hg prior to infusion (Fig. 12–3). Doses of dopamine as high as 24 μg/kg/min (alpha-adrenergic effects) to improve systemic hemodynamics in sepsis have also been studied and found to be ineffective.[73] Thus, clinical studies of dopamine use reported to date do not substantiate any useful alpha- or beta-adrenergic effects in burned patients. In some instances, because it produces pulmonary hypertension, dopamine may have deleterious effects on right ventricular function and

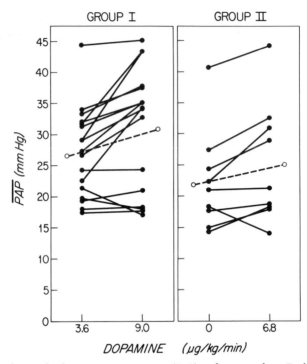

**FIGURE 12–3.** Relation of pulmonary artery pressure (PAP) to dopamine dose. Dashed line indicates mean change in PAP. Baseline PAP greater than 23 mm Hg was associated with increase in PAP during infusion of dopamine. (From Martyn JAJ, Farago LS, Burke JF: Hemodynamics of low-dose dopamine in nonseptic burned patients. Chest 89:357–360, 1986.)

pulmonary circulation. Whether dopamine has any beneficial renal effects via dopaminergic nerves is unknown.

Dopamine's inability to improve the hemodynamics in other nonburned critically ill patients has also been confirmed.[74, 75] In instances in which dopamine has been found to be ineffective, dobutamine has been shown to be effective.[74, 75] The molecular mechanisms by which these differences in pharmacological effects between dopamine and dobutamine are brought about are unknown. The chronic elevations of catecholamine observed following burns[60] may have caused a down-regulation and alterations in affinity of beta-receptors[76] and in turn the ineffectiveness of dopamine. The increased efficacy of dobutamine compared to dopamine may be related to the ability of dobutamine to increase cAMP in cardiac muscle by mechanisms other than through the beta-receptor.[77]

Confirming the down-regulation of beta-receptors is the observation that the application of topical epinephrine and neosynephrine to a burn wound to decrease bleeding and the subsequent absorption of the drugs into the systemic circulation have no ill effects on heart rate, heart rhythm, or blood pressure.[78–80] In one study plasma epinephrine concentrations were measured following the topical application of epinephrine.[81] Concentrations of catecholamines up to 10-fold higher than in normal plasma were observed in these patients. Some changes in heart rate were observed but no changes in blood pressure.[81] Although halothane anesthesia was used in some of the patients, the authors reported no associated arrhythmia. The levels noted in this study were higher than those observed in any other stress states[82] and would cause significant cardiovascular changes in normal patients.[83]

Numerous laboratory studies have documented the usefulness of cardiotonic and vasoactive substances such as verapamil, nitroprusside, and digoxin to improve cardiovascular function.[84–86] Clinical studies, however, have not confirmed the usefulness of these drugs. It should be pointed out that the binding of these drugs may be increased by the burn-induced inflammatory response and the release of alpha$_1$-acid glycoprotein, and higher than normal doses may be required to achieve a given effect.

## Neuromuscular Relaxants

Neuromuscular relaxants in clinical use can be classified into two categories: depolarizing relaxants, typified by succinylcholine, and nondepolarizing relaxants, typified by d-tubocurarine, metocurine, pancuronium, atracurium, and vecuronium. Depolarizing relaxants cause the depolarization of muscle before producing paralysis, whereas nondepolarizing relaxants competitively bind to acetylcholine receptor sites and prevent the interaction of the transmitter acetylcholine with the receptor sites at the neuromuscular junction. Muscle relaxants are frequently used in the operating room to produce paralysis for intubation and as an adjunct to anesthesia; for example, a relaxant would be used to prevent reflex movements during surgery under high-dose narcotic anesthesia. Muscle relaxants are also frequently used in nonsurgical situations, such as in the emergency room or in intensive care units, where muscle paralysis is used to facilitate rapid control of the airway for intubation. Finally, muscle relaxants are important and useful drugs in the intensive care setting to maintain effective mechanical ventilation in patients with respiratory distress syndrome, particularly in patients requiring high levels of positive end-expiratory pressure. Several studies have shown improved gas exchange and faster recovery with the use of muscle relaxants.[87, 88]

The main advantage of succinylcholine in normal patients is its rapid onset of action. In the case of burn trauma (and in some other pathological states), the potential exists for hyperkalemia, which, if severe enough, can lead to cardiac arrest.[89, 90] Although no cases of cardiac arrest can be attributed to succinylcholine within the first 24 hours after burn injury, abnormal elevations of plasma potassium levels have been known to occur within a few days post burn. With extensive muscle injury, such as that which occurs following electrical injury, hyperkalemic response to succinylcholine can occur. Generally, the more extensive the burn, the more likely the hyperkalemic response. Potassium levels greater than 6 mEq/L following succinylcholine administration, however, have been noted with third-degree burns covering less than 10 per cent TBSA.[91] The rise in potassium concentration may also be dose-related, but doses as small as 0.4 mg/kg can give rise to dangerous hyperkalemia (normal dose is 1 mg/kg).[90] Brown et al, however, have administered 0.1 mg/kg to burned patients with adequate paralysis in some patients and without a hyperkalemic response.[92] Despite this new information, succinylcholine should be avoided in burn patients because of the unpredictability of the response.

The rise in potassium level in susceptible patients occurs within the first minute, peaks at 2 to 5 minutes, and then declines over the next 10 to 15 minutes. Cardiac arrest usually occurs at potassium levels of 8 mEq/L or greater. Several methods have been advocated for ameliorating the hyperkalemic response, including pretreatment with hexafluorene, diazepam, and magnesium sulfate and the use of nondepolarizing muscle relaxants.[90] Although some success can be claimed for all of these methods in healthy individuals, no method has been shown to be universally effective, especially in burned patients; therefore, their reliability is suspect. If succinylcholine has been administered inadvertently, an important diagnostic sign of the hyperkalemia may be the peaking of the T wave with widening of the QRS complex on the electrocardiogram (Fig. 12–4). This change usually occurs at a plasma potassium concentration of 6 mEq/L or more. If cardiac arrest occurs, cardiopulmonary resuscitation must be instituted

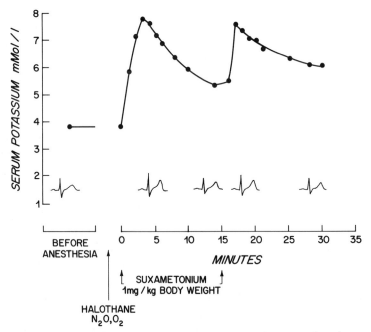

**FIGURE 12–4.** The change in potassium level in burned patients after 1.0 mg/kg. There is a rise in potassium-associated changes in T waves on EKG. (From Viby-Morgensen J, Hanel HK, Hansen E, et al: Serum cholinesterase activity in burned patients. Acta Anaesthesiol Scand 19:159–179, 1975.)

and incremental doses of calcium chloride or calcium gluconate administered until the electrocardiographic changes and cardiovascular functions revert to normal. Additional therapeutic maneuvers include the administration of bicarbonate, hyperventilation to increase blood pH, and the use of glucose with insulin. Indirect evidence suggests that the hyperkalemic response to succinylcholine may last up to two years in some individuals, although the magnitude of the response may not cause lethal cardiac arrest.[93] Therefore, succinylcholine may present a danger even after complete healing of burn wounds up to two years post burn.

Because succinylcholine is contraindicated in burned patients, the nondepolarizing relaxants have become the drugs of choice for induction of paralysis in patients with burn injury. Critically ill patients generally require smaller amounts of anesthetic drugs, yet burn patients are an exception. Numerous investigators have documented that the intravenous dose and plasma concentration required to achieve a given effect are usually markedly increased in patients with burns compared to those without burns.[31, 89, 94, 95] The rightward shift in the dose-response curve is related to both time after burn and magnitude of burn. Resistance to the neuromuscular effects of nondepolarizing relaxants usually is not seen in patients sustaining burns of less than 10 per cent TBSA. In patients with burns of more than 40 per cent TBSA, the dose must be increased 2.5- to fivefold. Thus, initial doses of *d*-tubocurarine, metocurine, pancuronium, atracurium and vecuronium would be 1.8, 0.8, 0.13, 2.0, and 0.13 mg/kg, respectively, for burned patients, compared to 0.51, 0.30, 0.05, 0.25, and 0.05 mg/kg, respectively, for patients without burns. Regardless of the high dose administered, recovery from paralysis is not seriously impaired, and the neuromuscular effect can be adequately reversed with the usual dose of antagonist drugs (atropine 0.03 mg/kg and neostigmine 0.06 mg/kg).

The ideal substitute for succinylcholine in patients with burns should produce rapid onset (within one minute) neuromuscular paralysis so that the drug can be used in emergency situations, such as intubation of patients with a full stomach, or for the relief of laryngospasm during anesthesia. Although 3.5 times the doses of *d*-tubocurarine, metocurine, and pancuronium described above for burns can be used to effect rapid paralysis, high doses may be associated with unwanted cardiovascular effects and will result in a prolonged recovery time from paralysis. The newer drugs atracurium and vecuronium offer some advantages over other relaxants because of their shorter duration of action and minimal cardiovascular effects.[94, 95] Vecuronium and atracurium are also pharmacokinetically distinct from the other nondepolarizing relaxants currently available, and they may, at least for the present, serve as useful alternatives to succinylcholine. Doses higher than those described above may have to be administered to initiate faster onset of paralysis, but the exact amount required has yet to be documented.

In the rodent model the hypothesis has been tested that thermal injury induces denervation-like phenomena, in which there is an increase in the number of nicotinic acetylcholine receptors at the neuromuscular junction at sites distant

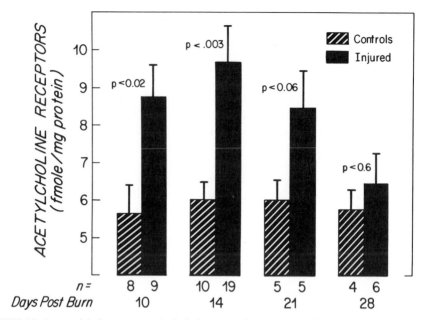

**FIGURE 12–5.** Acetylcholine receptor (AchR) changes with time in the diaphragm of the rat. At 10, 14, and 21 days, increases in AchR concentrations were seen. At 28 days the burned rats started gaining weight and had decreases in burn size, and the AchR concentrations in the diaphragm returned to control levels. (From Kim C, Martyn JAJ: Altered pharmacology of the burned patient. Clin Anesthesiol 1:649–661, 1987.)

from burn injury, and that these changes in acetylcholine receptor number contribute to aberrant responses to neuromuscular relaxants.[96, 97] These studies confirmed that there is in fact a 65 to 225 per cent increase in acetylcholine receptor concentration in the gastrocnemius and the diaphragm muscles (Fig. 12–5) following burn injury to the trunk. These studies further confirmed that the variability in the *d*-tubocurarine requirement is directly correlated with changes in acetylcholine receptor number induced by burn injury.[97] These laboratory studies have been complemented by electromyographic evidence of a denervation-like phenomenon in patients with burns,[98] including positive sharp waves and fibrillation potentials. The mechanisms by which these changes in skeletal muscles occur are unknown; however, since the effects are seen at sites distant from injury, neural and/or humoral mediators may be involved.

## SUMMARY

Pathophysiological alterations in burned patients result in many pharmacotherapeutic difficulties. The major factors responsible include changes in cardiovascular dynamics, protein binding, volume of distribution, and hepatic and renal function. All of these factors affect the pharmacokinetics of drugs. In addition, the continuous presence of humoral factors released as a result of the pathophysiological response to the trauma causes alterations in receptor number and affinity, as discussed for the adrenergic nervous system and the nicotinic acetylcholine receptor. Although not documented as yet, evidence appears to exist for changes in modulation of pain and pain perception. Thus, in addition to altered pharmacokinetics, altered pharmacodynamics complicate and confound drug therapeutics in burned patients. The mechanisms that induce these changes at distant sites are unknown. Pharmacotherapy in burns is complicated and should be closely monitored in terms of toxic effects and adequacy of response.

## REFERENCES

1. Demling RH: Burns. N Engl J Med 313:1389–1398, 1985.
2. Moncrief JA: Burns. N Engl J Med 288:444–454, 1973.
3. Aikawa N, Martyn JAJ, Burke JP: Pulmonary artery catheterization and thermodilution cardiac output determination in critical burn management. Am J Surg 135:811–817, 1978.
4. Turbow ME: Abnormal compression following circumferential burn. Cardiovascular response. J Trauma 13:533–541, 1973.
5. Maoti F, Sepulchre C, Miskulin M, et al: Biochemical and pharmacological properties of a cardiotoxic factor isolated from blood serum of burned patients. J Pathol 127:147–156, 1979.
6. Morgan RF, Martyn JAJ, Philbin DM, et al: Water balance and antidiuretic hormone response following acute thermal injury. J Trauma 20:468–472, 1980.
7. Harms BA, Bodai BI, Smith M: Prostaglandin release and altered microvascular integrity after burn injury. J Surg Res 31:274–280, 1981.
8. Williams RL: Drug administration in hepatic disease. N Engl J Med 390:1616–1622, 1984.
9. Klockowski PM, Levy G: Kinetics of drug action in disease states. XXIII: Effect of hypovolemia on the pharmacodynamics of phenobarbital in rats. J Pharm Sci 77:365–366, 1988.
10. Ziemniak JA, Watson WA, Saffle JR, et al: Cimetidine kinetics during resuscitation for burn shock. Clin Pharmacol Ther 36:228–233, 1984.
11. Glew RH, Moellering RC, Burke JF: Gentamycin dosage in children with extensive burns. J Trauma 16:819–823, 1976.
12. Martyn JAJ, Snider MT, Farago LF, Burke JF: Thermodilution right ventricular volume: A novel and better predictor of volume replacement in acute thermal injury. J Trauma 21:619–626, 1981.
13. Wilmore DW, Goodwin CW, Aulick LH, et al: Effect of injury and infection on visceral metabolism and circulation. Ann Surg 192:491–504, 1980.
14. Gump FE, Price JB, Kinney JM: Blood flow and oxygen consumption in patients with severe burns. Surg Gynecol Obstet 130:23–28, 1970.
15. Gregoretti S, Gelman S, Dimick AR: Lack of immediate effects of wound excision on hyperdynamic circulation. J Burn Care Rehab 9:180–183, 1988.
16. Aulick LH, Wilmore DW, Mason AD Jr, Pruitt BA Jr: Depressed reflex vasomotor control of the burn wound. Cardiovasc Res 16:113–119, 1982.
17. Daniels JC, Larson DL, Abston S, Ritzman SE: Serum protein profiles in thermal burns. I. Serum electrophoretic patterns, immunoglobulins and transport proteins. J Trauma 14:137–152, 1974.
18. Martyn JAJ, Abernethy DR, Greenblatt DJ: Plasma protein binding of drugs after severe burn injury. Clin Pharmacol Ther 35:534–536, 1984.
19. Bloedow DC, Hansbrough JF, Hardin T, Simons M: Post-burn serum drug binding and serum protein concentrations. J Clin Pharmacol 26:147–151, 1986.
20. Bowdle TA, Neal GD, Levy RH, Heimbach DM: Phenytoin pharmacokinetics in burned rats and plasma protein binding of phenytoin in burned patients. J Pharmacol Exp Ther 213:97–99, 1980.

21. Greenblatt DJ, Sellers EM, Koch-Weser J: Importance of protein binding for interpretation of serum or plasma concentrations. J Clin Pharmacol 22:259–263, 1982.
22. Kim C, Martyn JAJ: Altered pharmacology of the burned patient. Clin Anesthesiol 1:649–661, 1987.
23. Martyn JAJ, Greenblatt DJ: Lorazepam conjugation unimpaired in burn trauma. Clin Pharmacol Ther 43:250–255, 1988.
24. Bloedow DC, Goodfellow LA, Marvin J, Heimbach D: Meperidine disposition in burn patients. Res Comm Chem Path Pharmacol 54:87–99, 1986.
25. Medical News. Lidocaine-cimetidine interaction can be toxic. JAMA 247:3174–3175, 1982.
26. Czaja AJ, Rizzo TA, Smith WR, Pruitt BA: Acute liver disease after cutaneous thermal injury. J Trauma 15:887–894, 1975.
27. Greenblatt DJ, Shader RI, Abernethy DR: Current status of benzodiazepines. N Engl J Med 309:354–358, 410–416, 1983.
28. Martyn JAJ, Abernethy DR, Greenblatt DJ: Increased cimetidine clearance in burn patients. JAMA 258:1288–1291, 1985.
29. Loirat P, Rohan J, Bailet A, et al: Increased glomerular filtration rate in patients with major burns and its effect on pharmacokinetics of tobramycin. N Engl J Med 299:915–919, 1978.
30. Goodwin CE, Aulick LH, Becke RA, Wilmore DW: Increased renal perfusion and kidney size in convalescent burn patients. JAMA 244:1588–1590, 1980.
31. Martyn JAJ: Clinical pharmacology and drug therapy in the burned patient. Anesthesiology 65:67–75, 1986.
32. Eklund J, Gramberg PO, Liljedahl SO: Studies on renal function in burns. Acta Chir Scand 136:627–640, 1970.
33. Gombar CJ, Burak E, Harper N, Smith BR: Pulmonary clearance of vasoactive drugs: Oxidation of SK and F86466 in the isolated perfused rat lung. J Pharmacol Exp Ther 245:402–406, 1988.
34. Mehendale HM: Pulmonary disposition and effects of drugs on pulmonary removal of endogenous substances. Fed Proc 43:2586–2591, 1987.
35. Loft S, Boel J, Kyst A, et al: Increased hepatic microsomal activity after surgery under halothane or spinal anesthesia. Anesthesiology 62:11–16, 1985.
36. Feely J, Wilkinson GR, Wood AJJ: Reduction in liver blood and propranolol metabolism by cimetidine. N Engl J Med 304:692–695, 1981.
37. Sawchuck RJ, Rector TS: Drug kinetics in burn patients. Clin Pharmacokinet 5:548–556, 1980.
38. Brater DC, Bawdon RE, Anderson SA, et al: Vancomycin elimination in patients in burn injury. Clin Pharmacol Ther 39:631–634, 1986.
39. Gordon RC, Regamey C, Kirby WMN: Serum protein binding of aminoglycoside antibiotics. Antimicrob Agents Chemother 2:214–220, 1972.
40. Czaja AJ, McAlhany JC, Pruitt BA: Acute gastroduodenal disease after thermal injury: An endoscopic evaluation of incidence and routine history. N Engl J Med 29:925–929, 1976.
41. Curling TE: On acute ulceration of the duodenum in cases of burn. Med Chir Trans (London) 25:260–281, 1841.
42. Sevitt S: Duodenal and gastric ulceration after burning. Br J Surg 54:32–41, 1967.
43. Hastings PR, Skillman JJ, Bushnell LS, Silen W: Antacid filtration in the prevention of acute gastrointestinal bleeding: A controlled randomized trial in 100 critically ill patients. N Engl J Med 298:1041–1045, 1978.
44. Munster A: The early management of thermal burns. Surgery 87:29–39, 1980.
45. Martyn JAJ: Cimetidine and/or antacid for the control of gastric acidity in pediatric burn patients. Crit Care Med 13:1–3, 1985.
46. Watson WA, Russo J, Saffle JR, et al: Cimetidine in the prophylaxis of stress ulceration in severely burned patients. J Burn Care Rehabil 4:260–263, 1983.
47. McKlwee HP, Sirinek KR, Levine BA: Cimetidine affords protection equal to antacids in the prevention of stress ulceration following burns. Surgery 86:620–626, 1979.
48. Martyn JAJ, Greenblatt DJ, Hagen J, Hoaglin DC: Burn injury alters pharmacokinetics and pharmacodynamics of cimetidine in children. Eur J Clin Pharmacol 31:361–367, 1989.
49. Goudsouzian NG, Cote CJ, Liu LMP, Dedrick DF: The dose-response effects of oral cimetidine on gastric pH and volume in children. Anesthesiology 55:533–536, 1981.
50. Ostro MJ, Russell JA, Soldin JJ, et al: Control of gastric pH with cimetidine: Bolus versus primed infusion. Gastroenterology 89:532–537, 1985.
51. Oliveri M, Martyn JAJ: Ranitidine effectively controls gastric pH in burned patients (abstract). Proceedings of the American Burn Association, March 1989.

52. Martyn JAJ, Greenblatt DJ, Quinby WC: Diazepam kinetics following burns. Anesth Analg 62:293–297, 1983.
53. Abernethy DR, Greenblatt DJ, Divoll M, et al: Differential effect of cimetidine on drug oxidation (antipyrine and diazepam) vs. conjugation (acetaminophen and lorazepam): Prevention of acetaminophen toxicity of cimetidine. J Pharmacol Exp Ther 224:508–513, 1983.
54. Stanford GK, Pine PH: Post-burn delirium associated with the use of intravenous lorazepam. J Burn Care Rehabil 9:160–161, 1988.
55. Huang V, Figge H, Demling RH: Haloperidol complications in burn patients. J Burn Care Rehabil 8:269–273, 1987.
56. Perry S, Heidrich G: Management of pain debridement. Survey in U.S. burn units. Pain 13:267–280, 1982.
57. Perry S, Inturrisi CE: Analgesia and morphine disposition in burn patients. J Burn Care Res 4:276–279, 1983.
58. Gregoretti S, Vinik HR: Sufentanil pharmacokinetics in burn patients undergoing skin grafting (abstract). Anesth Analg 65:S64, 1986.
59. Demling RH: What are the functions of endorphins following thermal injury (discussion). J Trauma 24:S172–S176, 1984.
60. Wilmore DW, Long J, Mason D, et al: Catecholamines: Mediators of hypermetabolic response to thermal injury. Ann Surg 180:653–668, 1974.
61. White PF, Way WL, Trevor AJ: Ketamine: Its pharmacology and therapeutic uses. Anesthesiology 56:119–136, 1982.
62. Demling RH, Ellerbee S, Jarrett F: Ketamine anesthesia for tangential excision of burn scar: A burn unit procedure. J Trauma 18:269–270, 1978.
63. Coté CJ, Goudsouzian NG, Liu LMP, et al: Thiopental induction in burned children. A dose response study. Anesthesiology 55:A338, 1981.
64. Gronert GA, Schauer PJ, Gunther RC: Multiple halothane anesthesia in burn patients. JAMA 205:878–880, 1968.
65. Gregoretti S, Gelman S, Dimick AR: Total body oxygen supply-demand balance in burned patients under enflurane anesthesia. J Trauma 27:158–160, 1987.
66. Jim LJ, LaLonde C, Demling RH: Effect of anesthesia and positive pressure ventilation on early postburn hemodynamic instability. J Trauma 26:26–33, 1986.
67. Taylor JW, Hander EW, Skreen RL: The effect of central nervous system narcosis on the sympathetic response to stress. J Surg Res 20:313–320, 1976.
68. Thomson DA: Anesthesia and immune system. J Burn Care Rehabil 8:483–487, 1987.
69. Amos RJ, Amess JAL, Hinds CJ, Mollin DL: Incidence and pathogenesis of acute megaloblastic bone marrow change in patients receiving intensive care. Lancet 2:835–838, 1982.
70. Koenig A, Koenig UD, Binhold B: Differences in lymphocyte mitogenic stimulation pattern depending on anesthesia and operative trauma. Eur J Anaesth 4:17–24, 1987.
71. Cone JB, Ransom JM, Tucker WE, et al: Effect of dopamine on post burn myocardial depression. J Trauma 22:1019–1020, 1982.
72. Martyn JAJ, Farago LS, Burke JF: Hemodynamics of low dose dopamine in nonseptic burned patients. Chest 89:357–360, 1986.
73. Drueck C, Welsh GW, Pruitt BA: Hemodynamic analysis of septic shock in thermal injury: Treatment with dopamine. Am Surg 44:424–427, 1978.
74. Vincent JL, Reuse C, Kahn R: Effects on right ventricular function of a change from dopamine to dobutamine. Crit Care Med 16:659–662, 1988.
75. Molloy DW, Ducas J, Dobson K, et al: Hemodynamic management in clinical acute hypoxemic respiratory failure. Dopamine vs. dobutamine. Chest 89:5636–5640, 1986.
76. Motulsky HJ, Insel PA: Adrenergic receptors in man. Direct identification of physiologic regulation and clinical alterations. N Engl J Med 307:18–29, 1982.
77. Colucci WS, Wright RF, Braunwald E: New positive inotropic agents in the treatment of congestive heart failure. N Engl J Med 316:290–299, 1987.
78. Glasson DW: Topical epinephrine as a hemostatic agent. Plast Reconstr Surg 74:451–452, 1986.
79. Snelling CFT, Shaw K: The effect of topical epinephrine hydrochloride in saline on blood loss following tangential excision of burn wounds. Plast Reconstr Surg 12:830–836, 1983.
80. Carucci DJ, Pearce RSC, Innes DJ: Evaluation of hemostatic agents for skin graft donor sites. J Burn Care Rehabil 5:321–323, 1986.
81. Timonen RM, Pavlin EG, Haschee RH: Epinephrine level pre- and post-application of topical epinephrine during burn surgery. Anesthesiology 57:A138, 1982.

82. Cryer PE: Physiology and pathophysiology of human sympathoadrenal neuroendocrine system. N Engl J Med 303:436–444, 1980.
83. Stratton JR, Pfeifer MA, Ritchie JL, Halter JB: Hemodynamic effects of epinephrine: Concentration study in humans. J Appl Physiol 58:1199–1206, 1985.
84. Hilton J: Effects of verapamil on thermal trauma depressed cardiac output in the anesthetized dog. Burns 10:313–317, 1984.
85. Fozzard HA: Myocardial injury in burn shock. Ann Surg 151:113–119, 1961.
86. Moncrief JA: Effects of various fluid regimens and pharmacological agents on the circulatory hemodynamics of the immediate post burn period. Ann Surg 266:723–752, 1966.
87. Coggehill JW, Marini JJ, Newman JH: Improved oxygenation after muscle relaxation in adult respiratory distress syndrome. Arch Intern Med 145:1718–1721, 1985.
88. Pollitzer MJ, Reynolds EO, Shaw DG, Thomas RM: Pancuronium during mechanical ventilation speeds recovery of lungs of infants with hyaline membrane disease. Lancet 8216:346–348, 1981.
89. Martyn JAJ, Goldhill DR, Goudsouzian NG: Clinical pharmacology of neuromuscular relaxants in patients with burns. J Clin Pharmacol 26:680–685, 1986.
90. Gronert GA, Theye RA: Pathophysiology of succinylcholine hyperkalemia. Anesthesiology 43:89–99, 1975.
91. Viby-Mogensen J, Hanel HK, Hansen E, et al: Serum cholinesterase activity in burned patients. Acta Anaesthesiol Scand 19:159–179, 1975.
92. Brown TCK, Bell B: Electromyographic responses to small doses of suxamethonium in children after burns. Br J Anaesth 59:1017–1021, 1987.
93. Martyn JAJ, Matteo RS, Syzfelbein SK, Kaplan RF: Unprecedented resistance to neuromuscular blocking effects of metocurine with persistence after complete recovery in a burned patient. Anesth Analg 61:614–617, 1982.
94. Mills A, Martyn JAJ: Evaluation of atracurium neuromuscular blockade in pediatric burned patients. Br J Anaesth 60:450–455, 1988.
95. Mills A, Martyn JAJ: Vecuronium neuromuscular blockade in pediatric burned patients. Br J Clin Pharmacol 28:155–159, 1989.
96. Kim C, Fuke N, Martyn JAJ: Thermal injury to rat increases nicotine acetylcholine reception in diaphragm. Anesthesiology 68:401–406, 1988.
97. Kim C, Martyn JAJ, Fuke N: Thermal injury to trunk of rat causes denervation-like responses in gastrocnemius muscle. J Appl Physiol 65:1745–1751, 1988.
98. Mills A, Schriefer T, Martyn JAJ: Electromyographic studies in pediatric patients with burn injury. Anesthesiology 65:A294, 1986.

# 13

# Management of Pain

## PATRICIA F. OSGOOD and S.K. SZYFELBEIN

Pain in victims of burn injury has frequent and wide fluctuations in intensity, and its control presents a continuing challenge to those responsible for patient care.

Although some of the factors involved in the perception of pain have begun to be elucidated in recent years and new analgesic agents have multiplied, the management of pain in burned patients is still often unsatisfactory.[1] The contribution of severe protracted pain to the overall physiological response to trauma including immunodeficiency[2] is unknown, but, at the very least, it must intensify this process,[3] making better management of pain of the utmost importance.

It has been postulated that, in addition to the regulation of pain, it may benefit the patient to eliminate or reduce hormonally mediated metabolic stress responses to tissue injury by blocking specific neural pathways and receptors.[4] As yet there is little or no evidence to suggest that blocking of these responses in the burn victim would be of value.[4-6] The most effective suppression of the metabolic response is achieved by continuous regional anesthesia along with systemic, epidural, or subarachnoid opioid analgesia. Spinal routes of drug administration are generally avoided in burn patients, however, because of the risk of introducing infection; therefore, on practical grounds alone, these techniques would present difficulties.

## PROBLEMS ASSOCIATED WITH THE PAIN OF BURN INJURIES

The deficiencies of present analgesic practices for debridement and dressing changes in burned patients have been clearly documented by Perry and Heidrich.[7] Their survey of 181 staff members from 93 United States burn units showed that narcotics were the most commonly administered analgesics. Doses varied widely, with up to a 35-fold difference when route and relative potency were considered. Perhaps the most startling finding was that children were four times more likely than adults to receive no analgesic at all for this procedure, even though the extent of pain for both children and adults was judged to be the same (moderate). An earlier report[1] by the same group noted that, during therapeutic procedures, most patients suffered severe to excruciating pain after a moderate dose of narcotic. When at rest, however, pain in the burned patient may fall to comparatively low levels[1, 8] that can usually be controlled by relatively smaller doses of narcotic or even non-narcotic analgesics.

**201**

Although severity of pain was found to be unrelated to the extent or degree of burn in one study of 52 patients,[1] in a group of 42 burned children that we have studied, the total body surface area (TBSA) burned (Fig. 13–1) and particularly the depth of burn were directly related to the magnitude of the mean pain scores obtained during 104 burn dressing changes; comparison of the extent of third-degree burns with pain scores gave a correlation coefficient of 0.62, $P < 0.001$.[9] The widely held belief that third-degree burns give rise to no pain would thus seem untenable.

Another element that may prevent optimal pain control during painful procedures is the well-documented tendency of the burn nurse to underestimate

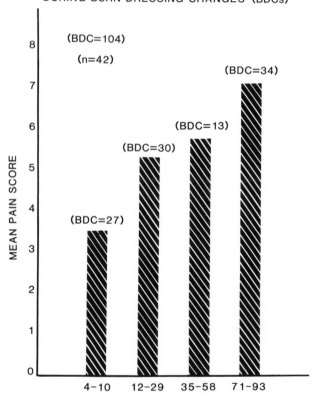

THE EFFECT OF BODY SURFACE AREA (BSA) BURNED

ON THE MEAN PAIN SCORES OF PATIENTS

DURING BURN DRESSING CHANGES (BDCs)

**FIGURE 13–1.** The mean pain scores of 42 acutely burned children (8 to 18 years old) during 104 burn dressing changes, ordered by the extent of body surface area involved. Scores were obtained at one-minute intervals at least (patients volunteered changes in scores occurring between the minute queries).

the intensity of a patient's pain at these times.[10-13] In assessing an individual's pain, therefore, the soundest course would seem to be an acceptance of the patient's own evaluation of his or her pain.[14]

## ENDOGENOUS MODULATION OF PAIN

A better understanding of the variability in pain perception among individuals and even in the same subject from day to day[15] has come with the recent elucidation of neural systems involved in pain modulation.[16, 17] A major impetus to this work was the discovery of stereospecific opioid binding sites (receptors) in the central nervous system (CNS)[18-21] and the endogenous opioid substances (endorphins) that combine with these receptors.[22-24]

At present, three families of endogenous opioid peptides are recognized, each having a distinct precursor molecule and anatomical distribution. Met- and leu-enkephalin, beta-endorphin, and dynorphin represent these three classes.[16] The binding sites for these peptides, as well as for exogenous opioid alkaloids (narcotics), include a number of subpopulations of opioid receptors; the most intensively studied of these have been designated mu, delta, and kappa.[25] Although narcotic compounds rarely act upon a single receptor, affinity for a particular receptor generally predominates. Thus, morphine is considered the prototypic mu agonist, whereas the enkephalin D-Ala$^2$-D-Leu$^5$-enkephalin (DADL) is a delta agonist and ethylketocyclazocine a kappa agonist. The existence of multiple receptors serving discrete neuronal pathways involved in the modulation of pain means that pharmacological agents specific to a given receptor may be more effective for a particular type of pain,[26-28] with the promise of even more selectivity and specificity in drugs of the future.

Recent work suggests the intriguing possibility that the analgesic, respiratory depressant, and dependence properties of opioid substances may be separated. Pasternak has recently (1986) presented a review of biochemical and pharmacological evidence showing that the central mu receptors may exist in two forms identified as $mu_1$ and $mu_2$. The $mu_2$ receptor is the classic morphine-selective site, whereas $mu_1$, although it has lower binding capacity, has far greater affinity for most opiates; these include not only morphine but the delta receptor–selective enkephalins and kappa-selective ethylketocyclazocine.[29] Studies in which the $mu_1$ receptor was inactivated with an irreversible antagonist (naloxazone or naloxonazine) revealed that $mu_1$ sites are involved in supraspinal analgesia while delta sites are prominent at the spinal cord level. The $mu_2$ receptor, in contrast, appeared to mediate effects such as respiratory depression and bradycardia.[30] As for dependence, the $mu_1$ receptor had a minor role in naloxone-precipitated withdrawal symptoms; these signs were attributed instead to a summation of effects stemming from a number of other receptor subtypes.[29, 31] Although other explanations are possible, the hypothesized multiple opioid subpopulations should provide a useful base in the search for better analgesic agents with the promise of improved pharmacological control of pain with minimal or no side effects.

Steps in this direction may include the synthesis of compounds acting primarily at the kappa receptor. Butorphanol (Stadol), for example, produces analgesia comparable to that of morphine but has limited respiratory depressant (ceiling) effects and little or no dependence liability. This agent has been used successfully for postoperative pain,[32] as has another kappa agonist (nalbuphine) for burn wound debridement.[33]

Endogenous opioids have been implicated in the analgesia that follows some forms of stress,[34] but nonopioid stress analgesia occurs as well.[35–37] Although the designation "stress-induced analgesia" has been questioned[16] because some seemingly non-noxious events produce analgesia while other aversive stimuli do not, it is a useful and frequently used phrase to describe an extremely interesting phenomenon.[38, 39]

The trauma of burn injury appears to involve at least one of these intrinsic pain systems, which may lead to an opioid form of analgesia. In the burned child, we have found an inverse association between plasma beta-endorphin immunoactivity (i$\beta$-EP) and pain levels on a given day.[8] A similar relationship has been seen in adult cancer patients.[40] In the rat, plasma levels of i$\beta$-EP increased markedly immediately following scald burn, and sensitivity to pain decreased (assessed by tail flick latency). These measures were both directly related to the TBSA of burn.[41] Since the increase in analgesia (tail flick latency) was prevented by the long-acting specific opioid antagonist naltrexone, this stress-induced analgesia appeared to be opioid in nature. The duration of these effects was limited: depending upon the size of burn, both i$\beta$-EP and tail flick returned to pre-burn levels in three to six hours (Fig. 13–2).

Normally, i$\beta$-EP plasma levels have a circadian variation[42] similar to that of cortisol (high in the morning, low at night). In children with burns of 60 per cent or more TBSA, however, these rhythms frequently seem to be lost for eight or more weeks after burn.[43] Cortisol levels tend to be uniformly high,[44] while i$\beta$-EP is most often low or undetectable (Fig. 13–3). Occasional spikes in i$\beta$-EP levels occurred immediately after surgical procedures or on days when body temperature was high (greater than 40°C or 104°F). Thus, it would appear that the hormonal response to burn injury is by no means uniform; patterns may be altered when day-to-day stressors are superimposed on the primary stress of burns.[43] Patients with smaller burns, however, seem to retain normal circadian variation in plasma i$\beta$-EP; nevertheless, these levels may vary markedly throughout the time of hospitalization.[8]

## TREATMENT OF PAIN

Despite the realization of the urgent need for improved means of pain control in burned patients,[7, 12, 45] there has been little systematic study of methods

EFFECT OF DIP IN 30°C WATER (CONTROL) OR SCALD BURN
ON β-ENDORPHIN PLASMA LEVEL AND TAIL FLICK LATENCY IN THE RAT

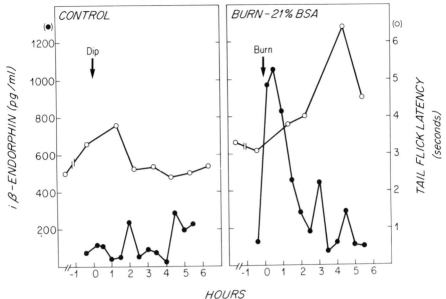

*HOURS*

**FIGURE 13–2.** The effect of scald burn or sham burn (tepid water) on plasma beta-endorphin levels (closed circles) and tail flick latency (a test of antinociception, i.e., analgesia) in the rat (open circles). Each rat (sham and burn) had approximately 20 per cent of the total body surface area exposed at 0 hours.

of alleviating pain in this group. Strategies for pain management during procedures such as tanking-debridement or burn dressing changes (BDC) range from hypnosis[46] to full anesthesia. Since all methods have drawbacks, there is no one generally accepted approach to pain control. Nevertheless, some form of pharmacological intervention underlies nearly all efforts to restrict pain.[7]

## Hypnosis

As a nonpharmacological means of modifying pain, hypnosis has an obvious appeal. A recent review of the limited literature on the use of hypnosis to reduce pain in burned patients noted, however, that, while most reports supported the efficacy of this technique, the design of these studies for the most part was so flawed (or lacking altogether) that no firm conclusions could be drawn as to the feasibility or utility of hypnotherapy in burn pain.[47]

## Anesthetic Agents

General anesthetics such as methoxyflurane,[48] ketamine,[49, 50] and nitrous oxide[51] have been advocated for their analgesic properties during BDC, but the need for repeated exposure over many weeks or months increases the probability

DIURNAL VARIATION OF PLASMA BETA-ENDORPHIN AND CORTISOL LEVELS

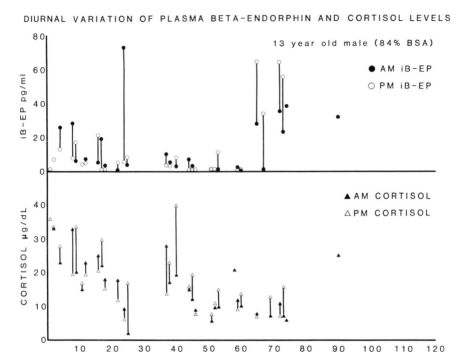

FIGURE 13–3. Variations in plasma beta-endorphin (iβ-EP) and cortisol levels in a 13-year-old boy with burns covering 84 per cent of the TBSA. Upper panel shows beta-endorphin levels (pg/ml); the bottom panel, cortisol (μg/dl). Closed symbols are morning levels (circles = beta-endorphins; triangles = cortisol) generally obtained between 7 and 8 A.M.; open symbols are evening levels (4:30 to 6:30 P.M.). Although patterns have varied widely among patients, there almost always have been periods when iβ-EP was low or undetectable (above, between post-burn days 37 and 61), as well as frequent inversions of the normal circadian rhythm of higher morning and lower evening iβ-EP and cortisol levels.

that the toxic effects of methoxyflurane and nitrous oxide may emerge[52–54] or, in the case of ketamine, that tolerance will develop.[49, 55] The very short action of ketamine (15 min) is also a disadvantage. In addition, the safe administration of these agents requires the presence of an anesthetist, making their routine use impractical. Moreover, the necessity for withholding nourishment prior to their administration disrupts the intensive nutritional support that is an important aspect of burn care. Thus, analgesic agents, particularly narcotics, are the preferred course for painful procedures.[7]

## Narcotic Agents

Because of the acceptability and ease of administering analgesics orally, preparations such as Percocet (5 mg oxycodone, 325 mg acetaminophen per tablet) are often used for BDC.[8] An evaluation of Percocet in a group of formerly burned patients returning for reconstructive surgery, however, revealed that the doses generally used for BDC (one or two tablets) rarely brought complete relief of moderate to severe postoperative pain (Fig. 13–4). Although virtually all of these patients agreed that their postoperative pain in no way compared in severity to the pain they had experienced during BDC, it is of interest that even the larger dose of Percocet reduced this postoperative pain by little more than half.

Morphine and meperidine, however, are the most widely used narcotic analgesics for pain control in both pediatric and adult burn patients.[12] Although both of these agents can be given orally, the intravenous (IV) or intramuscular (IM) route is more usual. Even with IV administration, however, the onset of the analgesic action and time to peak effect of these drugs are relatively slow and, thus, the sudden surges of pain that occur during a dressing change cannot easily be countered. Moreover, the- long duration of action, particularly of morphine (four to six hours), means that doses suitable for the extreme pain of

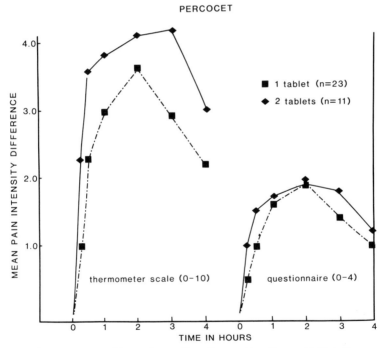

**FIGURE 13–4.** The time course of the analgesic effect of one and two Percocet tablets (5 mg oxycodone and 325 mg acetaminophen per tablet). Pain intensity difference is the initial pain score obtained using a 0 to 10 thermometer-like scale (left panel) or a standard pain questionnaire (right panel) minus subsequent scores obtained at 15 and 30 minutes and one, two, three, and four hours after drug administration. (Thus, the higher the mean pain intensity difference, the greater the pain relief.) Subjects were formerly burned children from 8 to 18 years old suffering from postoperative pain following reconstructive surgery. Closed square = one Percocet tablet (n = 23); closed diamond = two Percocet tablets (n = 11).

the dressing change will leave the patient oversedated and even, perhaps, with depressed respiration when the procedure has been completed, thus interfering with effective respiratory exchange and such activities as eating.

A further drawback of meperidine given in frequent, large doses over extended periods is the accumulation of the toxic metabolite normeperidine, which may lead to CNS excitation to the point of convulsions. Since milder symptoms (agitation and "shaky feelings") appear well before the more severe responses (tremor, twitching, seizures), immediate discontinuation of meperidine and substitution of another narcotic (e.g., morphine) when the earliest signs occur should prevent the development of the more adverse effects.[56]

The short-acting narcotics such as fentanyl have clear advantages in controlling the extraordinary discomfort of painful procedures. Their rapid onset of action allows the dose to be adjusted to the degree of ongoing pain, while their short duration of action prevents prolonged sedation. In our experience, patients given repeated single bolus doses or continuous IV infusions of fentanyl remain alert enough to give pain scores even during long dressing changes while their pain is generally kept at low levels (Figs. 13–5 and 13–6). For the former, an initial dose of 1 to 6 μg/kg is followed by 0.5 to 1 μg/kg doses as needed; for the latter, infusion rates of 0.03 to 0.05 μg/kg/min are begun 15 min before and continued throughout the BDC.

We have found a close correspondence of fentanyl plasma concentration and pain levels, as reflected by pain scores given at ± 3 min of blood sampling, most striking in individual patients (Fig. 13–7) but maintained when a group of subjects was combined ($r = 0.64$; $P > 0.001$, n = 35). When a procedure is expected to be exceptionally painful, the short-acting narcotics are an appealing alternative to the usual analgesics.

## Side Effects of Narcotics

Respiratory depression and muscle rigidity ("stiff chest") are side effects that must, of course, be kept in mind when administering narcotics.[57] Since they can be rapidly reversed by the specific opioid antagonist naloxone before they adversely affect the patient, concern for these possible side effects should not limit their use.

To counter respiratory depression, a dose of 40 μg naloxone is administered intravenously (a standard ampule containing 400 μl is diluted to 10 ml to make a 40 μg/ml solution). This dose is repeated at 30- to 45-second intervals until changes in pupil size and respiratory rate become evident; a return of the eyelid and cough reflexes, swallowing, or any purposeful movement, as well as monitoring of end-tidal carbon dioxide, also indicates the progress of reversal. In this way respiration can be restored without abolishing analgesia. Although it may rarely be needed, immediate access to naloxone allows the safe administration of narcotic agents.

Another often overlooked factor that should be considered when the burned patient is being given narcotics over extended periods is the high probability of

BURN DRESSING CHANGES WITH PERCOCET OR FENTANYL

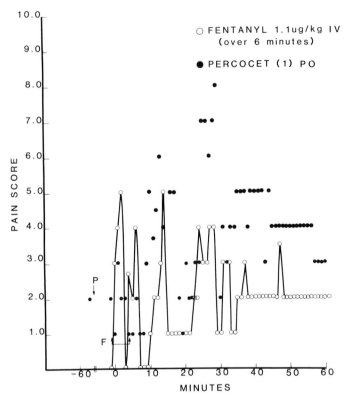

**FIGURE 13–5.** Moment-to-moment pain scores given by a 15-year-old boy with 58 per cent TBSA burns during burn dressing changes on two successive days (13 and 14 days post burn) in the presence of Percocet (one tablet) or a single dose of fentanyl (1.1 µg/kg IV). Pain scores were obtained with the thermometer scale described in Figure 13–4. Percocet scores = closed circles; fentanyl scores = open connected circles.

the development of tolerance to these drugs. In reviewing patients' records for analgesic regimens, Perry and co-workers[1] found no evidence that possible development of tolerance was ever taken into account. However, awareness on the part of attending medical personnel should make upward adjustments in dose easily accomplished. For this purpose, the daily assessment and documentation of a patient's pain are invaluable.[1]

## Analgesia for the Patient Being Mechanically Ventilated

For the patient being artificially ventilated and nourished, the long action of morphine is clearly advantageous. The high probability that a neuromuscular blocking drug will be administered to increase the efficiency of the respirator means that the patient can neither move nor speak, making it impossible to

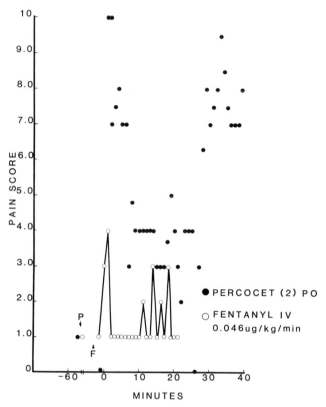

BURN DRESSING CHANGES WITH PERCOCET
OR CONTINUOUS INFUSION OF FENTANYL

**FIGURE 13–6.** Pain scores obtained from a 15-year-old boy with 20 per cent TBSA burns with the pain thermometer during a burn dressing change after two Percocet tablets (P; closed circles) or with a continuous infusion of fentanyl (F; open circles) of 0.046 μg/kg/min.

convey the extent of his pain. These drugs (e.g., curare) have no analgesic properties; therefore, an analgesic regimen that assures satisfactory pain control is imperative for such an individual. Unfortunately, no precise guidelines can be given for doses or blood levels of morphine necessary for good analgesia, since they vary among and within individuals[58]; moreover, narcotic requirements in the burned patient are increased.[54] These factors may help to explain the diversity in plasma concentrations found to give satisfactory analgesia. Plasma concentrations ranging from 13 to 57 ng/ml (median 19.6 ng/ml) were found to control pain in children with terminal malignancy.[58] In a group of children during surgery, the minimum concentration required to suppress clinical signs of pain was 65 ng/ml.[59] A study of adult burn patients showed adequate pain relief when plasma concentrations were approximately 50 to 100 ng/ml.[60] For nonburned

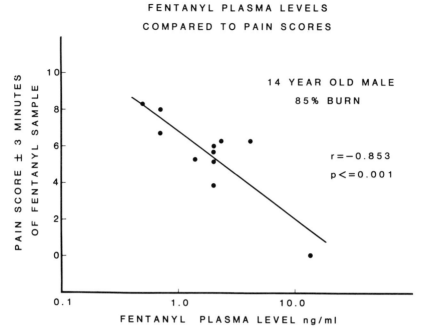

**FIGURE 13–7.** The logarithm of fentanyl plasma levels (ng/ml) compared to pain scores obtained with a thermometer-like scale at ± 3 minutes of blood sampling during two dressing changes in a 14-year-old boy with 85 per cent TBSA burns.

adults, an average concentration of 21 ng/ml sufficed for satisfactory relief of postoperative pain.[61]

Adequate blood levels of morphine are most easily maintained by continuous IV infusion, with supplementary doses superimposed prior to painful procedures. We try to maintain a background morphine plasma level of at least 20 ng/ml by continuous infusion of 0.03 to 0.2 mg/kg/hr (1 to 15 mg/hr) in mechanically ventilated burned children. Single doses of 0.05 to 0.2 mg/kg (1 to 15 mg) are given 15 to 20 min before any painful procedure (Fig. 13–8). For example, a 16-year-old male with 90 per cent TBSA burn, for a short time after his arrival on post-burn day 10, was maintained on an hourly single IV dose of 0.06 mg/kg morphine; the resulting plasma concentrations ranged from 2.8 to 36 ng/ml. To obtain more uniform levels, morphine was then continuously infused at rates of 0.03 to 0.06 mg/kg/hr, with a bolus dose of 0.06 mg/kg before dressing changes. Plasma concentration under these conditions and at the lowest infusion rate was 36 ng/ml and at the highest 41 ng/ml (on post-burn days 51 and 52). Between days 53 and 69, however, levels fell to consistently less than 5 ng/ml. On day 69 the infusion rate was increased to 0.12 ng/kg/hr with doses of 0.1 mg/kg before dressing changes; by the following morning (before dressing change) the morphine level was back to 29 ng/ml. In a subsequent patient, a male of 16 years with burns of 85 per cent TBSA, morphine was administered by continuous infusion

BLOOD CONCENTRATIONS OF MORPHINE

AFTER INJECTION OF A SINGLE DOSE

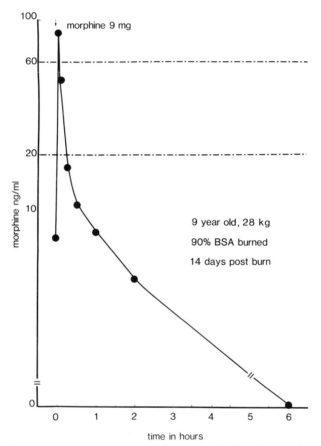

**FIGURE 13–8.** Plasma morphine concentrations following a single dose (0.32 mg/kg) in a 9-year-old boy of 28 kg with burns covering 90 per cent of the total body surface area (TBSA) at 14 days post burn. The dose was administered intravenously immediately after the point showing the morphine level at time "0" (7.4 ng/ml); a single dose of 0.18 mg/kg had been given 125 minutes before the depicted dose. The dashed lines denote the range of analgesic levels suggested by the literature.

along with single doses from the time of his admission until extubation and removal from a mechanical ventilator. Infusion rates were gradually increased from 0.06 to 0.12 mg/kg/hr, while plasma levels were generally between 20 and 40 ng/ml, except on day 20 when there was a fall to 14 ng/ml. On day 21 the rate was increased to 0.19 mg/kg/hr along with more frequent single doses of 0.06 mg/kg. Blood levels of morphine on this schedule ranged from 20 to 84 ng/ml (the last value was measured just prior to a dressing change). On the whole, it appeared that the analgesic management of this patient was better than that of the patient described earlier. Continuous infusion was clearly the better mode of administration of morphine in these patients.

Although tolerance to morphine usually develops, in our experience, dependence does not. Careful observation has revealed no withdrawal symptoms even after prolonged periods of morphine administration. However, doses of morphine are gradually reduced during the final days on a respirator, and this may ease the transition to an oral analgesic.

In summary, of the many avenues to better pain control in the burned patient, we would suggest the following:

1. For those patients on respirators, continuous infusion of morphine with supplemental single doses of the same or another narcotic prior to therapeutic procedures should provide satisfactory analgesia.

2. For those able to convey the severity of their pain, the need for reducing background pain can be readily ascertained and usually met by standard oral analgesics given as needed. Procedures such as tanking-debridement or burn dressing changes, however, present a far more difficult problem in these patients. One suggested regimen is the combination of the long-acting methadone for underlying pain with a short-acting narcotic (fentanyl or alfentanil) for the acute pain of therapeutic interventions.[45] Another similar strategy might be oral morphine or methadone with the relatively shorter-acting meperidine or even a narcotic–non-narcotic compound, such as Percocet, added prior to painful therapies. Whatever the plan, blind adherence to a fixed dosing schedule should be avoided; instead, an empirical approach, with a willingness to proceed by trial and error with the individual patient until adequate pain relief is obtained at these times, may be the most promising route, recognizing that methods currently available ensure no perfect solution.

3. It may be, in the future, that patient-controlled analgesic therapy will bring improved pain relief to the burned subject. With this system, a predetermined dose of IV analgesic is delivered by means of a pump activated by the patient himself as needed; accidental overdosing is prevented by allowing a maximum preset dose within an allotted interval. This method of self-administered analgesics has been shown to be safe and to give greater pain control in patients with postoperative pain following major surgical trauma, while the total amount of analgesia required has often been less than if given by conventional means.[61] Because analgesic needs vary widely among burned patients, patient-controlled analgesic therapy may offer a valuable strategy in the management of pain.[54]

Transcutaneous electrical nerve stimulation (TENS), another possible adjunct to pain management, has been recently found to be as effective as morphine in relieving pain during enzymatic debridement in burned patients.[62] Future prospects include transdermal narcotics and, for pediatric patients, fentanyl lollipops (Dr. Neil Schecter, personal communication).

The multiplicity of treatments vital to the survival and sustenance of a burned victim may lead to conflicting priorities that may sometimes relegate pain management to a low order of importance. Nonetheless, an awareness of the adverse effects of uncontrolled pain on the part of those involved in the care of the patient, as well as a knowledge of the many factors that may influence the perception of pain, may help prevent neglect of the problems of ameliorating pain.

## REFERENCES

1. Perry S, Heidrich G, Ramos E: Assessment of pain by burn patients. J Burn Care Rehab 2:322–326, 1981.
2. Winkelstein A: What are the immunological alterations induced by burn injury? J Trauma 24:S72–81, 1984.
3. Demling RH: What are the functions of endorphins following thermal injury? (Discussant) J Trauma 24:S172–176, 1984.
4. Kehlet H: Should regional anesthesia and pharmacological agents such as beta blockers and opiates be utilized in modulating pain response? J Trauma 24:S177–179, 1984.
5. Wilmore DW, Long JM, Mason AD, et al: Catecholamines: Mediator of the hypermetabolic response to thermal injury. Ann Surg 180:653–669, 1974.
6. Wolfe RR, Durkot MJ: Evaluation of the role of the sympathetic nervous system in the response of substrate kinetics and oxidation to burn injury. Circ Shock 9:395–406, 1982.
7. Perry S, Heidrich G: Management of pain during debridement: A survey of U.S. burn units. Pain 13:267–280, 1982.
8. Szyfelbein SK, Osgood PG, Carr DB: The assessment of pain and plasma beta-endorphin immunoactivity in burned children. Pain 22:173–182, 1985.
9. Atchison NE, Osgood PF, Szyfelbein SK, et al: The relationship of pain to the depth and extent of burn injury in the pediatric patient. Proc Am Burn Assoc 18:169, 1987.
10. Fagerhaugh S: Pain expression and control on a burn care unit. Nurs Outlook 22:645–650, 1974.
11. Walkenstein M: Comparison of burned patients' perception of pain with nurses' perception of patients' pain. J Burn Care Rehabil 3:233–236, 1982.
12. Perry SW: What objective measures are there for evaluating pain? (Speaker) J Trauma 24:S191–195, 1984.
13. Iafrati NS: Pain on the burn unit: Patient vs. nurse perceptions. J Burn Care Rehabil 7:413–416, 1986.
14. McCaffery M: Nursing Management of the Patient with Pain. Philadelphia, JB Lippincott, 1979, p 11.
15. Levine J: What are the functions of endorphins following thermal injury? J Trauma 24:S168–172, 1984.
16. Basbaum AI, Fields HL: Endogenous pain control systems: Brainstem spinal pathways and endorphin circuitry. Ann Rev Neurosci 7:309–338, 1984.
17. Terman CW, Lewis JW, Liebeskind JC: Endogenous pain inhibitory substrates and mechanisms. In Benedetti C, Chapman CR, Moricca G (eds): Advances in Pain Research. New York, Raven Press, 1984, pp 43–56.
18. Goldstein A, Lowney LI, Pal BK: Stereospecific and nonspecific interactions of the morphine congener levorphanol in subcellular fractions of mouse brain. Proc Natl Acad Sci USA 68:1742–1747, 1971.
19. Pert CB, Snyder SH: Opiate receptor: Demonstration in nervous tissue. Science 179:1011–1014, 1973.
20. Simon EJ, Hiller JM, Edelman I.: Stereospecific binding of the potent narcotic analgesic [³H] etorphine to rat-brain homogenate. Proc Natl Acad Sci USA 70:1947–1949, 1973.
21. Terenius L: Characteristics of the "receptor" for narcotic analgesics in synaptic plasma membrane fraction from rat brain. Acta Pharmacol Toxicol 33:377–384, 1973.
22. Hughes J, Smith TW, Kosterlitz HW, et al: Identification of two related pentapeptides from the brain with potent opiate agonist activity. Nature 258:577–579, 1975.

23. Li CH, Chung D: Isolation and structure of an untriakontapeptide with opiate activity from camel pituitary glands. Proc Natl Acad Sci USA 73:1145–1148, 1976.
24. Kakidani H, Furutani Y, Takahashi H, et al: Cloning and sequence analysis of cDNA for porcine β-neo-endorphin/dynorphin precursor. Nature 298:245–249, 1982.
25. Carr DB, Fisher JE: Opiate receptors, endogenous ligands, and anesthesia: A synopsis. In Estafanous FG (ed): Opioids in Anesthesia. Boston, Butterworth, 1984, pp 10–16.
26. Tyers MB: A classification of opiate receptors that mediate antinociception in animals. Br J Pharmacol 69:503–512, 1980.
27. Upton N, Sewell RDE, Spencer PSJ: Differentiation of potent μ and κ-opiate agonists using heat and pressure antinociceptive profiles and combined potency analysis. Eur J Pharmacol 78:421–429, 1982.
28. Yaksh TL: Multiple spinal opiate receptor systems in analgesia. In Kruger L, Liebeskind JC (eds): Advances in Pain Research and Therapy, Vol 6. New York, Raven Press, 1984, pp 197–215.
29. Pasternak GW: Commentary: Multiple mu opiate receptors: Biochemical and pharmacological evidence for multiplicity. Biochem Pharmacol 35:361–364, 1986.
30. Snyder SH: Drug and neurotransmitter receptors in the brain. Science 224:22–31, 1984.
31. Ling CSF, MacLeod JM, Lee S, et al: Separation of morphine analgesia from physical dependence. Science 226:462–464, 1984.
32. Caruso FS: Butorphanol: Clinical analgesic studies. In Foley KM, Inturrisi CE (eds): Advances in Pain Research and Therapy, Vol 8. New York, Raven Press, 1986, pp 253–257.
33. Lee J: Analgesic effects of nalbuphine hydrochloride (Nubain). J Burn Care Rehabil 8:316–317, 1987.
34. Akil H, Madden J, Patrick RL, Barchas JD: Stress-induced increase in endogenous opiate peptides: Concurrent analgesia and its partial reversal by naloxone. In Opiates and Endogenous Opioid Peptides. Amsterdam, Elsevier, 1976, pp 63–70.
35. Hayes RL, Bennett GS, Newlon PG, Mayer DJ: Behavioral and physiological studies of non-narcotic analgesia in the rat elicited by certain environmental stimuli. Brain Res 155:69–90, 1978.
36. Mayer DJ, Watkins LR: Multiple endogenous opiate and nonopiate analgesic systems. In Kruger L, Liebeskind JC (eds): Advances in Pain Research and Therapy, Vol 6. New York, Raven Press, 1984, pp 253–276.
37. Terman GW, Shavit Y, Lewis JW: Intrinsic mechanisms of pain inhibition: Activation by stress. Science 226:1270–1277, 1984.
38. Tricklebank MD, Curzon G: Stress-induced Analgesia. New York, Wiley, 1984.
39. Lewis JW, Terman GW, Shavit Y, et al: Neural, neurochemical, and hormonal bases of stress-induced analgesia. In Kruger L, Liebeskind JC (eds): Advances in Pain Research and Therapy, Vol 6. New York, Raven Press, 1984, pp 277–288.
40. Ventafridda V, Ripamonti C, Lodi F, et al: Pain intensity: Morphine and beta-endorphin plasma levels during chronic administration of oral morphine. In Foley KM, Inturrisi CE (eds): Advances in Pain Research and Therapy. New York, Raven Press, 1986, pp 95–102.
41. Osgood PF, Murphy JL, Carr DB, Szyfelbein SK: Increases in plasma beta-endorphin and tail flick latency in the rat following burn injury. Life Sci 40:547–554, 1987.
42. Dent RRM, Guilleminault C, Albert LH, et al: Diurnal rhythm of plasma immunoreactive beta-endorphin and its relationship to sleep stages and plasma rhythms of cortisol and prolactin. J Clin Endocrinol Metab 52:942–947, 1981.
43. Osgood PF, Atchison NE, Carr DB, Szyfelbein SK: Daily variation in beta-endorphin and cortisol plasma levels in the severely burned patient. Proc Am Burn Assoc 18:126, 1986.
44. Wise L, Margraf HW, Ballinger WF: Adrenal cortical function in severe burns. Arch Surg 105:213–220, 1972.
45. Hilberman M: Should regional anesthesia and pharmacological agents such as beta blockers and opiates be utilized in modulating pain response? (Discussant) J Trauma 24:S179–185, 1984.
46. Wakeman RJ, Kaplan JZ: An experimental study of hypnosis in painful burns. Am J Clin Hypn 21:3–11, 1978.
47. Paterson DR, Questad KA, Boltwood MD. Hypnotherapy as a treatment for pain in patients with burns: Research and clinical considerations. J Burn Care Rehabil 8:263–268, 1987.
48. Laird SM, Gray BM: Intermittent inhalation of methoxyflurane and trichloroethylene as analgesics in burn dressings procedures. Br J Anaesth 43:149–159, 1971.

49. Slogoff S, Allen GW, Wessels JV, Cheney DH: Clinical experience with subanesthetic ketamine. Anesth Analg 53:354–360, 1974.
50. White PF, Way WL, Trevor AJ: Ketamine—its pharmacology and therapeutic uses. Anesthesiology 56:119–136, 1982.
51. Baskett PJF: Analgesia for dressing of burns in children: A method using neuroleptanalgesia and entonox. Postgrad Med J 48:138–142, 1972.
52. Parbrok GD: Leucopenic effects of prolonged nitrous oxide treatment. Br J Anaesth 39:119–127, 1967.
53. Brodsky JB, Cohen EN, Brown BW, et al: Exposure to nitrous oxide and neurologic disease among dental professionals. Anesth Analg 60:297–301, 1981.
54. Martyn JAJ: Clinical pharmacology and drug therapy in the burned patient. Anesthesiology 65:67–75, 1986.
55. Demling RH, Ellerbe S, Jarrett F: Ketamine anesthesia for tangential excision of burn eschar: A burn unit procedure. J Trauma 18:269–270, 1978.
56. Inturrisi CE, Umans JG: Meperidine biotransformation and central nervous system toxicity in animals and humans. In Foley KM, Inturrisi CE (eds): Advances in Pain Research and Therapy, Vol 8. New York, Raven Press, 1986, pp 143–153.
57. Hill RG: The status of naloxone in the identification of pain control mechanisms by endogenous opioids. Neurosci Lett 21:217–222, 1981.
58. Nahata MC, Miser AW, Miser JS, Reuning RH: Analgesic plasma concentrations of morphine in children with terminal malignancy receiving a continuous subcutaneous infusion of morphine sulfate to control severe pain. Pain 18:109–114, 1984.
59. Dahlstrom B, Bolme P, Feychting P, et al: Morphine kinetics in children. Clin Pharmacol Ther 26:354–365, 1979.
60. Perry S, Inturrisi CE: Analgesia and morphine disposition in burned patients. J Burn Care Rehabil 4:276–279, 1983.
61. Dahlstrom B, Tamsen A, Paalzow L, Hartvig P: Patient-controlled analgesic therapy. Part IV: Pharmacokinetics and analgesic plasma concentrations of morphine. Clin Pharmacokinet 7:266–279, 1982.
62. Kimball KL, Drews JE, Walker S, Dimick AR: Use of TENS for pain reduction in burn patients receiving travase. J Burn Care Rehabil 8:28–31, 1987.

# 14

# Anesthetic Management of the Burned Patient

## J.A. JEEVENDRA MARTYN and S.K. SZYFELBEIN

Almost every organ experiences the systemic effects of burn injury. The skin serves many functions, including protecting against infection, preventing fluid loss, controlling body temperature, excreting some waste products, receiving sensory stimuli, producing vitamin D, and determining an individual's identity. In addition to the injury caused by direct inhalation of toxic chemicals, the respiratory system may be affected by the distant effects of cutaneous burn. The circulatory system may be on the verge of collapse from hypovolemia and sepsis. Renal function may be critically impaired. The burned patient is often agitated either because of hypoxia or because of severe pain. The extreme catabolic state usually requires specific nutritional management. Intravenous access may appear to be nonexistent. In spite of these problems, the burned patient usually has to be anesthetized a number of times. Each of the factors described above influences anesthetic and perioperative management.

The purpose of this chapter is to delineate general principles for providing a safe anesthetic to these critically ill patients. Although most of the problems that burn patients encounter (e.g., pain, fluid therapy) are discussed in other chapters, they are also briefly mentioned here whenever relevant. The anesthetic management of the patient for reconstructive surgery is not within the scope of this chapter.

## PATHOPHYSIOLOGICAL CONSIDERATIONS

### Airways

One of the most dramatic and life-threatening effects of thermal injury is the swelling and distortion of the upper airway. Patients are often intubated prophylactically for pulmonary toilet. Following intubation, patients should be sedated both for comfort and to prevent inadvertent extubation.

In addition to the direct effects of inhalation injury on the upper airway and lung tissue, a circumferential chest burn may create a corsette-like effect that decreases lung volume to the point of respiratory failure.[1] If the patient is being mechanically ventilated, peak airway pressures may rise progressively. If the patient is breathing spontaneously, the respiratory rate increases and tidal volume and functional residual capacity decrease. These changes in respiratory function can occur intraoperatively as well as in the intensive care unit. The final common problem is respiratory failure with worsening hypercapnia and hypoxemia. Similar impairment in excursion of the chest wall occurs in a circumferential burn of the abdomen, where increased intra-abdominal pressure slows the venous return to the heart.[2] Thus, in the presence of circumferential burns, longitudinal incisions must be made through the burn eschar to increase chest and abdominal wall compliance and thus improve pulmonary and cardiovascular function. The presence of bronchial secretions mandates the continuation of pulmonary toilet intraoperatively using aseptic techniques.

## Circulatory System

The massive efflux of fluid from the vascular compartment into both burned and nonburned tissue continues for a number of days after burn.[3] A variety of formulae have been described to aid in the resuscitation of the burned patient; these formulae should be used only as guidelines and should be adjusted according to the needs of the patient. During the first 24 to 36 hours after burn (the resuscitation phase), patients are usually hypovolemic, as evidenced by low urine volume (less than 0.5 ml/kg/min), low sodium excretion, and high hematocrit. During the next 7 to 10 days the edema fluid from both burned and nonburned areas is mobilized, and the patient may become hypervolemic, with resultant ventricular dysfunction.[4]

In the period after seven days of burn injury, patients may become hypovolemic because of increased renal losses due to a heightened glomerular filtration rate[5] and to tubular losses as a result of tubular dysfunction[6]; that is, adequate urine output may be seen even in the presence of hypovolemia. Thus, adequate and somewhat aggressive fluid replacement should occur prior to induction of anesthesia and should continue during the anesthesia; otherwise anesthetic administration in the face of hypovolemia may result in hypotension due to the combined effects of vasodilatation and cardiac depression by the anesthetic. The circulatory system may be compromised even prior to anesthesia by inadequate myocardial function due to burn disease[3, 7] or pre-existing systemic disease. Present experimental evidence supports the theory that, at least in burn trauma, colloid-containing solutions may have an advantage over crystalloids in terms of volume replacement in the burned patient, especially with regard to edema in nonburned areas.[3] The colloid/crystalloid controversy, however, continues.[8]

Cutaneous burn, when associated with other injuries, including visceral, electrical, or inhalation injuries, results in a need for resuscitation fluid volumes exceeding estimates based on per cent total body surface area (TBSA) burn.[9, 10] Low hematocrit or excessive volume requirements within the first 24 hours of burn should suggest the presence of such a co-existing injury.

## Renal Function

After thermal injury, renal function may be impaired owing to a variety of causes. Hypovolemia and/or myocardial dysfunction, with their resultant low cardiac output, may impair renal perfusion and produce acute tubular necrosis. An electrical burn or an ischemic or direct injury to an extremity may release myoglobin, which in turn may damage the renal tubules. In addition, treatment of burn wound infections may require the use of nephrotoxic antibiotics (see Chapter 16). Because of the many possible reasons for impaired function, anesthetic drugs must be chosen very carefully.

In most young, healthy patients who have been resuscitated adequately with no complications, cardiac output increases during the hypermetabolic phase, producing increased renal blood flow. Thus, renal clearance of many drugs such as antibiotics and cimetidine may be increased, particularly those eliminated by glomerular filtration.[5, 11] On the other hand, tubular function often continues to be depressed and, as indicated previously, can result in increased urine, sodium, and water excretion even in the presence of hypovolemia. Therefore, it is important to measure the quality as well as the quantity of urine. The reduced concentrating capacity of the tubules also contributes to diminished total water reabsorption. Even during hyperosmolar states, marked diuresis is common, suggesting inadequate renal response to antidiuretic hormone.[6] This finding emphasizes the limited value of urine volume measurement as a guide to renal function. Thus, when assessing glomerular and tubular function in the burned patient, creatinine clearance, urine volume, serum and urine osmolality, specific gravity, and sodium and potassium concentrations should be measured frequently.

## Electrical Injuries

The majority of electrical injuries occur to men, usually in an occupational setting. According to Joule's law, when a current passes through a conductor, the power (heat) is proportional to the amperage$^2$ × resistance; thus, bone and skin, which are poor conductors, very efficiently convert electrical energy to thermal energy. This accounts for the severe damage to periosseous muscle despite minimal damage to the outer tissue. The pathophysiology of electrical injury is discussed in Chapter 5.

A common immediate effect of an electrical injury is a loss of consciousness, which may be momentary or may persist for days.[9] Other immediate effects of electrical injury include seizures, cerebral edema/hemorrhage, and antidiuretic hormone disturbances. Concurrent injuries include broken bones and ruptured internal organs. Temporary quadriplegia is a rare immediate sequela of electrical injury. The intermediate effects occur three to five days after injury and commonly disappear within five days. These include temporary paralysis, pain in the trunk and extremities, headache, and autonomic disturbances such as painful arterial spasm and pupillary abnormalities. The late effects of electrical burn injury include a wide diversity of neurological sequelae that may involve one or more parts of the nervous system. Visceral complications include destruction of the abdominal wall and the underlying bowel, pancreatic necrosis, gallbladder disease, pseudodiabetic states, and coagulopathies.

## The Central Nervous System

The central nervous system (CNS) is vulnerable to several types of insult.[12] These include decreased oxygen delivery to the brain and may result from hypotension or from hypoxia secondary to altered pulmonary function. Direct effects of electrical injury may also alter the CNS function. Another major consideration is associated trauma. The patient who is injured in an automobile accident or by an object falling from a burning building may well have sustained a direct head injury in addition to inhalation and burn injury. If the airway is inadequate and the patient is suffering from hypoxia, no measure will restore normal CNS function until the airway problem has been corrected. The same is true of inadequate perfusion secondary to hypovolemia. Only after the inadequate airway has been corrected and circulating volume has been restored can the problem of direct CNS injury be addressed. Head injuries in burned victims test a physician's ability to control rises in intracranial pressure due to edema and, at the same time, to maintain cerebral perfusion pressure with adequate, sometimes massive, fluid resuscitation.

Severe psychological trauma may accompany burn injury. The event itself is surrounded with anger, guilt, and frustration, and the intensive care necessary for survival often consists of sleep deprivation, pain, and the administration of drugs that alter CNS function. The organic brain syndromes may be due to the combination of hypoxemia, carbon monoxide poisoning, drugs, and sepsis, resulting in encephalopathy.[12] Even the apparently comatose or sedated patient may be partially aware of his or her surroundings. Thus, the anesthesiologist must be acutely aware of the psychological health of the patient. Every move must be explained to the patient in an attempt to relieve fear and anxiety. The assistance of a psychiatrist or psychologist may help patients, parents, and staff to cope with the stresses of a major burn injury.

## PREOPERATIVE EVALUATION AND PREPARATION OF THE PATIENT

Early excision, wound closure, and grafting of the burn wound are now widely accepted procedures to improve the chances of patient survival.[13, 14] The early excision of burn tissue and rapid wound closure have been reported to eliminate post-burn immune system defects and to decrease fluid and protein losses.[3, 15] Therefore, it is now common practice for patients to undergo anesthesia and surgery following the initial stabilization and resuscitation. Patients are brought to the operating room early in the phase of burn injury, at a time when they are experiencing associated massive volume shifts, respiratory insufficiency, and unstable cardiovascular status, i.e., at a time when physical status is not optimal for maintenance of homeostasis during anesthesia. Nevertheless, every attempt should be made to return acid-base balance, oxygenation, and electrolytes to normal levels, as well as to update coagulation profiles, including platelet count.

When an anesthesiologist is consulting preoperatively, he or she must take into account the major physiological and psychological aberrations created by burn injury, in addition to the conventional concerns of any patient about to undergo surgery. The pertinent information should include time and extent of burn injury; when the patient last ate or drank; any history of allergies, problems with anesthetics, or blood transfusion; co-existing medical illnesses; recent drug history; and any family history of anesthetic misadventures.

The physical examination should include assessment of the airway, the presence of facial edema, and the adequacy of gas exchange. The cardiovascular system should be evaluated, noting pulse rate and rhythm, blood pressure, cardiac filling pressures (if available), and urine output. Neurological evaluation should include an assessment of the level of consciousness, orientation, and abnormalities of electrolytes.

Following evaluation, the anesthetic plan is based on a pathophysiological knowledge of the disease. Every patient with major burns has some or all of the problems listed in Table 14–1. Depending on the type and extent of surgery to be performed, the requisite amount of colloid and crystalloid fluid should be at hand for rapid infusion. (Perioperative fluid management is discussed in Chapter 15.) In the unintubated patient, preoperative visits should also include a close examination of the airway to ascertain possible difficulties with endotracheal intubation. Gastrointestinal function should also be closely monitored. Any evidence of gastrointestinal ileus should alert the anesthesiologist to the possible need for rapid induction of anesthesia in the unintubated patient. Rapid induction is not always necessary; it should not be assumed that patients who are being tube fed (which indicates normal gastrointestinal function) have empty stomachs even after a period of four to six hours of nothing by mouth.

### TABLE 14–1. Problems of Thermally Injured Patients

| | |
|---|---|
| Anemia | Immunosuppression |
| Airway deformity and obstruction | Limited intravenous sites |
| Altered drug response | Malnutrition |
| Circumferential burns | Metabolic aberrations |
| Coagulopathies | Monitoring difficulties |
| Coma | Multiple anesthetics |
| Electrical burns | Multiple organ failure |
| Hypoproteinemia | Pulmonary problems |
| Heat and water loss | Sepsis |

## PREOPERATIVE MEDICATION

Preoperative medication should be individualized for each patient, taking into account the factors previously discussed. Since many patients undergo frequent operations, they soon discover what they find pleasant or unpleasant. For example, one patient may desire oral premedication, another may prefer rectally administered methohexital, and a third would rather achieve sedation via an intravenous line. We rarely, if ever, use intramuscular injections; instead we rely on intravenous, oral, or rectal routes for premedication. Patients who previously have received multiple anesthetics often develop a tolerance to many anesthetic drugs and may require higher doses for premedication and induction.[16, 17] In the presence of an intravenous line, the critically ill burned patient will benefit most from the use of intravenous sedation titrated just prior to operating room transfer. A narcotic such as morphine is preferred because of its analgesic and sedative properties, which provide relief from the anxiety and pain associated with a trip to the operating room. Alternatively, a sedative such as lorazepam or midazolam may be used in combination with a narcotic such as meperidine or fentanyl. During transport, the anesthesiologist should maintain verbal contact with the conscious or even semiconscious patient, explaining every move. The unintubated patient should be warned that, upon waking from anesthesia, a tube may be present in the nose or mouth and that he or she may not be able to communicate as before.

Because of the increased incidence of stress ulceration in burned patients, antacid prophylaxis should be continued during the perioperative period.[7, 18] Cimetidine in normal doses is ineffective in burned patients. If patients have been on tube feeds and/or oral antacids (Mylanta), these should be stopped at least four to six hours prior to surgery, and the stomach should be aspirated prior to induction. In adults, at least 10 mg/kg cimetidine should be administered after the enteral feeding or antacids have been terminated.[5] In children, a 15- to 20-mg/kg dose is more appropriate prophylaxis.[19] Alternatively, ranitidine in the usual doses seems to be effective up to six hours after an intravenous dose.[20]

## INTRAVENOUS AND MONITORING LINES

Because of the critical and unstable nature of the patient and the massive volume losses associated with burn, close monitoring is essential. Intraoperative monitoring of major burns is similar to that of a patient undergoing any operation of similar magnitude. For every patient, inspired oxygen tension, temperature, electrocardiogram, expired carbon dioxide concentration, and blood oxygen saturation should be followed continuously. In the extensively burned patient, a blood pressure cuff may have to be placed over burned or recently grafted tissue, but great care should be taken to protect the underlying area, and cuffs must be sterilized before reuse.

Urinary catheters, arterial lines, and central venous or pulmonary artery catheters should be used in more critically ill patients. If an arterial line is not already present, it can be inserted after anesthesia has been induced. Direct, continuous arterial pressure measurements are the most accurate. We have used the radial, ulnar, dorsalis pedis, temporal, or femoral artery, depending upon the availability of nonburned areas. If all of these sites are burned, then it is appropriate to insert arterial lines through a burn wound in any of these sites after the area has been appropriately prepared. The arterial catheters are used for measuring blood pressure and for frequent blood sampling.

For major burn excision and grafting procedures, two large-bore intravenous lines, one of which preferably is a central catheter, should be established. The second venous line may be required for infusing drugs and measuring filling pressures. We have used the subclavian, internal jugular, and femoral veins quite extensively for these purposes. Sometimes it may be necessary to access the vessels through burned or surgically excised tissue. In these instances, the area through which the catheter is to be inserted should be thoroughly prepared with an antiseptic solution such as Betadine.

Some authors believe that the prolonged use (greater than 48 hours) of femoral venous lines should be avoided because of the risk of thromboembolism, even though this risk is small in burned patients.[21] Because of the high incidence of right-sided endocarditis, prolonged use of central venous and pulmonary artery catheters is discouraged unless clinically indicated.[22, 23] The prolonged use of intra-arterial catheters does not seem to cause any serious problems, provided that adequate preventive measures are taken.[24] The validity and usefulness of the flow-directed pulmonary artery catheter, however, are currently under question in a number of situations, including burns.[22, 23, 25] Thus, the routine use of pulmonary catheters in burned patients is discouraged, but in certain clinical situations these catheters provide useful information for therapeutic intervention. Invasive monitoring is as important as the vigilance and experience of the anesthesiologist in assessing the circulatory status of these patients during what is often a massive transfusion.

Monitoring clinical signs such as heart tones and urine output (quality and quantity), especially in children, is often more practical than monitoring pulmonary artery pressure. In patients with pre-existing cardiac and pulmonary disease, invasive monitoring of central pressures becomes more important. In patients with major burns and no cardiac or pulmonary disease, intra-arterial pressure monitoring alone should suffice. Every operating room should have immediate and easy access to blood gas analyses, hematocrits, and blood sugar, potassium, and ionized calcium levels. Since metabolic rate varies from patient to patient, monitoring oxygen saturation together with end-tidal carbon dioxide and expired oxygen tensions makes it possible to adjust fresh gas flows and ventilatory rates, particularly in patients in whom there is no access to an arterial line. Pulse oximetry has been a very useful addition to the monitoring of the critically ill burned patient. In addition to the fingers and toes, we have used the ear lobes, nares, tongue, and lips for monitoring oxygen saturation. Often no skin is available for the placement of EKG patches; in these instances, needle electrodes can be substituted. Alternatively, the EKG pads can be stitched onto the patient and used in both the operating room and the intensive care unit.

## INDUCTION AND MAINTENANCE OF ANESTHESIA

General anesthesia is usually the anesthetic of choice for patients undergoing burn surgery. In the face of sepsis, massive transfusion, and volume shifts, a well-controlled general anesthetic is often safer than a regional anesthetic, which may result in infection at the site of injection. In addition, sleep provides an escape from anxiety and the other psychological problems a patient might experience. Large burns most definitely require general anesthesia, as do electrical burns, owing to the fact that the extent of the electrical injury is often far greater than is appreciated preoperatively. Often the extent of the damage is evident only during exploration and debridement in the operating room.

The type of induction to be performed depends on the availability of intravenous access, the patient's age and desires, and the status of the airway and circulation. If an operation is to be performed in the acute resuscitation phase of injury, the major considerations for induction include the completeness of volume resuscitation and the presence or absence of airway damage. If the patient is experiencing facial edema and has not already been intubated, an awake intubation may be performed in the adult patient, although this procedure is not recommended in the child for psychological reasons. Children may be induced with incremental doses of diazepam or ketamine or with small doses of thiopental or narcotics and intubated following the administration of a nondepolarizing relaxant, provided that the child can be ventilated. Despite the clinical impression that ketamine is superior to thiopental in the hypovolemic patient, laboratory studies have not confirmed this impression.[26] Ketamine failed to show any superiority over thiopental when used in the minimal anesthetic dose for induction of anesthesia during hypovolemia. During the acute phase of thermal injury, halothane anesthesia and positive-pressure ventilation can decrease cardiac output significantly, despite normal filling or arterial pressures at the time of induction.[2, 27] Decreased cardiac output is usually in large part compensated for by decreased oxygen demands and increased oxygen extraction.[27] Fluid repletion should be continued during anesthesia, particularly in patients undergoing surgery within 24 hours of injury. Maintenance of anesthesia in these patients should not include anesthetic agents that cause myocardial depression.

Forty-eight hours after burn injury, fluid volume is usually better repleated. The patient is hypermetabolic, and cardiac output is increased 1.5- to three-fold. In the geriatric patient, this response is usually not very prominent; even though cardiac output is increased, older patients still can be quite sensitive to the effects of inhalational and other anesthetic drugs. Therefore, these should be administered with great caution. Gregoretti et al have documented that the administration of enflurane decreases cardiac output, oxygen delivery, and oxygen consumption.[28, 29] Despite the decreases in cardiac output during anesthesia, because metabolic requirements are also decreased, oxygen delivery is usually adequate, provided that hypotension is avoided. The administration of narcotics also decreases hypermetabolic and hyperdynamic circulation. These cardiovascular and metabolic changes revert to a hyperdynamic state with the discontinuation of anesthestic.[28, 29]

The repeated use of halothane in burned patients has been studied[30]; review of almost 2000 episodes of halothane anesthesia in 408 patients revealed no evidence of halothane hepatitis. Our experience in pediatric burned patients is quite similar. Little information is available on the repeated use of isoflurane or enflurane in burned patients, although one might anticipate no hepatic side effects with either of these anesthetics. The effects of long-term administration of nitrous oxide on bone marrow and the immune response also should not be ignored.[31] (The pharmacology and problems associated with anesthetics are reviewed in more detail in Chapter 12.)

Although anesthesiologists at the Shriners Burns Institute, Boston Unit, rarely use ketamine as the sole anesthetic, other institutions have used it with good results. With repeated use, narcotic or ketamine tolerance can develop.[16, 17, 32] Although definitive studies have not been performed, clinical impression suggests that burned victims have increased requirements for sedative, narcotic, and anesthetic drugs. The contributions made by altered target organ sensitivity, pharmacokinetics, and protein binding to the increased tolerance of drugs have not been completely defined; however, during sepsis or during the co-administration of drugs such as cimetidine, a physician must exercise caution, as both the kinetics and dynamics are altered. In summary, no single anesthetic agent or combination of agents is indicated or contraindicated in the extensively burned patient (with the exception of succinylcholine). Although ketamine has theoretical advantages in that it enhances circulatory dynamics, recent reports have suggested that the drug can produce hypotension in some septic patients.[32]

Burn injury creates a fascinating change in the response to neuromuscular blocking drugs. Depolarizing neuromuscular blockers such as succinylcholine produce life-threatening hyperkalemia.[33] Although this hyperkalemic response may not manifest itself until a few days after burn, we generally avoid the use of succinylcholine even in the first 24 hours. Burn injury greatly increases the need for nondepolarizing muscle relaxants, by as much as five times the dose and blood levels of an unburned patient.[33] (This subject has been reviewed in Chapter 12.) When rapid induction and intubation are necessary, high doses of atracurium or vecuronium may be useful, provided that the patient can be adequately ventilated following the administration of these drugs. The hemodynamic consequences of these high doses are unknown. The use of $H_1$ and $H_2$ histamine receptor antagonists may decrease the adverse hemodynamic consequences of high doses of neuromuscular relaxants as documented in nonburned patients.[34]

## OTHER CONSIDERATIONS

### Temperature Regulation

Damage to the skin due to a burn and the subsequent increase of blood flow to the burned area can cause heat loss through these areas to increase,[35] an effect that will be further enhanced by the inability of the skin blood vessels to constrict in response to the decrease in environmental temperature.[35] Thus, the patient should be covered with blankets during transport to the operating room; children are even more prone to hypothermia owing to their higher surface area–to-body weight ratio. The comfort temperature for the burned patient is much higher than normal (usually 75 to 80°F).[36] In the operating room the temperature should be raised to at least 75°F to decrease the possibility of convective and evaporative heat loss. Induction of general anesthesia decreases the metabolic rate, causes vasodilatation, and further compounds the problem of hypothermia.[37] Anesthetic drugs interfere with thermoregulatory control in several ways: (1) by blocking afferent input, (2) by lowering set point, and (3) by preventing efferent and afferent responses either centrally or peripherally.[37] For example, morphine produces hypothermia by depressing metabolic heat production.[38] These effects are mediated via the hypothalamus. Barbiturates also depress oxygen consumption and metabolism but by somewhat different mechanisms than morphine.[37] Inhalational agents promote surface blood flow and probably have some effect on the central thermoregulatory centers. Neuromuscular relaxants, by preventing the shivering response and lowering metabolic rate, will aggravate the occurrence of hypothermia during anesthesia.

After the induction of anesthesia, when the dressings are being removed and the patient is being evaluated, an Apollo radiant heat shield (Healthdyne, Inc., Marietta, GA) or radiant heat lamps may be placed over the body to maintain body temperature or to minimize temperature loss. Other adjuvants to prevent hypothermia include warming intravenous fluids, using warming blankets under the patient, and providing heated and humidified inspired anesthetic gases.

The intraoperative consequences of a decrease in temperature include depression of cardiac output and, if severe enough, ventricular fibrillation, abolition of hypoxic pulmonary vasoconstriction, movement to the left of the hemoglobin dissociation curve, release of catabolic hormones, including catecholamines, and reduction of hepatic and renal function.[37] The important postoperative consequences of hypothermia include shivering, delayed drug clearance, and masking of hypovolemia. Shivering can increase oxygen consumption by 400 to 500 per cent[39]; this further increases the already raised circulatory requirement in the burned patient. In addition, postoperative shivering can result in skin graft displacement and loss of graft. Therefore, every effort must be made to prevent decreases in body temperature. The hypothermic (less than 35°C) patient, particularly the very young and the very old, should not be extubated. Prevention of hypothermia should continue when the patients are transported from the operating room to the intensive care unit. Once again, heat loss can be prevented by covering the patient, changing the underlying wet sheets, and warming the infusions. The postoperative increase in oxygen consumption due to hypothermia can be prevented by the application of external warming techniques and the administration of meperidine.[39]

## Calcium Homeostasis

The marked fluctuations in the monovalent serum electrolyte composition which occur in patients after thermal injury have been well documented.[3, 7] Although some abnormalities in calcium metabolism, such as osteoporosis and heterotropic calcification, have been observed in patients hospitalized after trauma, the marked changes in the divalent cations, particularly depression of the total and ionized calcium levels during the acute and recovery phases of thermal injury, remain unclear. The fluctuations in both total and ionized calcium have been documented.[40] Significantly lower levels of calcium were observed immediately after burn injury and persisted as long as several weeks after injury. These levels can be further depressed acutely during the administration of solutions that bind calcium, including fresh-frozen plasma and albumin; the very low levels of calcium which result could cause electromechanical dissociation and circulatory collapse.[40]

The demonstration of marked hypocalcemia in the critically ill burned patient is consistent with previous reports that describe hypocalcemia with sepsis and with shock-like states.[41] The precise mechanisms involved in the development of hypocalcemia remain to be elucidated. In most patients, total protein concentrations are below normal. Although such changes could account for a lowering of total calcium, they cannot fully explain the ionized hypocalcemia because its measurement is independent of total protein content. However, as a result of burn injury, alterations could have occurred in protein structure which might result in increased binding of calcium. Other factors that might contribute to the hypocalcemia may include inappropriate response to parathyroid hormone, ionized hypomagnesemia, and increased calcium losses through burn wounds and urine.

The importance of normal calcium levels is related primarily to the role of calcium in both myocardial and peripheral vascular smooth muscle contraction. Even when arterial pressure is well maintained, marked disturbances in cardio-circulatory function may be present.[4, 41, 42] Because hemodynamic instability and cardiac arrest are often observed during rapid infusion of colloid substances such as albumin or fresh-frozen plasma, prophylactic administration of calcium chloride or calcium gluconate is encouraged.[41, 42] We empirically administer 1 mg of calcium chloride per kilogram of body weight per unit of citrated colloid or albumin to prevent such hemodynamic disturbances.

## POSTANESTHETIC MANAGEMENT

At the conclusion of the operation, a decision should be made regarding whether or not to extubate the patient based on his or her baseline condition, operative course, and plans for future care. Despite the measures taken to prevent it, hypothermia is one of the most common limiting factors that we have encountered. The shivering caused by intraoperative hypothermia and stormy emergence from anesthesia are common causes of early graft loss. Thus, adequate sedation and normothermia (greater than 36°C) should be established prior to extubation. Therefore, the recovery room bed should be made with warming blankets and prewarmed linen.

Great care must be taken to protect the very delicate, freshly grafted skin as well as the areas that have partially healed, because even slight abrasion or pressure can cause an area to slough. In some instances, therefore, emergence from anesthesia may be deferred by the administration of narcotics until the patient is suitably settled in his or her bed and the grafted areas are supported and protected. Significant intrapulmonary shunting may occur following anesthesia and surgery. Thus, if there is any potential for impairment of oxygenation or ventilation, the anesthesiologist should continue mechanical ventilation therapy in the postoperative period. Even in the extubated patient, oxygen supplementation should continue during transport from the operating room to the intensive care unit. If a halogenated anesthetic has been used as the primary drug, it is advisable to use a narcotic to prevent shivering and also to provide pain-free transport from the operating room. In the intensive care unit or in the recovery room, appropriate postoperative pain relief with systemic narcotics should be administered, since the stress induced by pain not only decreases the immune response but also further enhances the catabolic process.[43, 44] There is preliminary evidence to suggest that survival is better in patients appropriately sedated, narcotized, and mechanically ventilated to decrease the stress response compared with patients who did not undergo this regimen.[44]

## SUMMARY

The anesthesiologist is challenged on all fronts by the burned patient. Respiratory, circulatory, and other vital organ functions become dramatically altered, and the patient's psychological health may be equally affected. Care of the burned patient requires utmost co-operation from anesthesiologists, nurses, pediatricians, psychiatrists, surgeons, and family members. Successful anesthetic and intensive care management necessitates an understanding of the pathophysiology of injury and the co-operation of all individuals involved. By understanding, appreciating, and predicting preoperative, intraoperative, and postoperative problems, safe care can be provided for burned patients.

Attention should be focused on the decisive importance of preanesthetic management and the specific anesthetic problems of the burned patient. The choice of anesthetic should be related to the anesthesiologist's own experience, to the surgical procedure, and to the requirements of the surgeon. Most burned patients are well aware of the subtleties of their medical care and appreciate a kind and thoughtful approach. A smooth emergence from anesthesia cannot be overemphasized.

## *REFERENCES*

1. Demling H: Pulmonary dysfunction in the burned patient. J Burn Care Rehabil 7:277–283, 1986.
2. Turbow ME: Abdominal compression following circumferential burn: Cardiovascular responses. J Trauma 13:535–541, 1973.
3. Demling RH: Burns. N Engl J Med 313:1389–1398, 1985.
4. Martyn JAJ, Snider MT, Szyfelbein SK, et al: Right ventricular dysfunction following acute thermal injury. Ann Surg 191:330–335, 1980.
5. Martyn JAJ, Abernethy DR, Greenblatt DJ: Increased cimetidine clearance in burn patients. JAMA 258:1288–1291, 1985.
6. Eklund J, Gramberg PO, Kiljedahl SO: Studies on renal function in burns. Acta Chir Scand 136:617–640, 1970.
7. Moncrief JA: Burns. N Engl J Med 288:444–454, 1973.
8. Goodwin CW, Dorethy J, Pruitt BA: Randomized trial of efficacy of crystalloid and colloid resuscitation on hemodynamic response and lung water following thermal injury. Ann Surg 197:520–531, 1983.
9. Dixon GF: The evaluation and management of electrical injuries. Crit Care Med 11:384–387, 1983.
10. Navar PD, Saffle JR, Warden GD: Effect of inhalation injury on fluid requirements after thermal injury. Am J Surg 150:716–720, 1985.
11. Martyn JAJ: Clinical pharmacology and drug therapy in the burned patient. Anesthesiology 65:67–75, 1986.
12. Mohnot D, Snead OC, Benton JW: Burn encephalopathy in children. Ann Neurol 12:42–47, 1982.
13. Burke JF: Primary excision and prompt grafting as routine therapy for treatment of burns in children. Surg Clin North Am 56:477–494, 1976.
14. Demling RH: Improved survival after massive burns. J Trauma 23:179–184, 1983.
15. Echinard C, Sajdel-Sulkowska E, Burke P, Burke JF: The beneficial effects of early excision on clinical response and thymic activity after burn injury. J Trauma 22:560–565, 1982.
16. Perry S: Pain and anxiety in the burned patient. J Trauma 24:S191–S195, 1984.
17. Coté CJ, Petka AJ: Thiopental requirements may be increased in the children reanesthetized at least one year after recovery from extensive thermal injury. Anesth Analg 64:1156–1160, 1985.
18. Czaja AJ, McAlhany JC, Pruitt BA: Acute gastroduodenal disease after thermal injury: An endoscopic evaluation of incidence and routine history. N Engl J Med 29:925–929, 1976.
19. Martyn JAJ, Greenblatt DJ, Hagen J, Hoaglin DC: Burn injury alters pharmacokinetics and pharmacodynamics of cimetidine in children. Eur J Clin Pharmacol 36:361–367, 1989.
20. Oliveri M, Martyn JAJ: Rantidine pharmacokinetics and pharmacodynamics in burned patients. Proc Am Burn Assoc, 21:218, 1989.
21. Purdue GF, Hunt JL: Pulmonary emboli in burned patients. J Trauma 28:218–220, 1988.
22. Sasaki TM, Panke TW, Dorethy JF, et al: The relationship of central venous and pulmonary artery catheter position to acute right-sided endocarditis in severe thermal injury. J Trauma 19:740–743, 1979.
23. Echhrie M, Morgan AP, Moore FD: Endocarditis with the indwelling balloon-tipped pulmonary artery catheter in burn patients. J Trauma 18:664–666, 1978.
24. Gurman GM, Kriermerman S: Cannulation of big arteries in critically ill patients. Crit Care Med 13:217–220, 1985.

25. Robin ED: Death by pulmonary artery flow directed catheter (editorial). Chest 92:727–731, 1987.

26. Weiskoff RB, Bogetz MS, Roizen MF, Reid IA: Cardiovascular and metabolic sequelae of inducing anesthesia with ketamine or thiopental in hypovolemic swine. Anesthesiology 60:214–219, 1984.

27. Jim LJ, Lalonde C, Demling RH: Effect of anesthesia and positive pressure ventilation on early post-burn hemodynamic instability. J Trauma 26:26–33, 1986.

28. Gregoretti S, Gelman S, Dimick AR: Lack of immediate effects of wound excision on hyperdynamic circulation. J Burn Care Rehabil 9:180–183, 1988.

29. Gregoretti S, Gelman S, Dimick AR, Proctor J: Total body oxygen supply-demand balance in burned patients under enflurane anesthesia. J Trauma 27:158–160, 1987.

30. Gronert GA, Schaner PJ, Gunther RC: Multiple halothane anesthesia in burn patients. JAMA 205:878–880, 1968.

31. Amos RJ, Amess JA, Hinds CJ, Mollin DL: Incidence and pathogenesis of acute megaloblastic bone marrow—change in patients receiving intensive care. Lancet 2:835–838, 1982.

32. White PF, Way WL, Trevor AJ: Ketamine—its pharmacology and therapeutic uses. Anesthesiology 56:119–136, 1982.

33. Martyn JAJ, Goldhill DR, Goudsouzian NG: Clinical pharmacology of neuromuscular relaxants in patients with burns. J Clin Pharmacol 26:680–685, 1983.

34. Scott RPF, Savarese JJ, Ali HH, et al: Atracurium: Clinical strategies for preventing histamine release and attenuating hemodynamic response. Br J Anaesth 57:550–553, 1985.

35. Aulick LH, Wilmore DW, Mason AD, Pruitt BA: Depressed reflex vasomotor control of the burn wound. Cardiovasc Res 16:113–119, 1982.

36. Wilmore DW, Mason AD, Johnson DW, Pruitt BA: Effect of ambient temperature on heat loss in burn patients. J Appl Physiol 38:593–597, 1975.

37. Morley-Forster PK: Unintentional hypothermia in the operating room. Can Anaesth Soc J 33:515–528, 1986.

38. Taylor JW, Hander EW, Skreen R: The effect of central nervous system narcosis on the sympathetic response to stress. J Surg Res 20:313–320, 1976.

39. Henneberg S, Eklund A, Joachimsson A, Wiklund L: Effects of a thermal ceiling on postoperative hypothermia. Acta Anaesth Scand 29:602–606, 1985.

40. Szyfelbein SK, Drop LF, Martyn JAJ: Persistence of ionized hypocalcemia in burned patients. J Crit Care Med 9:454–458, 1981.

41. Drop LJ, Laver MB: Low plasma ionized calcium and response to calcium therapy in critically ill man. Anesthesiology 43:300–305, 1975.

42. Coté CJ, Drop LJ, Daniels AL, et al: Ionized hypocalcemia after fresh frozen plasma administration to thermally injured children. Anesth Analg 67:152–160, 1988.

43. Carli F, Itiaba K: Effect of heat conservation during and after major abdominal surgery on muscle protein breakdown in elderly patients. Br J Anaesth 58:502–507, 1986.

44. Demling RH: What are the functions of endorphins following thermal injury (discussion). J Trauma 24:S172–S176, 1984.

# 15

# Perioperative Fluid Requirements in the Thermally Injured Patient

## EDWARD G. PAVLIN

The nature of surgery for thermal injury has undergone great change in the past decade. Prior to 1978, most burns were treated with topical antibiotic therapy and an eschar allowed to form with daily "scrubbing." Those who survived came to the operating room for excision of scars. Often, the principal anesthetic problem was placement of an endotracheal tube in patients with contracting scars in the facial and neck region. The advent of early excision of the burn wound has necessitated that the anesthesiologist become much more aware of acute care of burn patients, including their peculiar and rapidly changing fluid requirements. We have had to contend with two aspects of fluid management; that secondary to the thermal injury itself and that secondary to the surgery of excising the burn wound.

The importance of fluid resuscitation in the immediate post-burn period (first 24 hours) is well appreciated and has been described elsewhere in this book. Familiarity with this early phase of treatment is important to the anesthesiologist because many patients come to surgery during this initial phase for treatment of other injuries sustained during the burn (e.g., open fractures, abdominal injuries, cranial injuries). While a small number of patients may undergo burn wound excision within hours of admission, the more common approach is to perform excision after 48 hours of stabilization and fluid resuscitation. In general, as much of the burn wound is removed as possible between the third and ninth day post injury during multiple visits to the operating room. This allows removal of most of the burn wound before bacterial burn wound sepsis begins. In our institution, the surgeons attempt to limit the amount of residual burn wound to less than 20 per cent total body surface area (TBSA) by nine days, with the concept that infection of this limited area of burn eschar is less likely to pose a threat to the life of the patient.[1] Thus, victims of major burn injury may be anesthetized three or four times in the early post-burn period.

Adequacy of fluid replacement is one of the most important problems associated with the perioperative management of such patients. The interlude in the operating room represents a period of intensive care during which the anesthesiologist must continue to provide the fluids normally required for that patient at that stage of his or her thermal injury. An appreciation of the natural history of the burn, as well as assessment of preoperative needs, is mandatory. Superimposed on this are the additional fluids required by the surgery itself.

## INSENSIBLE WATER LOSS

Since surgery involving burn wound excision typically starts on the third day post burn, or after the "immediate post-burn phase," the initial fluid resuscitation will have taken place. The period from the third through the nineteenth days is called the "early post-burn phase" and is characterized by fluid requirements that are quite different from those of the immediate phase. With the denaturing of the skin by heat, the ability of the skin to retain water is drastically reduced. The destruction of the stratum corneum and of lipids in the skin itself allows increased evaporation of water through the burn eschar. Normally, most evaporative water loss takes place through the lungs. The loss through burned skin adds considerably to that. A full-thickness burn has a surface vapor pressure similar to that of open water at the same temperature. A rule of thumb, elaborated by Artz et al, states that evaporative water loss in grams per hour is 25 + (per cent of TBSA burn × square meters of body area).[2] For example, a 70-kg patient (1.7 m²) with 50 per cent TBSA burn would lose 110 ml/hr of water through burned skin area. The rate of loss is modified by several factors: (1) A partial-thickness burned area loses water at a lesser rate; (2) loss is higher up to 10 days post burn and then diminishes; (3) dressings and auto- and homografting may diminish water loss. In the operating room, the wound is usually exposed and, therefore, loss may be maximal. Since the loss is salt-free, serum sodium concentration may be an important indicator of the preoperative state of hydration, with hypernatremia indicating requirements for increased water intake.

Since ventilation may be increased secondary to elevated metabolic rate, pulmonary free water loss may be elevated as well. Fever can accelerate the rate of loss.

In summary, with respect to replacement of insensible water loss in the operating room:

1. Note the fluid intake in the burn intensive care unit required to maintain normal urine output. This will be increased in the operating room because of increased wound exposure.

2. Serum sodium may be a useful aid in assessing fluid status preoperatively.

3. Heated and humidified inspiratory gases will diminish pulmonary evaporative loss.

4. Ultimately, a stable hemodynamic status and adequate urine output are the parameters of adequate fluid infusion. Our experience is that patients who seem to be adequately hydrated in the burn intensive care unit may become quite hypotensive on induction of anesthesia and may require rapid fluid infusion at this point.

## RED BLOOD CELLS

Anemia is a common finding in severely burned patients and may require attention in the preoperative period. In the immediate post-burn period, erythrocytes are damaged or destroyed by the heat[3] and are removed by the spleen in the first 72 hours. This decrease in red cell mass is not immediately apparent because of loss of plasma fluid and hemoconcentration. With fluid resuscitation, the deficit becomes more apparent. In the early post-burn period, when patients come to surgery, more red cell loss occurs. Causes of this are splenic clearance of damaged red cells, reduction in the rate of erythropoiesis,[4] and blood loss secondary to gastric ulcers, although this latter cause is now rare with the introduction of $H_2$-receptor antagonist therapy. Hemolysis may continue. The erythropoietic response to the anemia is diminished[5] for reasons that are at present unclear. The result is that patients with severe burns covering 25 per cent or more of TBSA may require red cell transfusion in the early post-burn phase, particularly before surgery for burn wound excision where blood loss can be anticipated. In the operating room, red cell transfusion may precede blood loss from the excision.

## HYPERALIMENTATION

Intravenous hyperalimentation may be utilized to meet caloric requirements when oral feedings are insufficient.[6] When high carbohydrate solutions are utilized, some potential complications may be observed. In the operating room, the hyperalimentation *must* be continued without interruption. Abrupt cessation has led to rebound hypoglycemia. We have interrupted hyperalimentation twice to administer blood in cases of very rapid exsanguination and have documented blood glucose of less than 35 gm/dl on these occasions. Sugar solution (10 per cent) or a bolus of 50 per cent glucose must be administered in the case of interruption.

## BLOOD LOSS (Excision)

As burn tissue is removed, variable rates of blood loss occur. The volume and rate of loss depend on the depth of the burn, the area excised, and the clotting profile of the patient.

Second-degree burns are usually excised tangentially in depths of approximately 6 microns. Either hand-driven or power dermatomes are used to sequentially remove very thin layers of burned skin until viable tissue is reached. Tissue is judged to be nonviable based on its gray shiny appearance—a judgment that calls for skill and experience on the part of the surgeon. The ultimate clinical sign of viability is the presence of profuse bleeding! Shallow and moderate-depth burns bleed briskly after one slice. Deeper burns may require one or more sequential excisions with the dermatome before diffuse capillary bleeding is encountered. If excision is deep enough, pulsatile flow may be encountered.

The rate of blood loss from the excision may be astonishingly and frighteningly high. Although rates vary between patients, we have encountered blood loss as high as 250 ml/minute! Excision of a second-degree burn consisting of 15 to 20 per cent TBSA may result in rapid loss of the equivalent of one circulating blood volume. The rate of loss may be so high that it often defies collection on sponges and accumulates under the drapes or on the floor. Furthermore, blood is not collected via a suction device, so there is no visual index of hemorrhage available. Blood loss is, therefore, estimated by observation of the surgical field and by observation of clinical signs (blood pressure and central venous pressure). While this is less than satisfactory, there is currently no other means for measurement that keeps up with the extraordinary rates of loss, although careful collection and weighing of blood clot and sponges may yield retrospective blood loss data. Obviously, the anesthesiologist must be prepared for severe hemorrhage. Deep (third-degree) burns may be fascially excised; that is, eschar and fat are removed from muscle fascia utilizing scalpel and cautery. Bleeding is pulsatile (arterial) or venous rather than of the diffuse capillary type. Although the rate of loss is considerably slower than that experienced in excision of burn wounds of moderate depth (second-degree), surgical time of actual excision is longer. Thus, although replacement at the rate of loss is more easily accomplished, cumulative blood loss may be significant.

Estimation of blood loss is quite difficult for the reasons described. We rely on visual estimation by the surgeon and anesthesiologist. Clearly, experience is a factor here. Continuous monitoring of arterial blood pressure and central venous pressure utilizing vascular catheters is of great help. During and after the excision, urine output and serial hematocrits may be utilized in determining further fluid requirements. We rarely utilize pulmonary artery catheterization unless other indications exist (heart failure, myocardial infarction).

Clearly, homologous blood transfusion may be life-saving in these circumstances of rapid hemorrhage. However, each unit administered poses well-known risks, including transmission of disease (notably hepatitis) and immunological complications ranging from fever and urticaria to acute hemolysis.

Autologous blood donation practiced before elective surgery and scavenging of shed blood do not have applicability in burn surgery. Furthermore, blood availability may be limited in some areas because of increased demand (cardiac and transplant surgery) and decreased donations. Ideally, then, transfusion of red cells should be sufficient to prevent morbidity secondary to anemia in the postoperative period but should be limited to minimize patient complications. The issue of the optimum hematocrit in perioperatively transfused patients has been the subject of a recent N.I.H. consensus conference on perioperative red blood cell transfusion.[7] Intra- and postoperative transfusion practice in the past has dictated that a hematocrit of at least 30 be maintained to forestall complications of decreased oxygen delivery. This value has undergone reassessment in light of clinical observations that patients who have refused blood transfusion for surgery and have had profound hemorrhage have survived the resulting anemia. There is some evidence that some patients with acute anemia with a hematocrit of less than 20 may do less well postoperatively. In addition, the combination of hypovolemic hypotension and anemia may be devastating. The consensus was that patients with hematocrits less than 20 usually require transfusion, while those with hematocrits greater than 30 seldom do.

The issue of optimum transfusion in the burned patient is more complicated for several reasons:

1. The increased metabolic rate secondary to the burn injury requires oxygen delivery dramatically above that of the normal postsurgical patient.

2. The decreased oxygen delivery of anemia may be compensated for by an increased cardiac output. In thermally injured patients, cardiac output may already be doubled secondary to the increased metabolic demand. The ability of the cardiovascular system to respond to a superimposed anemia is not clear.

3. In more normal patients, acute anemia may result in increasing red cell production, whereas burned patients may not demonstrate this response.

Thus, the optimum target hematocrit in the burned patient is speculative. We aim for a hematocrit in the 26 to 30 range, but patients must be carefully monitored for signs and measures of inadequate oxygen delivery. Hypovolemia in particular is treated aggressively in the presence of low red blood cell counts. Clearly, more studies are required on the optimum blood oxygen–carrying capacity in the hypermetabolic burned patient.

## ADMINISTRATION OF FLUIDS

Intravenous access may be limited by the area burned and by the multiple venipunctures these patients receive during their hospital stay. Because of fear of introducing infection into the blood, access through burned area is avoided unless no other alternative exists (as in the case of TBSA involvement greater than 90 per cent). If burned areas are used, intravenous cannulae should be removed as soon as possible. For an excision of 10 per cent TBSA or more, two large gauge (at *least* 16 gauge) cannulae are strongly recommended. Superficial veins on extremities are preferred, since extravascular infusion at high rates of flow may be detected more quickly and possibly with less physiological perturbations than via a central line. If a central line is required, femoral or internal jugular cannulae are inserted and removed postoperatively.

The very rapid infusion rates required necessitate a pressure administration set. The conventional pressure bags suffice, but the compressed air–powered Alton Dean Infusion Device is faster and more convenient. In the case of children of 15 kg or less, infusion is effected with a stopcock and 50-ml syringe placed distal to the blood warmer and proximal to the intravenous site. This allows rapid administration for children with circulating blood volumes of a liter or less and an accurate measure of fluid or blood administered, precluding inadvertent volume overload.

All intravenous fluid, whether blood products or crystalloid, should be warmed prior to infusion. Conventional contact fluid warmers are adequate for infusion rates up to 20 ml/minute but become progressively less efficient at higher rates of administration. At rates of 100 ml/minute, fluid is warmed from 21°C to just 27°C at the infusion site. Since the thermally injured patient is already prone to hypothermia, the inadequate warming of large volumes of fluid may contribute significantly to a decrease in core temperature in the operating room environment. A newer generation of fluid warmers utilizes the countercurrent principle of warming; water heated to 41°C is pumped through a cyclinder while blood flows down concentrically placed tubing within the cylinder. Heat transfer is very efficient, such that blood may be warmed to 37°C at administration rates of 800 ml/minute! Level One and Haemonetics produce and market this type of equipment.

## METHODS OF DECREASING BLOOD LOSS

A number of techniques exist to diminish loss of blood; each has its own advantages and disadvantages.

1. Tourniquets placed on the extremities and inflated during excision may eliminate some blood loss. Obviously this technique is not suitable for excision involving the trunk or head and neck. A disadvantage is that during tangential excision of a second-degree burn wound, capillary blood loss is utilized as a sign of viability of dermal tissue and a signal to stop excision.

2. Epinephrine-soaked dressings are placed on the excised wound after removal of the burned tissue. Combined with pressure, vasoconstriction from the 1/10,000 dilution of epinephrine limits postexcision bleeding. When this technique was first proposed, we had concerns regarding the possibility of ventricular arrhythmias and hypertension secondary to systemic absorption of epinephrine. Careful continuous monitoring of our first 30 patients revealed no such complications. A later study[8] showed that blood levels of epinephrine were extremely high and prolonged, but the systemic response was much less than expected. We have, however, eliminated use of halothane anesthesia if epinephrine dressings are to be used.

3. Induced hypotension has been described as useful in one case report.[9] We have some concerns regarding the use of controlled hypotension in patients with cardiac output and oxygen requirements that may be double those of a normal patient. A study utilizing full cardiac monitoring, including pulmonary artery catheter placement during pharmacological hypotension in severely burned patients, is still lacking.

4. Scavenging and processing of shed blood has become popular and efficacious during surgery in traumatized patients. In burned patients, however, we have found that the collection and washing of shed red blood cells, utilizing

a Cell Saver (Haemonetics), did not eliminate bacterial contamination of the shed blood by the burned tissue. We are, therefore, reluctant to utilize this collection technique.

5. Topical thrombin on the excised area has been utilized. This technique is very expensive and of questionable efficacy.

## COMPLICATIONS OF FLUID THERAPY

Complications arise from the techniques used for infusion and the volume infused relative to need. The issue of catheter placement in burned tissue is an important one because of the possibility of introducing bacteria into the blood. Our preferred sites for central catheterization are either the femoral or internal jugular veins. We avoid, at all costs, penetrating burned eschar for this access. In fact, access through excised areas is preferred. Six hours postoperatively, the catheter is removed.

Infusing large volumes of blood products during periods of rapid and largely unmeasured blood loss is fraught with the danger of volume overload. Blood pressure (often from an arterial cannula), occasionally central venous pressure, and urine output remain the mainstays of monitoring fluid requirements. Most patients who have received volume overload resulting in congestive heart failure have tended to be in day three to six post burn. In this period, fluid is being mobilized from the edematous tissue, increasing intravascular volume. Cardiac depression, possibly from a circulating "cardiac depressant factor," has been described in the immediate post-burn period.[2] This may persist into the early period as well, but this is speculative. Thus, at this stage of injury, burned patients may be more prone to pulmonary edema.

Another fluid infusion that must be taken into account is the subcutaneous saline placed to increase tissue tension to better enable the harvesting of autograft. This technique, which may result in infusion of volumes over 1 liter, is used particularly in elderly patients and in children. This fluid must be included in the total volume administered.

We have noticed that large-volume infusions in patients placed prone for surgery may result in sufficient edema of the loose tissues of the face and oropharynx to cause airway obstruction postoperatively.

## POSTOPERATIVE CONSIDERATIONS

The postoperative period is one of reassessment of fluid needs for the next 24 hours. It is during this period that complications of fluid therapy are most often detected and treated. During the surgery, fluid requirements and red blood cell replacement are estimated at a time of rapid change during hemorrhage and anesthesia. As the patient regains stability postoperatively, various compartmental fluid shifts may occur which will require attention. Hypothermia may mask a relative hypovolemia. Careful monitoring of hemodynamic parameters and assessment of urine output may reveal the need for increased intravenous fluids. Serial hematocrits are useful in reassessing red blood cell requirements brought about by hemorrhage during burn wound excision.

## REFERENCES

1. Heimbach D, Engrave L: Surgical Management of the Burn Wound. Orlando, FL, Grune and Stratton, 1984.
2. Artz CP, Moncrief JA, Pruit BA: Burns: A team approach. Philadelphia, WB Saunders Company, 1979.
3. Kimber RJ, Lander H: The effect of heat on human red cell morphology, fragility and subsequent survival in vivo. J Lab Clin Med 64:922, 1961.
4. Andes WA, Rogers PW, Beason JW, et al: The erythropoietin response to the anemia of thermal injury. J Lab Clin Med 88:584, 1976.
5. Robinson H, Monafo WW, Saver SM, et al: The role of erythropoietin in the anemia of thermal injury. Ann Surg 178:565, 1973.
6. Askanazi J, Carpentier YA, Elwyn DH, et al: Influence of total parenteral nutrition on fuel utilization in injury and sepsis. Ann Surg 191:40–46, 1980.
7. Perioperative red blood cell transfusion—consensus conference. JAMA 260:2700–2703, 1988.
8. Timmonen RM, Pavlin EG, Hashke RH, et al: Epinephrine levels pre and post application of topical epinephrine during burn surgery. Anesthesiology 57(Suppl):A138, 1982.
9. Szyfelbein SK, Ryan JF: Use of controlled hypotension for primary surgical excision in an extensively burned child. Anesthesiology 41:501–503, 1974.

# 16

# Renal Function in Burns

JOHN T. HERRIN

The renal consequences of thermal injury may be directly associated with changes in renal function in response to the metabolic and circulatory consequences of the burn injury; with changes occasioned by the effects of therapy; or with the results of complications such as infection, pigment release, hemoglobin, and myoglobin (Table 16–1). An outline of changes in renal function in relation to differential diagnosis and therapy follows.

In the initial 24 hours after a burn injury, there occurs a marked shift of volume from the intravascular compartment to the burned area and the interstitial space, especially muscle.[1] This shift in fluid is most prominent in the first few hours and is proportional to the extent and depth of the burns. Hence, the initial renal response is to hypovolemia and decreased effective circulation. Urine flow decreases while urine osmolality or specific gravity rises and the fractional excretion of sodium ($FE_{Na}$) (Table 16–2) and sodium concentration in urine decrease.[2, 3] This response follows any diminution of circulating blood volume such as dehydration or trauma and is the result of renal response to antidiuretic hormone (ADH) and aldosterone.[4] This hypovolemic response occurs most likely in the very early post-burn period or when there has been inadequate resuscitation. In many burned patients, however, urinary electrolytes, serum, and urinary osmolalities show wide variations not co-ordinated with plasma vasopressin or hemodynamic variables.[5] Electrolyte excretion, however, does correlate with urine output.[7] High urine sodium reflects tubular rejection of sodium with resultant osmotic or solute diuresis. The degree of tubular sodium rejection varies with the extent of burns and may decrease the reabsorption of water. Underlying changes in renal function may thus be obscured by differences in treatment which vary the sodium load.

Further variations may reflect the administration of sodium in resuscitation fluid, volume expansion, and, in some patients, inappropriate secretion of vasopressin (ADH). Inappropriate secretion of ADH has been described especially after the third day and may cause dilutional serum hyponatremia with accompanying high concentrations of urinary sodium.[8, 12] If resuscitation is adjusted to maintain an adequate urine flow and sodium excretion, adequate circulation will be maintained. If resuscitation is not sufficient to restore effective circulation, acute renal failure may follow. When renal damage is present, tubular response to ADH and aldosterone does not occur. For example, in acute tubular necrosis the urine osmolality is low and $FE_{Na}$ is greater than 2 to 3 per cent.

## TABLE 16–1. Renal Response to Thermal Injury

| | Days 1–2 | Days 4–7 | Days 7–35 |
|---|---|---|---|
| Renal Blood Flow Glomerular Filtration Rate | Increased—response to tissue products Varies within circulation Decreased in severe burns with pigment, myoglobin, carboxyhemoglobin, sepsis, acute renal failure | Increased Increased creatinine clearance varies with age, burn surface area Corollary—increase drug doses —cimetidine —aminoglycosides | Variable (Continues) increased |
| Tubular Functions Proteinuria | Variable = nil, transient tubular, mixed Albumin, IgG = glomerular Low MW, microglobulin/acid mucoprotein Beta$_2$-microglobulin (selective decrease in reabsorption with tubular damage) | Maximum proteinuria Tubular type | Clear |
| Sodium FE$_{Na}$ | Decreased—poor circulation —nonoliguric renal failure Increased—acute renal failure —syndrome of inappropriate antidiuretic hormone —tubular rejection of Na | Increased Na loss—soluble diuresis | Solute diuresis clearing Decreased FE$_{Na}$—sepsis Increased FE$_{Na}$—renal tubular damage |
| Water | P$_{osm}$ varies with burn area U$_{osm}$ not co-ordinated with P$_{osm}$ Decreased urine volume | Increased reabsorption, antidiuresis | Antidiuresis—less severe Variable diuresis |
| Endogenous toxins | C$_{osm}$/C$_{creat}$ varies with burn area Carboxyhemoglobin, hemoglobinuria—burn in enclosed space, acute renal failure Myoglobinuria—severe deep burn | Pigment release hemolysis/ escharotomy Antibiotic | |
| Therapeutic factors and complications | Resuscitation Antibiotic—sepsis Anesthesia | Antibiotic | Sepsis |

**TABLE 16–2. Fractional Excretion of Sodium**

$FE_{Na}$ is calculated by comparing excreted sodium to filtered sodium, i.e.,

$$FE_{Na} = \frac{\text{excreted sodium}}{\text{filtered sodium}} \times 100\%$$

$$FE_{Na} = \frac{U_{Na} \times V}{GFR \times P_{Na}} \times 100 = \frac{U_{Na}}{P_{Na}} \times V \times \frac{P_{creat}}{U_{creat} \times V} \times 100 = \frac{U_{Na}}{P_{Na}} \times \frac{P_{creat}}{U_{creat}} \times 100\%$$

where $FE_{Na}$ = fractional excretion of sodium; Na = sodium; creat = creatinine; GFR = glomerular filtration rate; U = urinary concentration; P = plasma concentration.

$$FE_{Na} = \frac{\text{sodium excreted in urine}}{\text{sodium filtered in urine}} \times 100\%$$

$$= \frac{U_{Na} \times V}{GFR \times P_{Na}} \times 100\%$$

$$= \frac{U_{Na} \times V}{P_{Na}} \times \frac{P_{creat}}{U_{creat} \times V} \times 100\%$$

$$= \frac{U_{Na}}{P_{Na}} \times \frac{P_{creat}}{U_{creat}} \times 100\%$$

Hemolysis and rhabdomyolysis are common in patients with extensive deep (third-degree) or electrical burns. In the presence of hypovolemia or hemoconcentration, particularly in the presence of low urine flow, the risk of pigment nephropathy with acute renal failure is high.[13, 14]

Two to three days after burn injury, as capillary integrity is restored, a diuretic phase occurs as fluid reabsorbed from the extracellular fluid space is mobilized and excreted.[15] Treatment in this phase adds such potentially compounding factors as anesthesia, primary excision in patients with large burns, respiratory tract burns, and respiratory therapy, all of which alter the expected response and usually tend to blunt the diuresis. After day four, there is an increase in the glomerular filtration rate with associated sodium diuresis and an initial inability to fully concentrate the urine.[7, 16]

It is convenient for discussion of the changes in renal blood flow, glomerular filtration, and tubular function to artificially divide time post burn and to regard renal functions as if they occur separately: first 48 hours after injury; 4 to 7 days after injury; and 7 to 35 days or longer after injury.

## THE FIRST 48 HOURS

The first 48 hours are characterized by acute phase injury. Fluid losses produce hemodynamic stress and therapy is characterized by fluid resuscitation to maintain the circulation.

## Change in Renal Blood Flow

If resuscitation efforts are delayed, there is hemodynamic compromise, notably hypovolemia and hemoconcentration. Renal blood flow and the glomerular filtration rate decrease, and there is an accompanying hormonally stimulated decrease in the fractional excretion of sodium and water. That decrease in urine flow is the expected normal response to dehydration or trauma. If hypovolemic stress is continued to full vascular compromise, there will be an initial decrease in tubular function followed by the onset of acute renal failure.[14, 17] This complication is rare in the 1980s.[1]

After this initial phase, adequate resuscitation is followed by an increase of blood flow or response to the products of tissue trauma and injury.[1, 18] Tissue elements, including histamine, bradykinin, prostaglandin, and free oxygen radicals, are released from burned or damaged tissue. These products lead to changes in renal blood flow and redistribution of intrarenal blood flow and the potential for cellular damage.[19, 20] The magnitude of this change in renal blood flow is proportional to the burn surface area.[7, 21]

## Change in Glomerular Function

The rate of glomerular filtration is proportional to effective circulating blood volume and to the resulting renal blood flow.[7, 15, 22] Glomerular ultrafiltration is produced by a number of factors, including transcapillary hydrostatic pressure, the ultrafiltration coefficient (a function of the barrier function of the basement membrane), plasma flow (proportional to renal blood flow), and concentration of plasma protein, which directly influences the colloid osmotic pressure.[22]

The increase in the glomerular filtration rate seen in the patient with burns may result from increases in transcapillary hydrostatic pressure, secondary to relative hypervolemia and hypertension common in the burned patient and increased renal blood flow.[15] If the concentration of plasma protein is low, colloid osmotic pressure is decreased, thereby increasing the relative transcapillary pressure. This results in an increased rate of glomerular filtration and decreased reabsorption of proximal tubular fluid, leading to solute diuresis and interference with the apparent renal function in the distal tubule, e.g., decrease in concentrating ability.[18]

## Changes in Tubular Function

### Protein Excretion

A spectrum of changes in protein excretion has been observed.[22, 23] In the initial phase (less than 48 hours after burn injury) a mild, transient glomerular lesion may be present, in which increased filtration pressure from such vasoactive substances as renin, angiotensin, and catecholamines leads to a glomerular proteinuria with excretion of relatively high molecular weight proteins such as albumin (80 kDa) and IgG (150 kDa).[22] An associated selective secretion of lower molecular weight proteins that pass easily through the glomerular filtration membrane will occur. These proteins, antichymotrypsin, alpha$_1$-acid glycoprotein, alpha microglobin (33 kDa), and beta$_2$-microglobulin (11.8 kDa), are normally reabsorbed and degraded by tubular epithelial cells. Their presence in patients having glomerular damage represents a limitation of reabsorption with overflow in urine. The pattern of proteinuria rather than pure molecular weight comparison is important.[23]

Heavy glomerular proteinuria is rare and is confined to those patients with glomerular damage from circulatory insufficiency with associated decrease in renal blood flow. Maximal proteinuria occurs later (four to seven days) and most commonly demonstrates a pattern of tubular proteinuria.[24] (This is discussed in greater detail under changes in Tubular Function—Four to Seven Days).

### Sodium

In the first two days after injury, fractional excretion of sodium decreases, presumably secondary to the hormonal actions of the renin-angiotensin-aldosterone system, which are a response to variations in effective circulatory status.[25] This is followed over the next few days by a gradually increasing rejection of sodium by the tubules, increasing the fractional excretion of sodium. This increase is proportional to the total burn surface area (TBSA) and is associated with a concomitant increase in the volume of urine flow, similar to a pattern seen in nonoliguric renal failure.[2, 26, 27]

### Water Handling by the Tubules

An increase in free water absorption occurs with antidiuresis. The magnitude of antidiuresis does not correlate with the extent of the burn or with plasma osmolality or ADH levels.[5, 15, 28] Since plasma osmolality is related to the TBSA of the burn, the changes observed in tubular function represent a lack of appropriate response to osmolar regulation.[6, 18, 28] Careful control of electrolyte and fluid balance, adequate water to excrete the osmolar load generated from injured tissue, and nutritional support are required. Continued replacement of lost sodium is necessary after the first 48 hours when empirical formulae are of less assistance in estimating fluid and electrolyte needs. Table 16–3 outlines guidelines for the administration of fluid and electrolytes. Measurement of serum osmolality is helpful in determining whether plasma water content is normal. Abnormalities are seen not only in overhydration or dehydration, but also in the presence of such foreign low molecular substances in the blood as glucose, urea, amino acids, mannitol, and products of the breakdown of burn tissue or substances observed from drugs or topical agents.[29–31]

Although osmolar clearance (Table 16–4) does not correlate with the extent of the burns, the ratio of osmolar clearance to creatinine clearance ($C_{osm}/C_{creat}$) is proportional to burn surface area.[16, 28] This osmotic diuresis with signs of tubular dysfunction is similar to the pattern seen in nonoliguric renal failure.[18, 27]

**TABLE 16–3. Guidelines for Administration of Fluid and Electrolytes**

**Intravenous resuscitation required**
  Adults burned greater than 20% TBSA
  Children burned greater than 10% TBSA
  Electrical injury
  Pigmenturia—hemoglobinuria, myoglobinuria
**Resuscitation formulae—1st 48 hours**
  Brooke formula
  Parkland formula
  Evans formula
  Monafo (hypertonic replacement) formula
**Monitoring: aim at following parameters**
  Urine flow 1.5 ml/kg/hr child; 50 ml/hr adult
  Urine sodium greater than 40 mEq/L (random)
  Urine osmolality less than 750 mOsm/L
  Serum sodium less than 140–155 mEq/L
  Serum osmolality 280–310 mOsm/L
  Hematocrit 30—45%
  Serum proteins (total) greater than 2.5 gm/dl day 1–2
            greater than 4.5 gm/dl after day 4

Alternative explanations of this pattern of osmotic diuresis include (1) decreased medullary osmolar gradient; (2) increased nonreabsorbable colloid in the tubular fluid from products of tissue destruction; (3) tubular cell injury in the burn patient; (4) diuresis from the osmolar load of administered substrates for nutrition—glucose or amino acids; or (5) diuresis from the vehicle for topical or intravenous medications such as glycerin or propylene glycol.[30, 31] Such products of cell breakdown could alter the function of the cells of the ascending loop of Henle or could redistribute blood flow from the cortex to the medulla.

After the first 48 hours, as the fractional excretion of sodium rises, the distal tubular fluid becomes less dilute (approaching isomolar), resulting in a decrease in the reabsorption of water and in the ability to fully dilute the urine, leading to an isosthenuric urine. It is possible that nonreabsorbable colloids, if formed, would produce an osmotic diuresis similar to that seen in patients with trauma or with carbohydrate or protein intolerance.[16]

The patient is at risk during this period of decreased concentrating ability and limited diluting ability, since he or she cannot respond to changes in the plasma osmolality. A higher water intake will be required to allow excretion of any increased osmolar burden if the risk of serum hyperosmolality is to be

**TABLE 16–4. Osmolar Clearance**

**Mathematical Definition:**

$$C_{osm} = \frac{U_{osm}}{P_{osm}} V$$

where $C_{osm}$ = osmolar clearance, $U_{osm}$ = measured urinary osmolality, $P_{osm}$ = measured plasma osmolality, $V$ = volume flow of urine in ml/min.
**Descriptive Definition:** Osmolar clearance is the theoretical volume of plasma cleared of osmotically active particles per unit time and is equivalent to the volume of urine, isomotic with plasma, which is necessary to excrete these particles.

avoided.[29] As this osmotic diuretic phase is entered, serum potassium decreases significantly and hypokalemia becomes a risk.

## FOUR TO SEVEN DAYS

### Glomerular Function

Most early phase studies of renal function cover this four- to seven-day period because it excludes the marked changes of fluid shifts during the first 48 hours post burn and resuscitation. Clinical studies are difficult to control in the earlier phase of injury because the first priorities are treatment and maintenance of circulation. During the later period, as circulation stabilizes, renal blood flow increases and is sustained at stable levels and glomerular function increases. Changes in glomerular function, measured as creatinine clearance (related to insulin clearance and iodothalamate clearance in burned patients after acute phase of one to two days), confirm that creatinine clearance is proportional to the patient's age. Although Martyn et al have shown a correlation of the increased creatinine clearance to increased TBSA of burn, such a correlation has not been seen in other studies.[16, 21, 32] In fact, Loirat et al found no relationship among creatinine clearance and fluid intake, TBSA burned, and temperature, despite elevated glomerular filtration in most patients studied.[32]

Increased cardiac output at this time varies with TBSA of burn, and serum hypoproteinemia and hypervolemia are expected to increase glomerular ultrafiltration with a consequent increase in creatinine clearance. Such clearance alters the effective level of those drugs excreted by filtration. Thus, cimetidine and tobramycin require higher dosages and monitoring of drug levels for optimal therapy.[21, 32] Additional factors of altered enzyme activity and target organ sensitivity change drug activity in patients with trauma and burns.

### Changes in Tubular Function

#### *Proteinuria*

Between days four and seven, while increased glomerular filtration is present, protein excretion reaches a maximum.[23, 24] This is usually of a mixed (glomerular and tubular) pattern and rarely reaches clinically significant levels of loss.[24] Infusions of exogenous serum albumin during this time have been observed to increase protein losses, particularly of serum albumin. This suggests that the apparent solute diuresis decreases tubular reabsorption, and even the presence of minor glomerular changes can overwhelm the reabsorptive mechanisms and lead to significant protein loss.

During this period the proportion of albumin to total protein excreted diminishes, producing an initially mixed glomerular and tubular pattern with gradual development of a pure tubular pattern.[23, 24]

Tubular proteinuria is characterized by excretion of low molecular weight proteins (less than 60 kDa) in electrophoresis, the appearance of kidney-derived proteins, Tamm Horsfall glycoprotein, secretory IgA, or the presence of enzymes of renal cell origin—glutamyl transferase and $N$-acetyl-BD glucosaminadase (NAG).

Tubular proteinuria is thought to occur as a result of toxic pharmacological or hormonal modulations of the cellular inflammatory response of renal tubular cells, leading to injury.[22] The degree of tubular proteinuria is proportional to the severity of the burn injury.[23, 24] It is noteworthy that this proteinuria occurs when tubular rejection of sodium is occurring, with the potential for interference in reabsorptive processes by solute diuresis.[16, 18, 33] Measurements of low molecular weight protein (beta$_2$-microglobulin) and enzyme excretion (NAG) may be used to monitor tubular damage.

Gradual clearing of tubular proteinuria over one to two weeks occurs in a selective fashion. Beta$_2$-microglobulin (11.8 kDa) returns to normal first, followed sequentially by reabsorption of microglobulin (30 kDa) and acid glycoprotein (40k Da).

### Sodium Excretion

Between days four and seven, sodium excretion shows elevated fractional excretion with an increase in volume of urine excreted in a pattern similar to that of the osmotic diuresis seen in nonoliguric renal failure.[16, 18]

### Water Excretion

Osmolar clearance and volume of urine appear to be highest between one and three days after the burn injury. Although they do not correlate with burn surface area, a relationship between osmolar clearance and burn surface area does become evident between days five and ten.

## SEVEN TO 35 DAYS OR LONGER AFTER INJURY

During this time the glomerular filtration rate remains relatively stable and elevated.[21, 32] Proteinuria gradually clears between one and two weeks, although some patients continue to show a healing tubular proteinuria (see Proteinuria under Four to Seven Days). Proteinuria may recur in the presence of further tubular damage from sepsis, aminoglycosides, or other toxins.[22]

## ACUTE RENAL FAILURE IN THE BURNED PATIENT

Oliguric renal failure is uncommon in the acute phase of the burn injury unless a delay in resuscitative effort occurs and leads to hemodynamically mediated renal failure. Renal functional changes are similar to those seen in other forms of shock or circulatory insufficiency. Acute tubular injury in oliguria or nonoliguric renal failure and pigment nephropathy may also occur. In earlier studies, renal failure in burns carried a heavy mortality, but the increasing vigor of early resuscitation and patient stabilization has produced better overall survival and more sustained renal output.[1, 17] Established renal failure, however, still carries significant morbidity and mortality, since the burned patient is in a severe catabolic state with an increased risk of infection, hyperpyrexia, and caloric deficit. This risk is particularly pertinent in oliguric renal failure.

The functional pattern of polyuric renal failure in the burned patient appears to differ from that of other forms of nonoliguric renal failure in that the fractional excretion of sodium in urine remains low while the urine-to-plasma osmolar ratio ($U_{osm}/P_{osm}$) remains above one.[7, 18, 34] Such a pattern suggests a reduced rate of glomerular filtration and reduced proximal renal tubular function while the function of the distal renal tubule remains intact. Polyuric renal failure differs further from nonoliguric renal failure in that its onset is late, often in the second or third week after the injury. This suggests that hypovolemia or pigmenturia (hemoglobinuria or myoglobinuria) which occur early are not prominent etiological factors. Low fractional excretion of sodium and high urinary potassium levels that have been demonstrated could be explained by high aldosterone activity on an intact distal tubule.[4, 25] Prerenal causes are excluded because of their lack of response to vigorous volume expansion (Table 16–5). The burned patient's limited ability to concentrate urine ($U_{osm}/P_{osm}$ less than 1.5) in the face of an increased plasma osmolality and a decreased glomerular filtration rate (rising blood urea nitrogen and serum creatinine in nonoliguric failure) suggests solute diuresis or the washout of medullary interstitial gradient.[33] Under these circumstances, ADH activity is reflected in volume flow of urine rather than in changes in urinary

### TABLE 16–5. Response to Volume Expansion

| | Untreated | Adequate Response | Renal Failure | | SIADH |
| | | | Oliguric | Nonoliguric | |
| --- | --- | --- | --- | --- | --- |
| Urine volume (ml/kg/hr) | 1 | 1.5 | 0.7 | 1.5 | 1 |
| Urine sodium (mEq/L [random]) | 20 | 40 | 40 | 20–30 | 80 |
| $FE_{Na}$ | 1% | 2% | 4% | 2% | 4% |
| Urine osmolality (mOsm/L) | 800 | Decreased | 250–350 | 200–250 | 400 |
| $U_{osm}/P_{osm}$ | 2 | 1.5 | 1.2 | 1.2 | 1.5 |
| Urinary potassium | 20–40 | 40 | 20–40 | 20–40 | Variable 40 |
| Serum sodium (mEq/L) | N | N | Decreased | | Decreased |
| Serum osmolality | 295 | 290 | Decreased | | Decreased |
| BUN (mg/dl) | 20 | 20 | 20 rising | 20 rising | 20 |

SIADH = Syndrome of inappropriate antidiuretic hormone; $FE_{Na}$ = fractional excretion of sodium; $U_{osm}$ = urine osmolality; $P_{osm}$ = plasma osmolality; BUN = blood urea nitrogen; N = normal.

osmolality.[4] Further, the pattern of urinary indices resembles that seen in patients with radiological contrast–induced renal failure, suggesting potential alteration of glomerular hemodynamics, although actual toxicity cannot be excluded.[35]

The picture of nonoliguric renal failure in the burned patient awaits fuller definition. A decreased rate of glomerular filtration may follow a change in the balance of afferent and efferent arteriolar resistance, which produces a relative decrease in filtration, even in the presence of normal or increased renal blood flow. Proximal tubular dysfunction with relative solute diuresis decreases the responsiveness of the distal tubule to ADH activity, limiting urinary concentration (and dilution). High levels of renin and aldosterone are associated with sodium reclamation and potassium excretion.[6, 16, 18, 21] Hence, creatinine clearance is the best guide to defining nonoliguric renal failure in the burned patient.

## EFFECTS OF THERAPY ON RENAL FUNCTION

Exposure to multiple therapeutic agents during burn therapy provides potential interference with renal function and the consequent production of true renal damage. Thus, the risk to the patient of potent new drugs needs to be balanced with potential benefits. This discussion aims at highlighting potential problems rather than being exhaustive. Examples of drugs with possible nephrotoxicity include the following:

1. Antibiotics: aminoglycosides, such as gentamicin, tobramycin, penicillin, cephalosporin, amphotericin, Sulfamylon[36]
2. Diuretics: furosemide, thiazides
3. Acetaminophen[37]
4. Nonsteroidal anti-inflammatory agents[38]
5. Silver nitrate
6. Hypertonic saline therapy[36–39]

## Antibiotics

### Aminoglycosides

GENTAMICIN. Renal failure induced by gentamicin is particularly prominent in the nonoliguric renal failure group of a general hospital population.[26] Patients on gentamicin almost invariably exhibit mild histological changes and less commonly show slight abnormalities of the glomerular filtration rate. The abnormalities ensuing from gentamicin toxicity follow proximal tubular damage; brush border antigens are initially excreted, leading to enzymuria and beta$_2$-microglobulinuria. Mild to moderate proteinuria is common. A few patients demonstrate a defective ability to concentrate urine, and some progress to nonoliguric renal failure. Oliguric renal failure after gentamicin therapy is rare and has an ominous prognosis.

Low sodium intake, water deprivation, metabolic acidosis, and constant gentamicin levels in the blood enhance gentamicin toxicity, while fluid expansion and alkalinization may protect against nephrotoxicity.[40] Gentamicin in combination with other antibiotics such as clindamycin, cephalosporin, amphotericin, furosemide (with volume depletion), and prostaglandin inhibitors increases toxicity and should be avoided, if possible. Tobramycin and amikacin are less nephrotoxic.[36]

PENICILLIN. Synthetic penicillin derivatives have been associated with interstitial nephritis.

CEPHALOSPORIN. Cephaloridine is the agent most reported as a cause of nephrotoxicity; it has a direct toxic effect on the kidney, leading to acute tubular necrosis.[41] Reduced dosage is suggested in renal impairment.

AMPHOTERICIN. Amphotericin produces renal vasoconstriction and reduced renal blood flow, and its chronic use causes tubular damage, potassium loss, and diminished concentrating abilities.[42] Acute renal failure is inevitable with large dose therapy, although alkalinization may provide some protection.

SULFAMYLON. When absorbed, Sulfamylon acts as a carbonic anhydrase inhibitor and may lead to systemic acidosis.

## Diuretics

Inappropriate or prolonged use of diuretics such as furosemide or thiazides can lead to volume depletion or electrolyte abnormalities. Diuretics may also potentiate the toxic effect of other agents such as antibiotics.

## Acetaminophen

Acetaminophen in ordinary doses produces metabolites by oxidative metabolism via the cytochrome P-450 mixed function oxidative system. These metabolites are conjugated by glutathione and rendered nontoxic. The ability to generate the protective compound is overwhelmed by overdosage, however, and renal tubular necrosis may follow.

## Nonsteroidal Anti-inflammatory Drugs

Nonsteroidal anti-inflammatory drugs reduce renal blood flow where renal perfusion is dependent on prostaglandin-mediated renal vasodilatation, particularly in situations of decreased renal perfusion.[38]

## Silver Nitrate

Silver nitrate, applied topically, leads to the precipitation of silver chloride at the skin, with subsequent loss of sodium and chloride and the systemic absorption of nitrate with potential hypochloremic alkalosis and hyponatremia. This occurs particularly when renal function is not normal or a marked deficit in chloride is present, which limits the reabsorption of potassium and sodium ions.

Further, a tendency to hyponatremia may occur if the dressings are occlusive and prevent water loss.

### Hypertonic Saline Resuscitation

Moncreif has recommended sodium replacement (sodium 224 mEq/L, potassium 5.9 mEq/L, chloride 147 mEq/L, acetate 77 mEq/L) at a rate of 2 ml per per cent burn per kilogram of body weight.[39] If this solution is used in the presence of mild renal insufficiency, hypertonicity rapidly occurs. Care must be taken to provide sufficient free water to maintain serum sodium at less than 160 to 165 mEq/L, and the circulation must be supported sufficiently to maintain a satisfactory urine output to allow excretion of the sodium load.

Early and vigorous resuscitation has been associated with better overall survival and a more sustained urine output, but the risks of fluid overload and respiratory insufficiency are present. Consequent respiratory therapy is linked to hormonal changes mediated by the kidney, which are related to sodium and water retention.

Anesthesia used in early excision procedures is also associated with the potentiation of water retention by opiates used in premedication and as pain medication, with the resulting decreased renal blood flow and increased release of ADH. Retention of sodium and water after renal vasoconstriction with increased renal vascular resistance also occurs with these inhalational anesthetic agents.[43]

## EFFECTS OF ENDOGENOUS TOXINS—PIGMENT NEPHROPATHY[13]

Myoglobinuria and hemoglobinuria, characteristic of burn injuries sustained within an enclosed area (hemoglobinuria) or of deep burns, pressure necrosis, or interference with blood supply to muscle (myoglobinemia), may have secondary effects on the kidney. Hemoglobinuria is usually seen in a burn sustained in an enclosed space and usually correlates with carbon monoxide exposure or poisoning or the detrimental effects of carboxyhemoglobin. The combined effects of pigment load and such abnormalities of oxygen carriage lead to interference with oxygenation and an increased risk of acute tubular damage and acute renal failure in these patients.

Myoglobinuria occurs in patients having severe burns or deep burns or in patients with muscle ischemia. This complication therefore occurs if impairment of the vascular supply to a muscle compartment is present.[14] Release of myoglobin may follow escharotomy.

Myoglobin and hemoglobin have direct effects on the kidney and produce nontraumatic acute tubular necrosis (ATN). In the burned patient, hypotension and hemoconcentration may exacerbate the renal effects of myoglobin released from damaged muscle.[45] Definitive diagnosis of myoglobinuria requires detection of myoglobin in the urine. Although counterimmunoelectrophoresis is definitive, it is not readily available. Presumptive diagnosis rests on orthotoluidine testing of blood and urine, absence of red blood cells in spun urinary sediment, and marked elevation of serum levels of creatinine phosphatase and other muscle enzymes.

The clinical course of pigment-induced acute renal failure is similar to that of other forms of acute renal failure. The release of creatinine from muscle, however, produces a more rapid rise in serum creatinine and higher average serum values.[45] The blood urea nitrogen:creatinine ratio in rhabdomyolysis is usually lower than in other forms of renal failure, since elevated creatinine reflects increased creatinine load from muscle damage as well as lowered renal function, while urea levels reflect only renal function. Increased administration of fluid to increase urine output, prophylaxis with mannitol, loop diuretics (furosemide), and alkalinization may prevent anatomical or physiological damage by blocking intraluminal precipitation of pigment, cellular swelling, and direct or indirect vasodilatation.[13] The risks of this therapy are congestive heart failure from an overdose of mannitol or toxicity from loop diuretics that are not excreted.

The hypercatabolic state linked to muscle injury complicates management and requires careful caloric, fluid, and electrolyte balance, with consideration of early dialysis.[46, 47]

## RENAL FAILURE IN ASSOCIATION WITH SEPSIS

Sepsis is a common and potentially lethal complication of burns. Initial interference in the effective circulating blood volume and renal blood flow leads to prerenal azotemia. If circulation cannot be restored by appropriate antibiotic therapy, fluid expansion, and pressor support, acute ischemic tubular damage ensues.[44, 48] For the burned patient, increased catabolism and the continuing risk of serious infection, present until skin coverage is attained, make renal failure particularly dangerous.

Therapy includes control of infection and maintenance of circulation. Early therapy by caloric and amino acid supplementation has been connected with improved prognosis. Early and vigorous dialysis with prophylaxis against gastrointestinal bleeding is necessary until renal function is restored.[46, 47]

## SPECIFIC FEATURES OF TREATMENT OF RENAL FAILURE

### Prophylaxis

Early and vigorous resuscitation with emphasis on maintenance of circulation and urinary output has been linked to a decreased incidence of oliguric renal failure in the early phase of burn injury.[15]

Recent experience with plasma exchange in patients failing resuscitation from burn shock suggests that such therapy may also be effective.[49, 50] In patients who do not respond to conventional volume therapy, plasma exchange has been associated with marked improvement in urine output, resolution of lactic acidosis, and marked reduction in fluid requirements, usually with a return to calculated requirements within two or three hours of treatment.

## Vigorous Caloric and L-Amino Acid (Protein) Supplementation

Such parenteral supplements can reduce the catabolic rate significantly, reduce the generation of urea, and lead to electrolyte stabilization. Ultrafiltration or continuous arteriovenous hemofiltration (CAVH) may be necessary to allow adequate fluid volumes to provide appropriate hyperalimentation.[46]

## Choosing a Mode of Dialysis and/or Ultrafiltration

Dialysis consists of two separate processes. The first involves solute clearance across a semipermeable membrane, and the second is the removal of fluid by ultrafiltration. The efficiency of each process depends on the area and characteristics of the membrane, the pressure differential across the membrane, the rate of flow of blood and dialysate along the membrane, and dialysate composition.

In clinical practice, the choice for the burned patient is among hemodialysis, peritoneal dialysis, and CAVH. Gradient dialysis, such as acute peritoneal dialysis and hemodialysis, is more efficient than CAVH in solute removal but tends to produce more marked changes in circulation. If the rate of generation can be diminished by concurrent use of parenteral hyperalimentation, CAVH may be adequate to balance fluid and control electrolytes.[46]

Intermittent hemodialysis is preferred in the presence of a marked catabolic state, provided that circulation is stable and that vascular access (preferably not through burned tissue) is possible.[47] Heparinization is necessary.

Peritoneal dialysis is less efficient, but when performed intermittently and continued over a full 24-hour period, it can provide clearances similar to those of hemodialysis with less interference with circulation. Ultrafiltration, however, is variable and less well controlled than in hemodialysis or CAVH.

CAVH can be used as extracorporeal therapy over a prolonged period and facilitates the removal of water and medium-sized solutes. Heparinization is necessary. Simultaneous removal of fluid and reconstitution of blood volume are carried out to produce control of fluid and electrolytes. Solute and urea clearances are low, and if the generation of urea is not controlled, supplemental hemodialysis is required.

The choice of replacement therapy in the burned patient, therefore, depends on catabolic rate, generation of urea, remaining urine output (renal function), and the need for fluid removal. Mechanical methods of solute and fluid control need to be co-ordinated with a full therapeutic regimen. The aim is to provide energy as calories and protein sufficient to control the rate of urea generation if renal failure therapy is to be successful in the burned patient.

## SUMMARY

In earlier studies, renal failure in burns was a prominent and highly toxic complication. The present increased vigor of early resuscitation has led to more stable circulation and sustained urine output; oliguric renal failure has become a rare consequence of burn injury. Similarly, attention to prophylaxis in the presence of potential pigment nephropathy has led to a decrease in the incidence of renal failure following myoglobinuria and hemoglobinuria.

There is, however, a series of alterations in renal function which result in an initial decrease in glomerular filtration and retention of sodium and water during the first one to two days of injury, consistent with hypovolemia. Following this early phase, glomerular filtration is elevated, with a possible increase in effective circulating blood volume and decreased serum protein level. The constellation of tubular abnormalities observed in the burned patient shows sodium loss and water retention, changes consistent with proximal tubular dysfunction and solute diuresis, and fairly well retained distal renal tubular function.

Polyuric renal failure or a nonoliguric renal failure in burns is characterized by similar changes in tubular function, but with decreased glomerular filtration. This effect may be secondary to the imbalance of renal afferent and efferent arterial pressures that may be the result of toxic products of the burn injury.

## REFERENCES

1. Demling RH: Burns. N Engl J Med 313:1389–1398, 1985.
2. Espinel CH, Gregory AW: Differential diagnosis of acute renal failure. Clin Nephrol 13:73–77, 1980.
3. Miller TR, Anderson RJ, Linas SL, et al: Urinary diagnostic indices in acute renal failure. A prospective study. Ann Intern Med 89:47–50, 1978.
4. Raymond KH, Stein JH: Efferent limb of volume homeostasis. In Brenner BM, Stein JH (eds): Body Fluid Homeostasis. Contemporary Issues in Nephrology, Vol 16. New York, Churchill Livingstone, 1987, pp 36–38.
5. Balogh D, Benzer A, Hackl JM, Bauer M: Sodium balance and osmolality in burn patients. Intensive Care Med 12:100–103, 1986.
6. Morgan RJ, Martyn JAJ, Philbin DM, et al: Water metabolism and antidiuretic hormone (ADH) response following thermal injury. J Trauma 20:468–472, 1980.
7. Eklund J: Studies on renal function in burns. II. Early signs of impaired renal function in lethal burns. Acta Clin Scand 136:735–740, 1970.
8. Collentine GE, Waisbren BA, Long GE: Inappropriate secretion of antidiuretic hormone as an accompaniment of burn injury in research burns. Transactions of the Third International Congress on Burns. Bern, Switzerland, Hans Huber, 1971.
9. Mahler D, Hanbran D, LeRoith D, Glick SM: Radioimmunoassay of ADH in the burn shock period: A preliminary report. Burn 5:269–273, 1978.
10. Shirani KZ, Vaughn GM, Robertson GL, et al: Inappropriate vasopressin secretion (SIADH) in burned patients. J Trauma 23:217–224, 1983.

11. Stark H, Weinberger AG, Ben-Bassat M: Persistent hyponatremia and inappropriate antidiuretic hormone secretion in children with extensive burns. J Pediatr Surg 14:149–153, 1979.
12. Bartter FC, Schwartz WB: The syndrome of inappropriate secretion of antidiuretic hormone. Am J Med 42:790–806, 1967.
13. Flanenbaum W, Gehr M, Gross M, et al: Acute renal failure associated with myoglobinuria and hemoglobinuria. In Brenner BM, Lazarus JM (eds): Acute Renal Failure. Philadelphia, WB Saunders Company, 1983, pp 269–282.
14. Mitchell RM, Freeman J: Crush syndrome: The management of hypovolemia and renal complications. Aust NZ J Surg 39:155, 1969.
15. O'Neill JTA, Pruit BA Jr, Moncreif JA: Studies of renal function during the early post burn period. In Mater P, Barclay TL, Konickova Z (eds): Research in Burns. Bern, Switzerland, Hans Huber Publishers, 1971, pp 95–99.
16. Eklund J, Granberg PO, Liliehahl SO: Studies on renal function in burns: I. Renal osmolal regulation: GFR and plasma solute composition related to age, burn surface area and mortality probability. Acta Clin Scand 136:627–640, 1970.
17. Sevitt S: Renal function after burning. J Clin Pathol 18:572–578, 1965.
18. Planas W, Wachtel T, Frank H, Henderson LW: Characterization of acute renal failure in the burned patient. Arch Intern Med 142:2087–2091, 1982.
19. Gump FE, Price JB, Kinney JM: Whole body and splanchnic blood flow and oxygen consumption measurements in patients with intraperitoneal infection. Ann Surg 171:321–328, 1970.
20. Wilmore DW, Goodwin CW, Aulick LH, et al: Effect of injury and infection on visceral metabolism and circulation. Ann Surg 192:491–504, 1980.
21. Martyn JA, Greenblatt DJ, Abernathy DR: Increased cimetidine clearance in burn patients. JAMA 253:1288–1291, 1985.
22. Coombes EJ, Shakespeare PG, Batstone GF: Urine proteins after burn injury. Clin Chem Acta 95:201–209, 1979.
23. Shakespeare PG, Coombes EJ, Hambleton J, Furness D: Proteinuria after burn injury. Ann Clin Biochem 18:353–360, 1981.
24. Jackson SH, Farmer AW, Slater RJ, DeleWolfe MS: Resolution of urinary or serum proteins by chromotography on DEAE cellulose columns with particular reference to urinary proteins after burn injury. Can J Biochem Physiol 39:881–889, 1961.
25. Bane JW, McCaa CS, et al: The pattern of aldosterone and cortisol blood levels in thermal burn patients. J Trauma 14:605–611, 1974.
26. Anderson FJ, Linas SL, Bearns AS, et al: Non-oliguric renal failure. N Engl J Med 296:1134, 1977.
27. Vertel RM, Knochel JP: Non-oliguric acute renal failure. JAMA 200:598–602, 1967.
28. Eklund J: Studies on renal function in burns: III. Hyperosmolal states in burned patients related to renal osmolal regulation. Acta Clin Scand 136:741–751, 1970.
29. Genarri FJ: Serum osmolality—uses and limitations. N Engl J Med 310:162–165, 1984.
30. Hershey SD, Gersel E: Hyperosmolality caused by percutaneously absorbed glycerin in a burned patient. J Trauma 22:150–252, 1982.
31. Kulick MI, Lewis NS, Bensal V, Warpeha R: Hyperosmolality in the burned patient: An analysis of an osmololal discrepancy. J Trauma 20:223–228, 1980.
32. Loirat P, Rohan J, Baillet A, et al: Increased glomerular filtration rate in patients with major burns and its effect on the pharmacokinetics of tobramycin. N Engl J Med 299:915–919, 1978.
33. Bricker N: On the pathogenesis of the uremic state. N Engl J Med 286:1093–1099, 1972.
34. Diamond JR, Yonurn DC: Non-oliguric acute renal failure associated with a low fractional excretion of sodium. Ann Intern Med 96:5970–6000, 1982.
35. Fang LST, Sirota R, Ebert TH, et al: Low fractional excretion of sodium with contrast media-induced acute renal failure. Arch Intern Med 140:531–533, 1980.
36. Coggins CH, Fang LST: Acute renal failure associated with antibiotics, anesthetic agents and radiographic contrast agents. In Brenner BM, Lazarus JM (eds): Acute Renal Failure. Philadelphia, WB Saunders Company, 1983, pp 283–320.
37. Duggin GG: Mechanisms in the development of analgesic nephropathy. Kidney Int 18:553–561, 1980.
38. Garella S, Matarese RA: Renal effects of prostaglandins and clinical adverse effects of non-steroidal anti-inflammatory agents. Medicine 63:165–181, 1984.
39. Moncreif JA: Burns. N Engl J Med 288:444–454, 1973.

40. Chin PJ, Miller GH, Long JF, Waltz JA: Renal uptake and nephrotoxicity of gentamicin during urinary alkalinization in rats. Clin Exp Pharmacol Physiol 6:317–326, 1979.
41. Foord RD: Cephaloridine, cephalothin and the kidney. J Antimicrob Chemother 1:119–133, 1975.
42. Bhathena DB, Bullock WE, NuHall CE, Luke RG: The effects of amphotericin B therapy on the intrarenal vasculature and renal tubules in man. Clin Nephrol 9:103–110, 1978.
43. Debodo RC: Antidiuretic action of morphine and its mechanism. J Pharmacol Exp Ther 82:74–85, 1944.
44. Habif DV, Papper EM, Fitzpatrick HF, et al: The renal and hepatic blood flow, glomerular filtration rate and urinary output of electrolytes during cyclopropane ether and thiopental anesthesia, operation and the intermediate post-operative period. Surgery 30:241–255, 1951.
45. Walsh MB, Miller SL, Kagen LJ: Myoglobinemia in severely burned patients: Correlations with severity and survival. J Trauma 22:6–10, 1982.
46. Bosch JP: Continuous arteriovenous hemofiltration (CAVH): Operational characteristics and clinical use. AKF Nephrol Lett 3:15–26, 1986.
47. Lazarus JM: Dialytic therapy: Principles and clinical guidelines. Hospital Practice, 17:11–133, 1982.
48. Kassirer JP: Clinical evaluation of kidney function—glomerular filtration. N Engl J Med 285:385–387, 1971.
49. Schnarrs RH, Cline CW, Goldfarb IW, et al: Plasma exchange for failure of early resuscitation in thermal injuries. J Burn Care Rehabil 7:230–233, 1986.
50. Warden GD, Stratta RJ, Saffle JR, et al: Plasma exchange therapy in patients failing to resuscitate from burn shock. J Trauma 23:945–951, 1983.

# 17

## Psychiatric Management of the Burned Patient

FREDERICK J. STODDARD

The experiences of being burned and needing acute and continuing treatment cause enormous biological, psychological, and social stress to burned patients and their families. Emergency personnel, nurses, house officers, and surgeons often provide psychiatric triage before a member of the mental health team becomes involved. It is essential that the burn team utilize recent findings about psychobiological assessment and psychosocial crisis intervention for these multiply traumatized patients and their loved ones. This chapter presents an approach to psychiatric management of the acute burn patient and identifies specific areas of early focus for improving psychological rehabilitation.

The need for services is highlighted by the fact that more than two million burns and more than 10,000 deaths occur annually.[1] Of these burns, 70 per cent occur in children under five, and more than 68 per cent are severe enough to require hospitalization of patients under 19 years of age.[2] The continuing serious threat of burns from nuclear explosions, accidents, and war means that much larger numbers of burn victims could need treatment at any time. In the Middle East military burn casualties are common today and overwhelm the meager resources for treatment.

Adults, adolescents, infants, and their families who endure burns experience profound biological and social stress. Families are thrown into turmoil and crisis because of the injury and hospitalization. The tragedy is increased if others are burned or killed. It is especially stressful when the home is destroyed or abuse or neglect is involved.[3-5] Usually preventable accidents, explosions, scalds, firesetting, housefires, and self-immolation may be causes of subsequent feelings of blame, responsibility, and guilt.[6, 7]

### ASSESSING COPING STRENGTHS AND RISK FACTORS

Burns cause intense (although not generally chronic) pain, disability, and disfigurement. Most burn patients experience confusion, anxiety, and depression that benefit from psychiatric intervention.[8] Many authors have asserted that burn victims have a high rate of pre-burn psychiatric morbidity, including personality and conduct disorders, family disruption, divorce, alcohol and drug abuse, and self-destructive behavior.[9] Because of the disturbances after severe burns, burn specialists are particularly interested in pre-burn psychopathology, coping strengths, and stressful life events. Much evidence is emerging that the post-burn coping strengths of most burn victims are stronger and more effective than was earlier recognized.[10] There is also evidence that pre-burn risk factors are very important.

These studies include large numbers of severely burned patients, but their methodologies are partially flawed; e.g., all but two lack control groups. Nevertheless, the most significant findings are that burned children are likely to have been unwanted,[11] to have depressed mothers,[12] or parents with marital conflict, to be neglected, and to cause their own burns.[13] Approximately 4 to 5 per cent of childhood burns are due to abuse, but some centers have a much higher incidence. These findings established the importance of preventive family mental health interventions in childhood burn prevention and the need for psychiatric intervention after the burn for pre-existing disorders.

There have been three well-designed studies of pre-burn risk factors in adult patients. About 50 per cent of adult patients suffer from an illness that places them at increased risk.[14-16] These include alcoholism, drug abuse, schizophrenia, manic-depressive illness, arteriosclerotic heart disease, chronic obstructive pulmonary disease, and senility.[17] These findings point to measures that may prevent such burns and to the need for intensive post-burn medical, psychiatric, and substance abuse treatment of these adults, even those with small burns.

## CARING FOR THE DYING PATIENT AND THE FAMILY

The burned patient who is dying presents an enormously tragic and stressful situation to the family and staff. Martin et al,[18] in one of the few papers on this, described families' reactions to deaths of seven children from burns and emphasized how staff responses could increase or decrease these intense reactions. The reactions included isolation, despairing anger, feelings of helplessness, intense guilt, severe depression, constant emotional preoccupation with the dead child even years later, and marital estrangement. They explained how difficult it was to approach many of these families after the death.

The situation is complex, since a number of patients who survive have been told they would not.[19] The survival rate in the United States for acute burns increased from 81 per cent for 1965–1971 to 86 per cent for 1972–1975 to 90 per cent for 1976–1979, owing primarily to improvements in life support measures, grafting, and infection control.[2, 20] Nevertheless, when death is probable, it is ethically and emotionally highly stressful. Questions commonly are asked, "Why are we saving this patient?" "Are my efforts worthwhile?" "Will life be worth living even if he or she survives?" Medical personnel, with or without family participation, are required to make such decisions, although their inner feelings may conflict with whatever decision is made. Imbus and Zawacki[21] proposed to interview patients not expected to live during the lucid predelirium phase to tell them of probable death and to inform them that they may choose not to have the heroic treatments available. In our experience, although some patients are indeed lucid, their metabolism and mental state are acutely disturbed and they tend not to be able to understand or make meaningful choices from among the various treatment courses.

From a psychiatric and an ethical viewpoint, it is most important to sustain open communication among patient, family, and the entire burn team so that the ethical choices, fears of the treatment, fears of death, anticipatory grief, and grief can be worked through rather than denied or avoided.[22]

Wachtel et al,[23] in a very thoughtful and ethically sensitive study, reported on 24 patients whose prognoses were judged very poor by several prognostic indices. During a five-year period they offered a change in treatment regimen from curative to comfort care to patients aged 14 to 88 with a mean burn size of 66 per cent (range 18–95 per cent). Eleven received comfort care and did not survive. Thirteen patients received aggressive care, of whom five survived with severe deformity and disability and one committed suicide. They report that this last patient was most troubling to them, as he "had originally accepted comfort care, had second thoughts and ultimately survived." Recognizing and describing such difficult problems, they present a process for arriving at such a decision and a detailed protocol for administering comfort care. They did not weigh considerations of limited resources or distributive justice in their decisions, but felt that "we may be entering an era in which the rights and benefits available to individuals will be increasingly diminished in favor of those of the society as a whole." This protocol for comfort care should be considered when physicians and burn teams attempt to deal with the ethical dilemmas of treating very severely burned patients, and, even if not considered, some families may choose such an option.

## PSYCHOBIOLOGICAL RESPONSES TO ACUTE BURNS

Although acute reactions to burns may be characterized as a single acute phase, there are several different acute psychobiological reponses. Most common are acute post-traumatic stress disorder, burn delirium, pain syndromes, sleep disorders,[24] and acute grief. In this author's view, the hypermetabolic response to burn injury[25] is a probable contributor to these phenomena, first in a pseudomanic state (hypercatecholaminergic delirium) with anxiety and delirium and then in a state of depression (steroid/catecholaminergic depletion) with depressive mood, interpersonal withdrawal, and decreased appetite.[96] Additional important factors in altered mental states after burns are infection, opiates, benzodiazepines, anesthetic agents, and altered fluid and electrolyte balance. This subject is discussed below under burn delirium, but mental state may be affected with or without delirium.

## Post-Traumatic Stress Disorder (PTSD)

Post-traumatic stress disorder criteria have recently been revised,[26, 27] but the syndrome was described much earlier in literature and medical writings.[28, 29] The essential criteria for diagnosis of PTSD are, in part:

the development of characteristic symptoms following a psychologically distressing event that is outside the range of usual human experience. The stressor producing this syndrome would be markedly distressing to almost anyone, and is usually experienced with intense fear, terror and helplessness. The characteristic symptoms involve re-experiencing the traumatic event; avoidance of stimuli associated with the event or numbing of general responsiveness and increased arousal. The diagnosis is not made if the disturbance lasts less than one month. The most common traumata involve a serious threat to one's life or physical integrity; a serious threat or harm to one's children, spouse, or other close relatives and friends; sudden destruction of one's home or community; or seeing another person who has recently been or is being seriously injured or killed as a result of an accident or physical violence.[27]

The causes of PTSD in burn victims can include all or some of those physical, psychological, and social stressors.[30] Adler[31] described the characteristic anxiety, depression, apathy, and intense autonomic arousal in adult burn victims after the Cocoanut Grove fire in 1943. Hamburg and Hamburg[32] at Brooke Army Hospital reported an intensive study of 12 out of 400 adult burn patients. They found that psychological coping mechanisms to deal with the unbearable reality of burns form a continuum, varying in degree at any one time, and include delirium, illusion-delusion-hallucination, denial, regression, constriction, and suppression. In one recent comparative study, there is evidence that adults with electrical burns manifest more severe post-traumatic symptoms than psychiatric, chronic pain, or blepharospasm groups. The most severe symptoms are dreams, flashbacks, panic attacks, depression, and refusal to return to work even when cleared surgically.[33] Tucker found that 23 per cent of burned adults in rehabilitation manifest PTSD.

In a study of burned young Israeli soldiers, Solnit and Priel[33] found that affective regression could be adaptive and serve to assist emotional coping with such severe trauma. Stoddard[34] similarly found adaptive regression, including temporary loss of recently acquired developmental gains, to be an important consideration in treatment of burned children.

Benians[12] in his 2 1/2-year study of 105 acutely burned children with follow-up identified 33 per cent with persistent severe disturbances, such as refusal to eat and resistance to nursing procedures, and only 10 per cent with no evident disturbance; he also found that children who were not visited regularly by their parents deteriorated emotionally and physically. In an outcome study of burned children ages 7 to 19, Stoddard et al found that 23.3 per cent of a representative sample of 30 children studied to date manifest a full PTSD syndrome, 30 per cent manifest a partial syndrome, and others manifest severe post-burn depression or anxiety disorders different from PTSD.[36, 94] PTSD is a very active area of psychiatric research in both children and adults.[37–40]

Psychiatric management of PTSD is planned according to the stage of burn treatment and the degree of intensity of symptoms. Primary aspects of treatment include encouraging the patient to talk about what is being experienced, reassuring the patient and family about the usually transient nature of the acute symptoms, and giving appropriate reality-oriented clarifications and explanations in language the patient can understand. Benzodiazepines are usually helpful in relieving acute anxiety and sleep disorders. Regular brief psychotherapeutic interventions by the psychiatrist or other mental health team members facilitates nursing and medical management.

## Burn Delirium

Delirium, a transient derangement of cerebral function, is an organically caused mental disorder whose essential features include a reduced ability to maintain attention to external stimuli and disorganized thinking as manifested by rambling, irrelevant, or incoherent speech. The syndrome also involves a reduced level of consciousness, sensory misperceptions, disturbances of the sleep-wake cycle and level of psychomotor activity, disorientation to time, place, or person, and memory impairment. The onset is relatively rapid, and the course typically fluctuates. The total duration is usually brief. "Other terms which essentially describe the same phenomenon are burn encephalopathy and burn coma. It includes perceptual disturbances (illusions or hallucinations), speech incoherence, sleep disorder, altered motor activity, disorientation and memory impairment, and a rapid fluctuating course."[41]

Management of delirious patients generally consists of controlling and preventing impulsive behavior while correcting the organic cause.[42, 43] Burn delirium was studied by Blank and Perry,[8] who found that 34 of 189 burn patients (18 per cent) met the DSM-III criteria and an additional 6 per cent had some symptoms; they concluded that psychological as well as medical interventions were important because of the increased severity of post-traumatic psychological reactions in those who had been delirious. Antoon et al[44] studied 140 consecutively admitted children with burn injuries, 20 of whom had a diagnosis of burn encephalopathy. The symptoms that they described ranged from hallucinations, personality changes, and delirium to seizures and coma. They found hypoxia in nine of 20 cases, hypovolemia in one, sepsis in four, hyponatremia in four, and cortical vein thrombosis in one. They described all of their patients as having virtually complete recovery in follow-up. Andreasen et al[45] studied 13 delirious burned adults and, on follow-up, found evidence of long-term neurological impairment. During the acute phase, 70 per cent had cognitive and neurological disturbances. In 90 per cent there were EEG abnormalities present before the development of symptoms. One year after burn trauma, 17 per cent continued to have minimal deficits and diffusely abnormal EEGs. The minimal neurological deficits included decreased concentration, labile mood, and decreased memory function. Haynes and Bright[46] reported 10 cases of burn coma associated with 21 to 54 per cent second- and third-degree burns. Symptoms included lethargy, coma, slurred speech, muscular incoordination, nystagamus, and ataxia. EEGs revealed diffuse slowing, and symptoms correlated with gram-negative sepsis; recovery was complete without residua. The most common EEG abnormality is diffuse nonspecific slow waves.[47] Hughes et al[48] found slow-wave abnormalities in 88 per cent of 49 recordings done in 40 acutely burned patients. EEG abnormalities were maximal at 3 to 11 days post burn. Peterson et al[49] studied 58 acute and chronic burn patients and found a 67 per cent incidence of EEG abnormality and 100 per cent abnormality in burns over 40 per cent of total body surface area (TBSA). According to Jefferson and Marshall,[47] the EEG abnormality should be useful in differentiating the behavioral changes of an anxiety disturbance from those of delirium. The etiologies of burn delirium may include fluid or electrolyte imbalance, cerebral edema, respiratory insufficiency, infection, renal or cardiovascular insufficiency, drug toxicity, sleep deprivation, and pre-existing disorders.

Treatment is directed toward the causative factors[95] but should usually be supplemented with appropriate psychotropic medications (benzodiazepines, e.g., Dalmane, or antipsychotics, e.g., haloperidol). Specific psychotherapeutic interventions are usually very helpful. Providing familiar personal objects, reassurance from fears, orientation to time, place, and person, and consistency of staff are helpful. Since sensory overload may contribute to delirium, decreased light intensity, noise levels, and nursing and medical intrusions during sleep periods are helpful. Since altered biorhythms contribute to delirium, a regularized sleep-wake cycle helps the patient return to familiar biological and psychological patterns, thereby decreasing stress.

## Managing Pain

Pain is the most severe recurrent experience endured by the burned person which the physician and burn unit staff can treat effectively. Psychiatric staff have a very important role here. The child's or adult's pain is shaped by the extent and depth of burn, stage of healing, age and stage of emotional development, cognition, responsiveness to analgesia, pain threshold, and interpersonal and cultural factors.[35]

Hypnosis has a significant role in relieving pain of awake, alert, and co-operative burn patients. Bernstein,[50] Gardner,[51] Spiegel and Spiegel,[52] and others[53, 54] have reported patients who had major or total pain relief with hypnosis and self-hypnosis. Fortunately, children and adolescents are more hypnotizable than adults. The Hypnotic Induction Profile (HIP) is a useful quick method of estimating the degree of hypnotizability.[54] Relaxation techniques, resembling natural childbirth methods, are quite similar and are in wide use. These include specific methods such as Benson's relaxation audiotapes and yoga. Such methods have also been found to decrease physiological stress responses such as elevated pulse and blood pressure due to excessive anxiety. Other activities in common use, which resemble hypnosis in relieving pain, are viewing or listening to pleasant television or radio programs or being read a story. Even an intubated medical patient with facial dressings can select a favorite book or program with assistance. For an infant, being held, cuddled, and rocked appears to have a hypnotic effect.

Studies have documented the effectiveness of other specific interventions: the presence of a supportive person, adequate opiate analgesia,[55, 56] encouraging patient control and participation in burn care,[57, 58] relaxation techniques, transcutaneous electrical nerve stimulation (TENS), and biofeedback.[59] Many of these methods have in common the important fact that another person cares enough to attempt to lessen the pain—a powerful analgesic in itself.

Pain control poses a number of problems. Despite recent studies, there is still the problem that the patient's report of excruciating pain is often underestimated by busy, emotionally burdened staff; as a result, inadequate analgesic medication is given, a problem by no means limited to burn pain. The problem of undermedication is most prevalent with adolescents, for whom fear of drug dependence may inappropriately influence treatment. A related problem is that the patient's specific pain experience may be misunderstood; e.g., even a small wound may elicit intense pain. This is especially so for anxious patients, those who are confused and alone, or those with pre-existing emotional disorders. A final problem is staff overconfidence in a particular mode of pain relief, such as medication, to the exclusion of another, such as patient understanding and participation. It is to be hoped that, as described in Chapter 13, measurement of patients' self-perceived pain and endorphin levels will permit greater targetting of psychological and pharmacological treatments specific to the patient's pain threshold and personality.[60, 61]

## Managing the Grieving Patient

Lindemann and Cobb, in classic papers, described the syndrome of acute grief for the first time based on their work with burn victims of the Cocoanut Grove fire.[62, 63] This is a common syndrome in burned adults, children, and their families. Lindemann described it in this manner:

> Sensations of somatic distress occurring in waves lasting from twenty minutes to an hour at a time, a feeling of tightness in the throat, choking with shortness of breath, need for sighing, an empty feeling in the abdomen, lack of muscular power, and an intense subjective distress described as tension or mental pain. The patient soon learns that these waves of discomfort can be precipitated by visits, by mentioning the deceased, and by receiving sympathy. There is a tendency to avoid the syndrome at any cost, to refuse visits lest they should precipitate the reaction, and to deliberately keep from thoughts all references to the deceased.
>
> Five points—somatic distress, preoccupation with the image of the deceased, guilt, hostile reactions, and loss of patterns of conduct—seem to be pathognomonic for grief.

He added that a sixth characteristic, appearance of traits of the deceased in the behavior of the bereaved, is displaced to their own bodies and activities by identification. He clarified that the syndrome is a separation reaction. It is seen in many burn patients suffering separation from loved ones, home, and work, and loss by death. In addition, grief reactions occur after losses of previous body image, as in facial burns, and loss of digits, hands, or limbs.[64]

Furman, in her extensive study of children who have lost a loved one, emphasizes the emotional burdens of professionals aiding grieving children.[65] These burdens, and the need to share them, are even heavier among burn unit staff who have many tasks in addition to caring emotionally for the grieving person.

The grieving process varies from individual to individual, with intermittent numbness and distress.[66] Generally relevant factors in aiding the grieving person are understanding the pre-existing personality, facilitating the patients' awareness of the death including its cause and the burial, assisting the patients' fears of their own deaths, and assisting the experiences of alternating detachment from and identification with the lost person. Intervention with grieving children needs to be geared to their cognitive level, as elaborated by Koocher.[67]

It is generally desirable that information about the death of a loved one be shared as early as possible, when a relative is present, when the patient is able to respond verbally (optimally, not intubated or delirious), and when a mental health professional will remain available to work verbally through the grief with the patient for at least several sessions.

## MANAGING THE FAMILY

Families affect how a burn happens, and they also affect hospital adjustment.[68] Familial risk factors, especially poverty, pre-existing psychopathology, and medical illnesses, play a major role in the occurrence of burns in infants, children, and adults. Burns also occur in well families without such risk factors. Like patients, family members pass through phases of adaptation. They are often shocked and confused and afraid of what has happened and of the burn unit and hospital environment.[69] Forming a therapeutic alliance with family members begins with as flexible a response as possible, allowing them to be expressive in their own language, maintaining control or withdrawing, while encouraging participation as they learn about burn care.[70] Marital stress is often pre-existing and may be exacerbated by the trauma.

Social supports sustain burn patients, and the family, when there is one, is the key continuing support.[71-73] Absence of a spouse or family is probably a risk factor for a poorer emotional outcome.[33, 74] Cases of child abuse or neglect legally mandate filing a referral to a state agency. Most families are grief-stricken and require time with emphathetic staff members to share their confusion, fear, grief, and anger. One recent study found greater stress in parents of burned children than in those of other children undergoing surgery. Another study differentiated responses of wives into poor relators, good relators, and over-relators and found that the over-relator arouses guilt and anger in staff.[75] Various studies have identified post-burn depression in family members for up to six months, with lasting post-traumatic symptoms in at least 15 per cent.[76–78] The consultant advises staff on dealing with stressed or mentally ill relatives and may provide direct care or refer them. Group and individual meetings are effective in supporting and educating families about scarring, skin grafts, and the psychological after-effects of burns.[70, 79, 80]

Preparation of families for discharge begins once the acute phase is past. There may be significantly altered relationships because the burn patient no longer feels as competent, attractive, or sexually desirable. Counselling helps to overcome interpersonal strains and isolation. It is particularly essential and effective for those with burns affecting their work, leisure activities, or sexual functioning. Appropriately caring and protective family responses, rather than over- or underprotectiveness, can be very helpful and can make social re-entry shared and somewhat less stigmatizing.

## PSYCHOPHARMACOLOGICAL MANAGEMENT

To support essential treatment of acute and recovering burn patients, sound choices of psychotropic drugs must be made quickly, based on general knowledge and the limited information available.[45] A few studies have been done. Medication has an essential place in the management of pain, anxiety, aggression, delirium, ICU psychosis, drug and alcohol withdrawal, depression, and pre-existing mental disorders in burn patients. Many have an acute disorder requiring rapid treatment, but delirium, depression, and sleep disorders can also develop gradually.

Life-threatening conditions such as agitated delirium, severe suicidal or aggressive behavior, acute organic brain syndrome, or toxic disorders require rapid assessment and often initial physical restraint, followed by chemical restraint, if appropriate.[81] Medical assessment should include the history of medication use, drug abuse, or other medical disorder, including CNS injury or CNS depression. Before medication is used, its benefits should be weighed against such risks as the possibility of obscuring evidence of changes in physical or mental states needed for accurate diagnosis. Although some authors and burn units de-emphasize the role of medication for burn patients, including young children, the high levels of distress found in acutely burned patients[82] and their medical histories indicate a serious need for improved management of psychotropic medications. Careful psychiatric assessment and diagnosis are advised when possible to individualize the approach. Four classes of psychotropic drugs may be necessary in burn patients:

**ANALGESICS.** Morphine and meperidine are most commonly used for debridement and burn wound pain. They may induce delirium or cause excessive sedation, dysphoria, sleep disorders, or nausea and should be decreased if necessary. Undermedication is a more common problem.[83] Degree of pain relief has been found to correlate with levels of plasma beta-endorphin[61] and morphine.[84] Withdrawal effects include yawning, rhinorrhea, abdominal cramps, and insomnia.

**ANTI-ANXIETY AGENTS.** Diazepam is often effective in alleviating anxiety associated with pain, but lorazepam (Ativan) is metabolized more rapidly and may be preferable. Recent experience with clonazepam (Klonopin) indicates that its long duration of action potency and pain-relieving properties are helpful in some patients. These agents may, in some patients, induce sedation, paradoxical excitement, and suicidal ideation; withdrawal may produce tremor, dysphoria, insomnia, and weight loss. Martyn et al studied diazepam kinetics in severely burned adults and found reduced clearance and extraordinary levels of accumulation, especially in those also receiving cimetidine.[85] The metabolism of lorazepam is unimpaired in burned patients.[86] Despite increased attention, anxiety has been inadequately evaluated and undertreated pharmacologically in acutely burned patients.

**ANTIPSYCHOTIC AGENTS.** Small doses of chlorpromazine or promethazine may be helpful in alleviating anxiety and pain during debridement. Larger doses of antipsychotics may be necessary as chemical restraints for agitated delirious patients including adolescents, those who are violent or self-destructive, and those with pre-existing psychoses. Intravenous haloperidol in low doses for two to three days aids in the management of acute severe delirium because of fewer extrapyramidal side effects than oral or intramuscular administration, few cardiovascular risks,[87] and demonstrated effectiveness.[88] The severe dystonias and akithesias induced by haloperidol led one group to discourage its use in burn patients,[89] however. In our experience, concurrent or rapid use of anti-Parkinsonian agents, such as Cogentin, or short-term or reduced dosage reduces these problems. Long-term and oral or intramuscular use of haloperidol causes extrapyramidal effects more often; for this reason, benzodiazepines may be preferable. Lithium carbonate or carbamazepine (Tegretol) may be indicated for control of manic-depressive (bipolar) patients, but the risk of severe lithium toxicity in metabolically unstable patients discourages its use. Similarly, phenothiazines or haloperidol in high doses may be necessary for schizophrenic or borderline psychotic patients, but side effects and the patient's medical condition influence the choice of drug. Like haloperidol, but less commonly, the phenothiazines may cause dyskinesias. They also may cause hypotension, weight gain, and galactorrhea, among other side effects.

**ANTIDEPRESSANTS.** These drugs have two uses in burn patients. One is pain relief. Low doses of amphetamine, Ritalin, or tricyclic antidepressants may enhance opiate-induced analgesia and decrease the dose needed. The other use is for relief of depression late in burn treatment. Antidepressants are contraindicated in early burn treatment because of their potential cardiovascular complications, although Doxepin has recently been successfully used. After stabilization, however, tricyclics or other antidepressants (e.g., trazodone) are effective in lessening severe depressive symptoms, but discussion with the anesthesiologist about this is necessary if the patient requires further anesthesia and surgery.

Anticholinergic side effects of tricyclic antidepressants, such as dry mouth, blurred vision, and constipation, are more common at the beginning of treatment. Monitoring should include regular EKGs and measurement of pulse, blood pressure, and blood levels of the drug(s).[90]

Drug interactions and side effects should be considered in managing a psychotropic drug.[91] Bioavailability may be affected; for example, antacids can reduce the absorption of oral chlorpromazine or benzodiazepines. Drug metabolism is affected by competition for hepatic binding sites, serum protein-binding sites, or receptor sites, as in the reduction of diazepam clearance by cimetidine. Drug excretion, as for example of lithium carbonate, is commonly affected by overhydration or dehydration, the use of diuretics, or salt restriction. The specific needs and metabolic sensitivities of children[92] and the elderly[93] to psychotropic agents should be given special consideration.

## OUTCOME STUDIES

Since this is a text on acute care, only brief mention is made of outcome. Recent outcome studies have been attempting to resolve many questions: What types of adjustment do burn victims have? What mental disorders? Were there pre-burn disorders? What helps? How does becoming burned and disfigured affect personality development and self-esteem? Can patients function? Are they more or less impaired than control or comparison groups? Research of large samples of patients has provided surprising results that tend to contradict beliefs previously held firmly by many experienced professionals.

Of the large studies of adults, most burned in adulthood, as many as 70 to 85 per cent seem to have adequate self-esteem. Smaller studies revealed impairment in 60 to 75 per cent. A summary of the adult outcome studies suggests that a majority of adult victims have adjusted well to their burns over the long term, but that some, such as those with facial burns, experience social rejection and impaired self-esteem, and they tend to withdraw. There is *no* evidence of a higher-than-average suicide rate, possibly because of the interpersonal supports that are mobilized as a result of the burn injury. It is often suggested that severely burned persons lost to follow-up probably have poor outcomes, but this has not been substantiated. These results, while not as conclusive as controlled diagnostic studies, do not confirm speculations of severe emotional disorders or emotional disability (e.g., psychosis or severe depressions) in most burned adults.

Long-term studies of children and adolescents have found higher estimates of disorder, including those with comparison groups. Although some of the results are conflicting, for example, some found many emotional problems while others found few, conclusions may be drawn. First, all studies reveal some children and some families to be functioning well. In particular, more recent studies are more positive, probably reflecting the effectiveness of early studies in calling attention to the unmet needs of burn patients. While social supports are certainly very important, less is known about the inherent personality strengths, coping skills, and temperamental traits that improve outcome. More is known about pre-existing risk factors such as low social class, mental illness, and family disruption. There is no evidence that most burned children or adolescents are chronically depressed or suicide risks. The effects of severe disfigurement and the locations of burns are not yet clear, and most studies do not find definite correlations. Many of these patients do work, marry, and bear children. It appears that many patients with small burns are at psychological risk and that some with large burns do well. This may be due to more intensive surgical and psychosocial interventions to help the severely burned.

## MANAGING STRESS AND PREVENTING STAFF BURNOUT

Effective burn consultation by a mental health team (psychiatrist, psychologist, social worker, and psychiatric nurse clinician) occurs within the overall burn team. The challenges and opportunities for consultants are great because it is an interdisciplinary team that must work together closely. Professional and personal backgrounds of physicians, nurses, physical and occupational therapists, dieticians, social workers, and other staff differ widely. As Ravenscroft has described, there is stigma and awe associated with burn unit work which may make the team isolated and defensive, as well as proud and protective. "To a degree, the staff are identified with and take on some of the medical-surgical notoriety and social ostracism experienced by their burn patients who are perceived by outsiders as difficult, dirty, frightening and grotesque."[9]

The psychiatric consultant's empathic availability makes him or her vulnerable to emotional flooding and doubt that he can offer much help in such massive personal disaster and painful treatment.[9] Yet these personal reactions of anxiety and sadness and the tendency to withdraw are similar to those of patients, parents, and new staff and will serve as the most valid empathic guide for the psychiatrist in understanding the emotional stresses and reactions experienced in the burn unit and during ongoing work. The psychiatrist must be attuned to his or her own and others responses, since the tensions, conflicts, and crises around much of burn treatment are expectable, frequent, and, in part, iatrogenic.

There are other specific stresses. Surgeons, anesthesiologists, and operating room nurses spend long hours operating on infected, disfigured patients who commonly have a high risk of major complications or mortality. The ward nursing staff inflicts pain with dressing changes and burn baths, eliciting angry, accusatory, and depressive reactions from patients and family. Other sources of stress are concern for survival of the patient, loss of body parts or functions, loss of physical attractiveness, and grief aroused by dying patients. The intermittent anxieties generated by such traumatic experiences may escalate and contribute to staff burnout.

Staff reactions affecting patient care include loss of professional control such as harsh or overly permissive responses, avoidance of talking with the patient or family, and anger at or withdrawal from team colleagues. There is also use of distancing, inappropriate bedside discussion, use of denial to avoid necessary conflict (for example, regarding decisions for or against continued life support), gallows humor, and temporary depressive episodes. These reactions should be anticipated as adaptive in some situations but carry the risk of becoming maladaptive, especially when not recognized or discussed with superiors. Several steps are encouraged in order to prevent staff burnout:

1. Maintain regular formal and informal group and individual meetings of the mental health consultant with burn team members to help them acknowledge, bear, and understand their thoughts, feelings, and actions.

2. If individual guilt or depression or group demoralization increases, this must be faced rather than denied or avoided.

3. Staff burnout can be alleviated by more intense psychiatric consultation, decreased admissions of the severely burned when possible, in-service education about staff tensions and burnout, and encouraging staff reassignments or changes where necessary while acknowledging the contributions of those taking on different roles.

## SUMMARY AND CONCLUSIONS

This chapter presents approaches to management of emotional trauma and psychiatric disorder experienced by the burn patient and family. The arduous treatment and rehabilitation process of infants, children, and adolescents places extreme stress on their families and staff because of their dependency and immaturity. Burned adults may provide even more stress to their families because of the high incidence of pre-existing substance abuse, psychopathology, medical illness, and the threat to their capacity to return to work. Geriatric burn patients present special emotional and metabolic challenges, and they are at a higher risk of dying. Care of the dying patient and family requires special emotional consideration that may be difficult to provide on an acute unit. The following 10 principles are recommended for the management of severely burned patients:

*An integral member of the burn team should be a psychiatrist consultant familiar with the principles of consultation-liaison psychiatry; this consultant should be funded and work closely with the surgical and nursing staffs and collaborate with psychologists and social workers.

*Anticipate staff stress and design a program of stress reduction to improve the quality of care and to prevent staff burnout.

*Obtain a past history of mental disorders from the patient, family, and friends.

*Diagnose specific emotional reactions or disorders, most commonly pain syndromes, delirium, post-traumatic stress disorder and other anxiety disorders, grief, and depression.

*Alleviate pain based on the patient's self-ratings and put the patient in control as much as possible.

*When a patient is critically ill or dying, team communication should be especially close to support the patient, family, and team members and to reduce stress. Ethical issues should be discussed within the team, and some units may choose to develop a comfort care alternative.[23]

*Plan individualized psychiatric and psychological treatment from admission through rehabilitation.

*Institute treatment with appropriate hypnosis/relaxation/techniques, individual and family therapy, and pharmacotherapy.

*Begin verbal preparation of the patient and family for rehabilitation early in treatment.

*Review, assess, and study the quality of psychiatric care being provided.

These principles are based on discussion in this chapter of psychiatric assessment and treatment of acute burns, including general aspects of burn management, the dying patient, delirium and pain, psychopharmacology, and approaches to family crises. Also presented are the results of outcome studies and constructive interventions to assist staff in adapting to the challenges and stresses of work on the burn unit.

## REFERENCES

1. Herrin J, Crawford J: The seriously burned child. In Smith C (ed): The Critically Ill Child: Diagnosis and Medical Management. 2nd ed. Philadelphia, WB Saunders Company 1985, 1977, pp 21–69.
2. Feller I, Tholen D, Cornell RG: Improvements in burn care, 1965 to 1979. JAMA 244:2074–2078, 1980.
3. Rapkin C (ed): The Impact of Fire on the Family in The Social and Economic Consequences of Residential Fires. Lexington, MA, Lexington Books, 1983, pp 137–210.
4. Deitch EA, Staats M: Child abuse through burning. J Burn Care Rehabil 3(2):89–94, 1982.
5. Hight DW, Bakalar HR, Lloyd JR: Inflicted burns in children. JAMA 242(6):517–520, 1979.
6. Kolko DJ, Kazdin AE, Meyer EC: Aggression and psychopathology in childhood firesetters. J Consult Clin Psychol 53(3):377–385, 1985.
7. Stoddard FJ, Pahlavan K, Cahners SS: Suicide attempted by self-immolation in adolescents. Adolesc Psychiatry 12:251–265, 1985.
8. Blank K, Perry S: Relationship of psychological processes during delirium to outcome. Am J Psychiatry 141:843–847, 1984.
9. Ravenscroft K: The burn unit. Psychiatr Clin North Am 5:419, 1982.
10. Knudson-Cooper M: What are the research priorities in the behavioral areas for burn patients? J Trauma 24:S198–201, 1984.
11. Martin HL: Antecedents of burns and scalds in children. Br J Med Psychol 43:39–47, 1970.
12. Benians RC: A child psychiatrist looks at burned children and their families. Guys Hosp Rep 123(2):149–154, 1974.
13. Galdston R: The burning and healing of children. Psychiatry 35:57–66, 1972.
14. MacArthur JD, Moore, FD: Epidemiology of burns: The burn prone patient. JAMA 231(3):259–263, 1975.

15. Noyes R, Frye SF, Slymen DJ, et al: Stressful life events and burn injuries. J Trauma 19(3):141–144, 1979.
16. Vogtsberger KN, Taylor ER: Psychosocial factors in burn injury. Texas Med 80:43–46, 1984.
17. Kolman PBR: Incidence of psychopathology in burned adult patients. J Burn Care Rehabil 4(6):430–436, 1984. Of special note in this article is a listing of references on premorbid alcohol and drug problems.
18. Martin HL, Lawrie JH, Wilkenson AW: The family of the fatally burned child. Lancet ii:628–629, 1968.
19. Bedell SE, Pelle D, Maher PL, Cleary PD: Do-Not-Resuscitate orders for critically ill patients in the hospital: How are they used and what is their impact? JAMA 256(2):233–237, 1986.
20. Burke JF, Bondoc CC, Quimby CC: Primary burn excision and immediate grafting: A method shortening illness. J Trauma 14:389–395, 1974.
21. Imbus SH, Zawacki BE: Autonomy for burned patients when survival is unprecedented. N Engl J Med 297:308–311, 1977.
22. Waller DA, Todres D, Cassem NH, Anderton A: Coping with poor prognosis on the pediatric intensive care unit. Am J Dis Child 133:1121–1125, 1979.
23. Wachtel TL, Frank HA, Nielsen JA: Comfort care: An alternative treatment programme for seriously burned patients. Burns 13(1):1–6, 1987.
24. Hartmann, E: The Nightmare: The Psychology and Biology of Terrifying Dreams. New York, Basic Books, 1984, pp 189, 213.
25. Molnar JA, Wolfe RR, Burke JF: Burns: Metabolism and nutritional therapy in thermal injury. In Sneider HA, Anderson CE, Coursen DB, et al (eds): Nutritional Support of Medical Practice. 2nd ed. Philadelphia, Harper & Row, 1983, pp 261–262.
26. Diagnostic and Statistical Manual of Mental Disorders. 3rd ed. (DSM-III) Washington, DC, American Psychiatric Association, 1980, p 236.
27. Diagnostic and Statistical Manual of Mental Disorders, 3rd ed, Revised (DSM-III-R). Washington, DC, American Psychiatric Association, 1987, p 247.
28. Kardiner A, Spiegel H: War Stress and Neurotic Illness. New York, Hoeber, 1947.
29. Grinker RR, Spiegel JP: Men Under Stress. New York, Blakiston, 1945.
30. Van der Kolk B: Post-Traumatic Stress Disorder: Psychological and Biological Sequelae. Washington, DC, American Psychiatric Press, 1984.
31. Adler A: Neuropsychiatric complications in victims of Boston's Cocoanut Grove disaster. JAMA 123:1098–1101, 1943.
32. Hamburg DA, Hamburg B, DeGoza S: Adaptive problems and mechanisms in severely burned patients. Psychiatric 16:1–20, 1953.
33. Solnit A, Priel B: Psychological reactions to facial and hand burns in young men—Can I see myself through your eyes? Psychoanal Study Child 30:549–566, 1975.
34. Stoddard FJ: Coping with pain: A developmental approach to treatment of burned children. Am J Psychiatry 139:736–740, 1982.
35. Manusi-Ungaro HR, Tarbox AR, Wainwright DJ: Posttraumatic stress disorder in electric burn patients. J Burn Care Rehabil 7:521–525, 1986.
36. Stoddard FJ, Norman DK, Murphy JM: An outcome study of DSM-III disorders in severely burned children and adolescents compared to matched controls. J Am Acad Child & Adol Psychiatry, July, 1989.
37. Horowitz MJ: Stress Response Syndromes. 2nd ed. New York, Jason Aronson, 1986.
38. Childrens' Reactions to Severe Stress. J Child Psychiatry 25:299, 1986 (special section).
39. Pynoos R, Eth S: Posttraumatic Stress Disorder in Children. Washington, DC, American Psychiatric Press, 1985.
40. Stoddard FJ: Acute stress disorders in infants and young children. Paper presented at Meeting of International Society of Burn Injuries, Denver, 1984.
41. Op. cit, footnote 26, 18:100–103.
42. Lipowski ZJ: Delirium: Acute Brain Failure in Man. Springfield, IL, Charles C Thomas, 1980.
43. Murray GM: Confusion, delirium and dementia. In Hackett TP, Cassem NH (eds): Massachusetts General Hospital Handbook of General Hospital Psychiatry, Second edition, Littleton, MA, PSG Publishing Inc, 1987, pp 84–115.
44. Antoon AY, Volpe JJ, Crawford JD: Burn encephalopathy in children. Pediatrics 50:609–616, 1972.
45. Andreasen NJ, Norris AS: Long term adjustment and adaptation mechanisms in severely burned adults. J Nerv Ment Dis 154:352–362, 1972.

46. Haynes BW, Bright R: Burn coma: A syndrome associated with severe burn wound infection. J Trauma 7:464–475, 1967.
47. Jefferson JW, Marshall JR: Burn Delirium. Neuropsychiatric Features of Acute Medical Disorders. New York, Plenum Press, 1981, pp 296–299.
48. Hughes JR, Cayaffa JJ, Boswick JA: Seizures following burns to the skin: III. Electroencephalographic recordings. Dis Neuro Syst 36:443–447, 1975.
49. Peterson I, Sorbye R, Johanson B, et al: An electroencephalographic and psychiatric study of burn cases. Acta Chir Scand 129:359–366, 1965.
50. Bernstein NR: Observations on the use of hypnosis with burned children on a pediatric ward. Int J Clin Exp Hypn 13(1):1–10, 1965.
51. Gardner G: Hypnosis with children. Int J Clin Exp Hypn 22(1):20–37, 1974.
52. Spiegel H, Spiegel D: Trance and Treatment: Clinical Uses of Hypnosis. New York, Basic Books, 1978.
53. Schafer DW: Hypnosis use on a burn unit. Int J Clin Exp Hypn 23:14, 1975.
54. Wakeman RJ, Kaplan JZ: An experimental study of hypnosis in painful burns. Am J Clin Hypn 21:1, 1978.
55. Marks RM, Sachar EJ: Undertreatment of medical inpatients with narcotic analgesics. Anal Intern Med 78:173, 1973.
56. Perry S, Heidrich G, Ramos E: Assessment of pain by burn patients. J Burn Care Rehabil 2:322, 1981.
57. West DA, Shuck JM: Emotional problems of the severely burned patient. Surg Clin North Am 58(6):1189–1204, 1978.
58. Kavanagh C: Psychological intervention with the severly burned child: Report of an experimental comparison of two approaches and their effects on psychological sequelae. J Am Acad Child Psychiatry 22(2):145–156, 1983.
59. Blimenthal JA: Relaxation therapies and biofeedback. In Psychiatry. Haupt JL, Brodie HKH (eds): Philadelphia, JB Lippincott, 1986, pp 273-285.
60. Shires GT, Black EA (eds): Pain and anxiety in the burn injured. J Trauma 24(Suppl):5168–5197, 1984.
61. Szyfelbein SK, Osgood PF, Carr DB: The assessment of pain and plasma beta-endorphin immunoactivity in burned children. Pain 22:173–182, 1985.
62. Lindemann E: Symptomatology and management of acute grief. Am J Psychiatry 101:141–148, 1944.
63. Cobb S, Lindemann E: Symposium on management of Cocoanut Grove Burns at Massachusetts General Hospital. Ann Surg 117:814–824, 1943.
64. Stoddard FJ: Body image development in the burned child. J Am Acad Child Psychiatry 21(5):502–507, 1982.
65. Furman E: Studies in childhood bereavement. Can J Psychiatry 28(4):241–247, 1983.
66. Osterweis M, Solomon F, Green M (eds): Bereavement Reactions Consequences and Cures. Washington, DC, National Academy Press, 1984.
67. Koocher GP: Children's conceptions of death, new directions for child development. Bribace R, Walsh M (eds): Children's Conceptions of Health, Illness, and Bodily Functions. San Francisco, Jossey Bass, 1981, pp 85–99.
68. Bowden ML, Jones CA, Feller I: Psychosocial Aspects of a Severe Burn: A Review of the Literature. 1979 Supplement to the International Bibliography on Burns. Ann Arbor, MI, National Institute on Burn Medicine, 1979, p 16.
69. Ravenscroft K: Psychiatric consultation to the child with acute physical trauma. Am J Orthopsychiatry 52:301, 1982.
70. Rivlin E, Forshaw A, Polowyi G, Woodruff B: A multi-disciplinary group approach to counselling the parents of burned children. Burns 12(7):479–483, 1986.
71. Cobb S: Social support as a moderator of life stress. Psychosom Med 38:300–314, 1976.
72. Davidson TN, Bowden ML, Feller I, et al: Social support and postburn adjustment. Arch Phys Med Rehabil 26:274–278, 1981.
73. Klein SB: Measuring the impact of chronic childhood illness on the family. In Grave GD, Pless IB (eds): Chronic Childhood Illness: Assessment and Outcome. Washington, DC, DHEW Publ NG (NIH) 76–877, 1976.
74. Jackson DM: The psychological effects of burns. Burns 1:70–74, 1974.
75. Reddish P, Blumenfield M: Psychological reactions in wives of patients with severe burns. J Burn Care Rehabil 5:388–390, 1984.

76. Reddish P, Blumenfield M: A typology of spousal response to the crisis of a severe burn. J Burn Care Rehabil 7(4):328–330, 1986.
77. Cella DF, Perry SW, Kulchycky S, et al: Longitudinal study of psychological adjustment in relatives of burn patients. Abstracts of American Burn Association Meeting, Washington, DC, May 1, 1987.
78. Poag ME, Cella DF, Perry SW, et al: Specific stress responses in parents during pediatric burn hospitalization. Abstracts of American Burn Association Meeting, Washington, DC, May 1, 1987.
79. Cahners SS: Group Meetings benefit families of burned children. Scand J Plast Reconstr Surg 13:169, 1979.
80. Bernstein N: Emotional Care of the Facially Burned and Disfigured. Boston, Little, Brown, 1976, pp 184–212.
81. Bassuk EL, Panzarino PJ, Schoonover SC: General principles of pharmacologic management in the emergency setting. In Bassuk EL, Birk AW (eds): Emergency Psychiatry. New York, Plenum Press, 1984, pp 61–73.
82. Perry S, Heidrich G: Management of pain during debridement: A survey of US burn units. Pain. 13:267–280, 1982.
83. Perry SW: Undermedication for pain on a burn unit. Gen Hosp Psychiatry 6(4):308–316, 1984.
84. Perry SW, Inturiss CE: Analgesia and morphine disposition in burn patients. J Burn Care Rehabil 4:276–280, 1983.
85. Martyn JAJ, Greenblatt DJ, Quinby WC: Diazepam kinetics in patients with severe burns. Anesth Analg 62:293–297, 1983.
86. Martyn JAJ, Greenblatt DJ: Lorezepam conjugation unimpaired in burned patients. Clin Pharmacol Ther 43:250–255, 1988.
87. Sos J, Cassem NH: The intravenous use of haloperidol for acute delirium in intensive care settings. In Siedd MH, Rudewald G (eds): Psychic and Neurological Dysfunctions after Open Heart Surgery. Stuttgart, Georg Thieme Verlag, 1980, pp 196–199.
88. Lerner T, Lwow E, Levitin A, Belmaker RH: Acute high dose parenteral haloperidol treatment of psychosis. Am J Psychiatry 136(8):1061–1064, 1979.
89. Huang V, Figge H, Demling R: Haloperidol complications in burn patients. J Burn Care Rehabil 8(4):269–273, 1987.
90. Task force on the use of laboratory tests in psychiatry: Tricyclic antidepressants—Blood level measurements and clinical outcome: An APA task force report. Am J Psychiatry 142(2):1155–1162, 1985.
91. Hollister L (ed): Drug side effects and interactions. American Psychiatric Association Annual Review, Vol 6. Section VI: Psychopharmacology. Washington, DC, American Psychiatric Press, pp 698–822, 1987.
92. Biederman J, Jellinek MS: Psychopharmacology in children. N Engl J Med 310:968–972, 1984.
93. Georgotas A, Cooper T, Kim M, Hapworth W: The treatment of affective disorders in the elderly. Psychopharmacol Bull 19:226, 1983.
94. Stoddard FJ, Norman DK, Murphy JM: A diagnostic outcome study of children and adolescents with severe burns. J Trauma 271:471–477, 1989.
95. Stoddard FJ, Wileus T: Delirium. In Jellinek MS, Herzog DB (eds): Handbook of Psychiatric Management of the Pediatric Inpatient. (in press).
96. Gold PW, Goodwin FK, Chrousos GP: Clinical and biochemical manifestations of depression. Relation to the neurobiology of stress. N Engl J Med 319(6):348–353, and 319(7):413–420, 1988.

# Minimizing the Potential for Infection in the Hospitalized Burned Patient:

## *Architectural, Engineering, and Environmental Considerations*

GARY C. DU MOULIN

The loss of normal host defenses in the hospitalized, thermally injured patient signals a protracted battle to prevent infection of the wound.[1, 2] The burned area, while initially sterile, within a short period of time develops a succession of microflora, initially gram-positive and ultimately gram-negative.[2, 3] The sources of bacteria that initially colonize and infect the burned area are the patient's own microorganisms, skin flora followed by fecal flora.[4] The gastric environment provides a secondary source of organisms, which become increasingly abundant as the patient undergoes antacid prophylaxis.[5] The patient is also exposed to organisms transmitted by direct contact with contaminated staff, visitors, or patient equipment. Finally, the inanimate environment, comprising contaminated air, water, food, floors, walls, and ceilings, contributes bacteria and fungi that tend to be resistant to antibiotics.[6-8] The environment of the severely burned patient cannot be made bacteria-free all through the healing process. Those who care for burned patients should understand those factors that can minimize the potential for infection through sound therapeutic management and a thorough understanding of the complex microbial environment to which patients are exposed.[9, 10] Measures to prevent infection include early wound closure, prevention of septic complications, adequate nutrition, and control of the external environment.[11-13] This chapter examines control of the external environment from the standpoint of burn unit function and design and places into perspective those elements that can be practically instituted in the protection of the burned patient.

## ATMOSPHERE OF THE BURN UNIT

### Ventilation

Ventilation systems in burn units have been and continue to be a controversial issue.[14] While there is evidence in the literature showing that fungal and viral infection have been transmitted to patients via nonexistent or faulty air-handling systems, there is not a great deal to suggest that expensive sophisticated ventilation systems are necessary to prevent bacterial or fungal colonization and subsequent infection of burned areas. Centralized, filtered, unrecirculating air-handling systems with an efficient preventive maintenance program should keep airborne organisms to a minimum. The major elements for ventilation systems in critical care areas are air pressure differential between the patient's room and the rest of the unit, filtration of air including the efficiency of filtration, and the rate at which the air is replaced. Air pressure differential in a patient's room can be under either positive or negative pressure with respect to the rest of the unit.[15, 16] Since the ultimate goal is to protect the patient from exogenous airborne bacteria, positive-pressure ventilation should be chosen. In units in which a patient has a contagious infection, one would choose exhaust ventilation or negative pressure. Some rooms come equipped with both negative and positive ventilation, and the type of pressure can be reversed by tripping a switch on the wall.[15] However, this design feature should be discouraged.

The air ventilating a patient's room should be filtered. High-efficiency particle arresting (HEPA) filters are well suited for this purpose and are extensively used. These devices are capable of removing from the air particles that are greater than $0.3 \mu$ in size with a greater than 99.97 per cent efficiency.

Ventilation should be provided at a rate ranging from 8 to 20 exchanges per hour.[35] Twelve exchanges of air per hour through HEPA filters is considered optimal.[17]

The most sophisticated form of ventilation offered to burn patients is the laminar air flow room, usually used in conjunction with HEPA filtration.[16, 18-21] This form of air handling comprises the movement of filtered air in a unidirectional laminar distribution, usually at a velocity between 30 and 50 feet per minute. This produces low turbulence and sterile air. The environment of laminar air flow is very expensive and not necessarily shown by itself to significantly decrease burn infection. Some air sampling studies have shown that cross-infection is markedly reduced. The use of laminar air flow facilities has been associated with increased nursing requirements as well as psychological disturbances in patients maintained in these nearly-sterile environments.[21]

Window air conditioning units are discouraged in favor of centralized units because of the latter's better record of preventive maintenance by hospital environmental staff and the former's need for individual attention. The direct connection of the window units to the outside concentrates and disseminates fungal spores into the patient's room.[7] Filtered unrecirculated air conditioning in conjunction with a well-run maintenance program is sufficient to minimize airborne contamination.

Two additional facts must be kept in mind for those designing ventilation systems for burn units. Fresh air intakes on hospital exterior walls or roofs must be placed away from the areas where trucking and kitchen exhausts can accumulate and be drawn back into the hospital. Fresh air intakes should also be located far from effluents from ventilation discharge outlets, incinerators, and boiler stacks. In those institutions upon which heliports have been built, rotor wash from arriving and departing aircraft can wreak havoc on intake filters, with subsequent contamination of the entire air-handling system.[22]

Microbiological contamination of compressed air and other gases has been demonstrated.[23] In one investigation, lower levels of bacteria were found in air generated from oil-free compressors. We purge all gas outlets as part of an ongoing program in all patient's rooms that are either newly constructed or recently renovated. Compressed air in tanks or from wall sources should be checked periodically by air samplers but especially during cross-connection testing procedures prior to the opening of new units.

It is important to remember that proper functioning of the ventilation system in burn units requires the cooperation of a well-trained maintenance staff. Adjustments in air changes, frequency of cleaning, and changing of filters are required and will have a direct effect upon the welfare of the patient. It is important to have someone on the burn unit staff who is knowledgeable about ventilation issues and can maintain a working rapport with maintenance personnel.

## Temperature and Humidity[22–27]

A number of studies have examined the effects of temperature and humidity on evaporative water loss from burned epidermis and the concomitant expenditure of heat and increase in metabolic rate.[25, 26] It has become clear through these studies that the patient's environment has a significant effect upon burn wound healing as well as on the morbidity and mortality associated with serious burns.[24, 28–31]

A number of investigators have examined the effects of alterations in temperature and humidity on the rate of healing and survival.[24, 27–29, 31] The most comprehensive of these studies involves the comparison of humidity/temperature combinations in a burned rat model.[28] While mortality was highest in burned animals subjected to combinations of extremes, that is, high temperature/high humidity (32°C, > 60 per cent relative humidity [RH]) and low temperature/low humidity (20°C, < 30 per cent RH), the most favorable climate appears to be that with high temperature (32°C) and a low relative humidity (< 30 per cent RH) during eschar formation. Low temperature settings (22°C) and high humidity (> 60 per cent RH) were found to promote a faster separation of eschar. Wilmore studied eight burned patients for 24-hour periods in each of two ambient temperatures, 25°C and 33°C. In both ambient temperatures hypermetabolism was present, as well as higher core and skin temperatures than in healthy controls. However, in those patients with large thermal injuries (> 60 per cent of total body surface area), there was a decreased metabolic rate in the higher ambient temperature environment.[27] It is therefore crucial to design into burn units the capability of independent humidity and temperature controls for each bed so that appropriate adjustments can be made as the healing of the burn evolves.

## Treatment Space

The single patient cubicle should now be considered mandatory in the design of burn care units.[32, 33] Physical separation contributes to a decrease in the spread of endogenous flora but also serves as a constant reminder and barrier to cross-contamination by unit personnel. Each cubicle or room should be separated from general unit activity by an anteroom or vestibule. It is in this anteroom that space should be provided for the storage of barrier gowns, gloves, and masks. A sink should be located at the entrance to the patient care area.

The room itself should provide a minimum of 120 square feet per bed. As much as 260 square feet per bed has been allowed in some units.[34] It is important to utilize the space efficiently and to keep the floor clear of equipment such as patient monitors and IV poles; new or renovated units should maximize the use of wall or ceiling fixtures for these devices. The area should be large enough to accommodate the patient's bed, equipment, and supplies. Accumulation of extraneous materials should be kept to a minimum, and those supplies not immediately needed should be stored in cabinets with doors. All horizontal surfaces should be made of durable materials that can be easily disinfected. It is essential in burn unit design to be able to keep clean storage physically separated from dirty storage and waste.

## Lighting[26, 32, 35]

Natural illumination is dependent upon the architecture of the facility and whether or not the unit is part of a new institution where energy-efficient glass is available and commonly employed. Windows to the outside world give a psychological boost to the burned patient during protracted hospitalization. In addition, windows from nursing stations into patient's rooms facilitate better management without the necessity of constantly entering the patient's room to check on developing conditions.[32] Fluorescent lighting should be installed to afford uniform illumination (20 lumens). Lights should not be situated above the patient's eyes. The walls of the unit should be of neutral colors so that examination of the patient's complexion or wound is not distorted. Lighting should be controlled not only in each patient's room but also at the nurse's station so that visits to the patient's room to adjust lighting can be minimized from an infection control standpoint and also to avoid disturbing the sleep of patients.

## WET AND MOIST ENVIRONMENTS OF THE BURN UNIT

Water provides a basic life support need for microorganisms. Even in supplies treated by reverse osmosis, deionization, or distillation, gram-negative organisms can proliferate to levels of $10^5$ to $10^7$ organisms per milliliter.[36] Tap water arising from either ground water or surface water sources undoubtedly supports a teeming microflora. The distribution system provides mechanisms that increase the number of organisms. Water reaching taps of burn unit sinks and ice machines will contain species of bacteria that can include members of the genera *Pseudomonas, Flavobacterium, Acinetobacter, Alcaligenes, Achromobacter, Aeromonas,* and *Serratia.* In addition, many species of nontuberculous mycobacteria, such as *M. avium* complex, are now commonly isolated from hospital water supplies.[37]

Even when sterile water is used in vaporizer or humidification equipment, endogenous microorganisms from the patient's own flora contaminate these devices and proliferate.[38] Production of aerosols from contaminated equipment or poorly designed sinks presents a direct hazard to the burned patient.[39]

In the design of burn units there are a number of factors that can be employed to lessen contact of the burned patient with contaminated water. The most accessible water sources, e.g., sinks and toilets, should be chosen for their lack of aerosol production. Toilets can be located within a cabinet that can be opened and the toilet swiveled out for use. Sinks can be designed with faucets that minimize aerosol formation or splashing. In our institution, cut-off valves have been incorporated into certain sink drains to facilitate filling with phenol-based disinfectants. This serves to eliminate enormous numbers of bacteria that accumulate over a 24-hour period, minimizing the risk of contaminated splashback onto the hands of medical personnel. Despite the thoroughness and frequency of hand washing, sterile gloves should immediately be put on in anticipation of manipulating the burned area. Nebulizer reservoirs are to be filled with sterile water, preferably in small volume reservoirs that are allowed to run dry before refilling. Bottles of sterile water should be dated upon opening and discarded within 24 hours. Cut flowers and plants, of course, have no place in the burn unit.

Hydrotherapy[30, 40–42] is a contested adjunct to the management of the burned patient but can represent a serious potential for infection. Hydrotherapy is not practiced at the Massachusetts General Hospital or the Shriners Burns Institute in Boston. All the conditions that encourage cross-infection are inherent in this form of therapy. These include a perpetually moist environment, a succession of patients who require therapy on a daily basis, and burn unit personnel. Patients shed enormous numbers of organisms into the water; $5.0 \times 10^6$ colony-forming units per milliliter were removed from water in a Hubbard tank following one such treatment.[42] It has long been stated that daily removal of eschar, the use of an antimicrobial agent in the water, and meticulous cleaning following each use will minimize the risk. However, outbreaks caused by both gram-negative and gram-positive organisms are still being reported.[40, 41] Cross-contamination of hydrotherapy water with *Enterobacter cloacae* was responsible for bacteremia in 15 patients in one burn center.[41] In an outbreak of methicillin-resistant *Staphylococcus aureus,* six of ten patients receiving hydrotherapy became colonized when a nurse who was a nasal carrier disseminated organisms by direct contact as well as by contaminating the hydrotherapy water. Organisms were subsequently recovered during air sampling studies and from surface swabs of the Hubbard tank and other areas of the hydrotherapy room.

Minimizing the risk of cross-infection of a hydrotherapy room can take a number of forms. Modification of the Hubbard tank—specifically, removal of the agitator, a piece of equipment usually difficult to disinfect—is one avenue of approach. Hypochlorite can be added to the water, although plastic liners are becoming more popular to separate each patient from a potentially contaminated hydrotherapy tank surface. The tanks should be completely disinfected, drained, and dried thoroughly at the end of each day, and it is important that microbiological checks be carried out on a frequent basis to give some indication of cleaning efficiency. Above all, disinfection and drying should be stressed. Personnel should wear disposable axillary-length gloves and aprons or gowns for each patient treatment, particularly if a common hydrotherapy team is used in a particular unit.

## PATIENT MANAGEMENT AND EQUIPMENT

### Nursing[42, 43]

The design of the burn unit should be such that effective infection control techniques can be carried out. Transmission of infection from staff to patients is probably the most important route and has been the cause of numerous outbreaks of infection reported in the literature.[40, 43, 44] It is clear in these studies, which describe lowered infection rates in new versus old units, that effective infection-control techniques are being practiced, and observance of these techniques is made easier by improvements in unit design, such as sink placement and the increased visibility into the patients' room by use of glass.[17, 33] Continuing education in infection control will be a mainstay in optimizing care, especially for new employees and those personnel who visit the unit periodically, such as x-ray technicians and respiratory therapists.

Hand washing has been uncontested as the most important infection-control practice.[45] In studies evaluating hand-washing practices, it was shown that physicians in an oncology unit washed less frequently but more thoroughly than a nursing cohort.[46] In general, any hand-washing protocol did not significantly reduce the number of bacteria. Between $10^4$ and $10^5$ colony-forming units were present even after vigorous hand washing with soap containing 0.5 per cent parachlorometaxylenol. The predominant organisms isolated were coagulase-negative staphylococci with increased antimicrobial resistance. Fifty per cent of staff members carried gram-negative bacilli even after hand washing. One reason for these organisms remaining was the lack of attention to the subungual region, which supports a lush microflora. Typical hand-washing practices concentrate only on the dorsa and palms. Disinfection of hands using brushes and more effective disinfectants has led to significant reductions of bacteria.[45, 47] It is, therefore, crucial that gloves be donned upon the entrance to a patient's room, and removed and discarded after care has been given, followed by hand washing.

Clothes-borne transmission is another way to spread infection, and this route has been extensively studied.[48] While there is no evidence to suggest that sterile garb is required, it is necessary upon entrance to a patient's room to don disposable hair covers, masks, shoe covers, and barrier gowns that are freshly laundered.

Owing to the condition of burn patients, the nurse/patient ratio should ideally be 1:1 during the day shift and 1:2 during the night shifts.[49] It has been demonstrated that outbreaks of nosocomial infection have taken place in units that are understaffed or that have had to assign temporary employees who lack proper infection control training and tend to abandon aseptic techniques. In the long run, minimizing infection and supporting stringent infection control protocols prevent outbreaks that add to morbidity and mortality of patients in burn units. In addition, outbreaks place an additional stress upon the staff, who are forced to adopt cohorting policies.[50] This type of patient care is very expensive. The search for the culprit among the staff by hand or nasal cultures only serves to demoralize the unit personnel. The key to successful burn unit operation rests on the caliber of nursing personnel. It is their function to maintain a calm, efficient decorum within the unit, to offer education to visitors in infection control, and to see to it that the burned patient receives adequate rest during regular periods of night and day without disturbance by staff and visitors.

## Bedding

Bedding has been a major problem in burn units from the standpoint of infection. The air-fluidized bed as well as conventional bedding becomes grossly contaminated.[43, 51] The situation is worsened when chemicals such as silver nitrate or phenolic disinfectants damage the mattress covers, allowing infectious materials to seep into the mattress. Since the heavily infected burned patient can shed up to $10^{11}$ organisms per gram, it is important to choose bedding that will stand up to effective decontamination on a regular basis.

## Food

Dairy products, fresh fruits and vegetables, and uncooked or unprocessed meats contain large numbers of bacteria, including enteric bacteria—*Pseudomonas*, *Klebsiella*, *Staphylococcus*, and *Streptococcus*. There is no evidence to suggest, however, that contaminated food presents a significant infectious hazard to the burned patient; proper nutritional support of the patient remains the crucial objective. It is sensible to design diets that contain pasteurized milk and sterile water or tap water that is changed at frequent intervals. Meat and vegetables should be cooked and served promptly. A microwave oven in the unit is useful in food preparation for patients who can manage solid foods.

## Disinfection

There are a number of good references that describe protocols for decontaminating the equipment necessary for the care of burned patients.[47] There are three major groups of disinfectants to be considered, each with advantages and disadvantages. The glutaraldehydes are effective against bacteria, viruses, and tubercle bacilli and offer good penetration. They come in liquid form and, with sufficient length of exposure, can be considered effective agents for sterilization. It must be remembered that they can be irritating to skin and tissues and exhibit an activity of about two weeks. The second major group of disinfectants are the phenolic compounds. These are active against bacteria even in the presence of organic material; however, they can also be irritating to skin and mucous membranes and can be absorbed by rubber components of medical devices. The third major group are the alcohols, primarily the isopropyl and methyl alcohols. These chemicals kill vegetative forms of bacteria and tubercle bacilli; however, the alcohols are very easily inactivated by blood and proteinaceous materials and are inactive against bacterial spores and viruses.

## ALTERATION OF PATIENTS' BACTERIAL FLORA

### Antacids and Cimetidine Therapy for Stress Ulcer Prevention

The stomach has been overlooked as an organ that can sustain a large microbial population.[5] Although the number of gastric microorganisms is small under normal conditions, increasing evidence suggests that this equilibrium can be quickly altered by several factors, including disease or medication, and result in intense microbial activity. This is particularly relevant in the prevention of stress ulcers resulting in gastrointestinal bleeding, a common problem in the early stages of hospitalization of the burned patient.[52] Accumulation of a reservoir of organisms has the potential to cause a wide range of infections, with aspiration and pulmonary infection presenting the greatest risk to the burn patient.

We studied the gastric and upper airway flora of 60 consecutive patients treated with antacids or cimetidine in a respiratory/surgical intensive care unit.[53] In 52 patients (87 per cent), one or more organisms were cultured simultaneously from both the upper airways and the stomach. In 17 of these patients, the sequence of transmission was apparent. Eleven patients in this group showed clear evidence of upper airway colonization by stomach microorganisms, predominantly gram-negative bacilli, including *E. coli*, *Klebsiella pneumoniae*, *Citrobacter freundii*, *Enterobacter cloacae*, and *Enterobacter aerogenes*. Gram-positive bacteria colonized the upper airways on four occasions: *Streptococcus viridans*,

*Staphylococcus epidermidis*, and *Corynebacterium* species. *Candida* species originating from the stomach colonized the upper airway on seven occasions.

In three patients, the upper airways were the reservoir for subsequent gastric colonization by *E. cloacae*, *Staphylococcus aureus*, and yeast. In three patients who spent an average of 33 days in our intensive care unit, organisms were transmitted in both directions. All were gram-negative bacilli. Gastric-to-airway colonization was caused by *E. coli*, *E. cloacae*, *K. pneumoniae*, and *Serratia liquefaciens*. Airway-to-stomach colonization was caused by *Serratia marcescens*, *Pseudomonas aeruginosa*, and *Pseudomonas fluorescens*. Sixty-two per cent of the patients were colonized by gram-negative bacilli, whereas only 18.3 per cent were colonized by gram-positive organisms or yeast. The mean time spent in the intensive care unit before airways colonization by gram-negative bacteria was six days.

Gram-negative pneumonia developed in 31 patients (52 per cent) in the intensive care unit. None of the eight patients whose stomach and upper airway flora were different developed pneumonia.

The use of cimetidine increases the risk of pneumonia.[54] Antacid therapy allows the stomach to return periodically to an acid environment, with concomitant killing of bacteria between doses. Cimetidine maintains a higher pH for considerably longer periods of time, although the accompanying reduction of gastric acid output limits the volume of potentially contaminated material that can be aspirated. The use of aluminum sucrose sulfate (sucralfate) has been proposed as a means of preventing gastrointestinal bleeding with reduced gastric overgrowth.[55]

Two studies have undertaken the comparison of microbial growth and gastric pH in patients receiving sucralfate and cimetidine. Both studies[56, 57] showed an absence of microbial and pH changes in the sucralfate-treated groups. Morris[56] demonstrated significantly greater bacterial counts and higher pH in patients taking cimetidine. Previous studies have shown a correlation between antacid administration and increased microbial growth.[53, 58] Furthermore, Tryba, in his study of the relative efficacy of sucralfate, antacids, and cimetidine in the prevention of acute stress bleeding, showed that the frequency of pulmonary infections was lower in the sucralfate-treated group than in the other two treatment groups.[55]

## Intubation

The introduction and maintenance of the tracheal tube in the seriously burned patient constitutes an invasion of host defenses and unquestionably alters the environment of the upper respiratory tract so as to favor colonization and subsequent infection by bacteria.[59] At least 15 per cent of all nosocomial infections involve the respiratory tract.[60] At our institution, patients with pneumonia due to *P. aeruginosa* have a mortality rate of 70 per cent, whereas patients with pneumonia due to other gram-negative organisms have a mortality of 33 per cent.[61]

Nosocomial tracheobronchitis and pneumonia are mediated by a number of basic interactions involving the condition of the patient's host defense mechanisms, the type of therapeutic intervention, the length of hospitalization, and the virulence of the endogenous and exogenous bacteria that abound within the hospital setting.

There is substantial evidence to show that tracheal intubation increases the number of patients who become infected.[60, 62–64] The reasons for this are clear when one realizes that two of the three major defense mechanisms are bypassed by intubation of the trachea. The nasopharyngeal functions of filtering, humidification, and warming inspired air are no longer operational, and the integrity of normal mucus flow on the bronchial epithelium is interrupted by contact with the cuff and shaft of the tube. These defects are magnified by attenuation of the normal cough reflex and lack of glottic closure. Despite aggressive attempts to manipulate the airway in an aseptic manner, most efforts have been futile, and gram-negative bacilli continue to dominate in respiratory infections in the burn care unit.

In a prospective study examining bacterial infection, 28 patients were studied following intubation with tracheal tubes. Of these, seven developed tracheobronchitis and three developed pneumonia, constituting an infection rate of 36 per cent, twice that found in studies of respiratory infection in general.[65] Most patients first became colonized within 48 hours of intubation. In another prospective study involving 213 patients, 36 of 56 patients (64 per cent) who were intubated became colonized with gram-negative bacilli, whereas 59 of 157 patients (38 per cent) who were not intubated became colonized with gram-negative bacilli ($P < 0.001$).[60] Neither inhalation therapy nor smoking made a difference in the rate of infection. Colonization with gram-negative bacilli was correlated with the use of antimicrobial drugs. Reinarz quantitated bacteria recovered in tracheal secretions shortly after intubation and found in a majority of the patients more than $10^5$ colony-forming units per milliliter of tracheal aspirate.[66] He believes that meticulous care of the endotracheal tube can delay gram-negative colonization for up to 48 hours. This approach seems unrealistic because most patients remain intubated for much longer periods of time. After 72 hours of intubation no degree of care prevents gram-negative colonization.[67]

The final mechanical barrier protecting the trachea remains the cuff of the tracheal tube. Schwartz has studied the environment of the endotracheal tube and describes a new anatomic "dead space" created when the cuff is inflated.[68] Secretions containing bacteria pool here and cannot be effectively removed by standard suctioning techniques. When the cuff is deflated for repositioning or prevention of circulatory embarrassment, these secretions spill directly into the trachea. Benefits are derived, in Schwartz's view, from the use of the low-pressure cuff, which eliminates the need for routine cuff deflation. When repositioning or removal is indicated, direct laryngoscopic observation aids in the removal of accumulated contaminated secretions.

Evidence is accumulating to show that injury to tracheal mucosa as a result of intubation causes selective adherence of gram-negative bacilli, particularly *P. aeruginosa*. In studies done with ferrets, placement of an endotracheal tube caused significant desquamation of tracheal epithelial cells, leaving basement membrane exposed. Subsequent challenge with *P. aeruginosa* and examination by scanning electron microscopy showed adherence of bacteria only to desquamated areas.[69] These areas provide the matrix for bacterial colonization and growth, which, if allowed to continue, inevitably provides a sufficient inoculum for the development of pneumonia.

## Antibiotic Prophylaxis

In order to protect our patients, we must somehow effectively interrupt contamination and subsequent colonization by bacteria. The use of prophylactic antibiotics to prevent colonization and pneumonia has been a controversial approach. We have found it to be of immense help in the intensive care unit setting, particularly during times when outbreaks of specific pathogens appear imminent.

We evaluated two modes of polymyxin B administration in an attempt to lower rates of upper airway colonization by gram-negative bacilli, particularly *P. aeruginosa*.[70, 71] In the first mode we used polymyxin every alternate two months for 22 months.[71] The second mode involved using polymyxin B continuously for a seven-month period.[70] Polymyxin B, prepared as a 0.5 per cent solution with physiologic saline, was administered in a total dose of 2.5 mg/kg/day in six divided doses. Each dose was given as an aerosol to the posterior pharynx. If the trachea was intubated, half of the dose was injected directly into the endotracheal tube. When polymyxin was being given, all sputum specimens were obtained using sterile techniques at least three hours after a polymyxin dose. We carefully monitored the rates of upper airway colonization, the incidence of acquired pneumonia, and the mortality rates of patients admitted to our respiratory-surgical intensive care unit. The incidence of upper airway colonization with *P. aeruginosa* was 1.6 per cent during polymyxin treatment cycles and 9.7 per cent during placebo cycles when patients received only physiologic saline ($P < 0.01$). Three patients acquired *Pseudomonas* pneumonia during polymyxin cycles, whereas 17 acquired *Pseudomonas* pneumonia during the placebo cycles ($P < 0.01$). Overall mortality and use of systemic antibiotics were similar in both polymyxin- and placebo-treated groups. In the second treatment mode, when polymyxin was used continuously in 292 patients for seven months, only one case of acquired *Pseudomonas* pneumonia occurred; however, ten others acquired pneumonia due to polymyxin-resistant organisms, suggesting that the aerosol used continuously to prevent airway colonization selects for resistant gram-negative bacteria.[70]

Since the time of these studies, acquired pneumonia in our unit has decreased to 1.9 per cent from a high of 6.5 per cent when polymyxin aerosolization was seen as a necessary measure. This marked decrease in acquired pneumonia is, we believe, attributable in part to improvements in hygiene and fluid balance, decreased numbers of tracheostomies, and tracheal tube designs that cause less trauma to mucosal surfaces. Earlier control of impending respiratory failure, improved nutrition, and reduction in gastrointestinal bleeding also contribute to an increased survival in the intensive care unit.

The factors responsible for the changes in the incidence of airway colonization for patients in the respiratory-surgical intensive care unit and their more favorable prognosis are many. Overall improvement in patient care includes more aggressive approaches to invasive monitoring to attain optimal fluid balance and good tissue perfusion. Nutritional status is supported by scrupulous attention to daily caloric intake either by the gastrointestinal route or by hyperalimentation.

Fewer patients have a tracheostomy performed for prolonged respiratory failure. Our increasing conservatism regarding tracheostomy is in part a reflection of the improvement in design of endotracheal tubes. Tracheostomy in burn patients is associated with a pulmonary sepsis rate of 78 per cent, whereas burn patients without tracheostomy have a pulmonary sepsis rate of 12.5 per cent.[72] A greater proportion of patients are being ventilated on admission to the respiratory-surgical intensive care unit. The frequency of patient contact is reduced by having the major ward rounds in a conference room rather than at the bedside. Improved techniques for routine disinfection of respiratory support equipment and the availability of newer antibiotics also contribute to the decreased rate of pulmonary sepsis.

## CONCLUSIONS

It is incumbent upon personnel who treat the thermally injured patient to be actively involved in the planning and design of new or renovated construction of burn care facilities. By minimizing the potential for infection in these patients, the time and effort of those who will ultimately be working in these environments will be well spent and enormously satisfying.

## REFERENCES

1. Lawrence JC: The bacteriology of burns. J Hosp Infect 6(Suppl B):3–17, 1985.
2. Settle JAD: Infection in burns. J Hosp Infect 6(Suppl B):19–29, 1985.
3. Moncrief JA: Medical progress. Burns. N Engl J Med 288:444–454, 1973.
4. McManus AT, McManus WF, Mason AD Jr, et al: Microbial colonization in a new intensive care burn unit. A prospective cohort study. Arch Surg 120:217–223, 1985.
5. du Moulin GC, Hedley-Whyte J: The stomach as a bacterial reservoir: Clinical significance. Intern Med Specialist 3:47–55, 1982.
6. Ayliffe GAJ, Lowbury EJL: Airborne infection in hospital. J Hosp Infect 3:217–240, 1982.

7. Lentino JR, Rosenkranz MA, Michaels JA, et al: Nosocomial aspergillosis. Am J Epidemiol 116:430–437, 1982.
8. Vidotto V, Caramello S, Lucchini A: Sources of fungal contamination in a burn-care unit. Mycopathologia 95:77–80, 1986.
9. Maejima K, Deitch E, Berg R: Promotion by burn stress of the translocation of bacteria from the gastrointestinal tracts of mice. Arch Surg 119:166–172, 1984.
10. Sasaki TM, Welch GW, Herndon DN, et al: Burn wound manipulation–induced bacteremia. J Trauma 19:46–48, 1979.
11. Arturson G: Pathophysiology of the burn wound. Ann Chir Gynaecol 69:178–190, 1980.
12. Donati L, Lazzarin A, Signorini M, et al: Preliminary clinical experiences with the use of immunomodulators in burns. J Trauma 23:816–831, 1983.
13. Murphy RC, Kucan JO, Robson MC, Heggers JP: The effect of 5% mafenide acetate solution on bacterial control in infected rat burns. J Trauma 23:878–881, 1983.
14. Barton FL, Branthwaite MA, English ICW, Prentis JJ: Atmospheric contamination in intensive therapy units. Anaesthesia 28:160–163, 1973.
15. Gaya H: Infection control in intensive care. Br J Anaesth 48:9–12, 1976.
16. Khanam T, Branthwaite MA, English ICW, Prentis JJ: The control of pulmonary sepsis in intensive therapy units. Anaesthesia 28:17–28, 1973.
17. Goldmann DA, Durbin WA Jr, Freeman J: Nosocomial infections in a neonatal intensive care unit. J Infect Dis 144:449–459, 1981.
18. Burke JF, Quinby WC, Bondoc CC, et al: The contribution of a bacterially isolated environment to the prevention of infection in seriously burned patients. Ann Surg 186:377–387, 1977.
19. Demling RH, Moylan JA, Ellerbe S, Jarrett F: Experience with laminar airflow in the management of major burns. Wisconsin Med J 76:S149–S150, 1977.
20. Demling RH, Perea A, Maly J, et al: The use of a laminar airflow isolation system for the treatment of major burns. Am J Surg 136:375–378, 1978.
21. Pizzo PA: The value of protective isolation in preventing nosocomial infections in high risk patients. In Dixon RE (ed): Nosocomial Infections. New York, Yorke Medical Books, 1981, pp 256–262.
22. Gardner S, Abzug MJ, Cymanski M, et al: Heliport-associated nosocomial mucormycoses in oncology patients. Abstracts of the 26th Interscience Conference on Antimicrobial Agents and Chemotherapy, New Orleans, 1986, p 233.
23. Oberg G, Bjerring P: Comparison of microbiological contents of compressed air in two Danish hospitals. Effect of oil and water reduction in air-generating units. Acta Anaesthesiol Scand 30:305–308, 1986.
24. Aulick LH, McManus AT, Pruitt BA Jr, Mason AD Jr: Effects of infection on oxygen consumption and core temperature in experimental thermal injury. Ann Surg 204:48–52, 1986.
25. Jelenko C III: Collective review. Systemic response to burn injury: A survey of some current concepts. J Trauma 10:877–884, 1970.
26. Russell JT, Stewart AW, Kessler A: The design and function of an intensive care unit. S Afr Med J 42:931–933, 1968.
27. Wilmore DW, Mason AD, Johnson DW, Pruitt BA Jr: Effect of ambient temperature on heat production and heat loss in burn patients. J Appl Physiol 38:593–597, 1975.
28. Farkas LG, McCain WG, Birch JR, James J: The effects of four different chamber climates on oxygen consumption and healing of severely burned rats. J Trauma 13:911–916, 1973.
29. Farkas LG, Bannantyne RM, James JS, Umamaheswaran B: Effect of two different climates on severely burned rats infected with Pseudomonas aeruginosa. Europ Surg Res 6:295–300, 1974.
30. Headley BJ, Robson MC, Krizek TJ: Methods of reducing environmental stress for the acute burn patient. Phys Ther 55:5–8, 1975.
31. Kaufman T, Alexander JW, Nathan P, et al: The microclimate chamber: The effect of continuous topical administration of 96% oxygen and 75% relative humidity on the healing rate of experimental deep burns. J Trauma 23:806–815, 1983.
32. Ollstein RN, Symonds FC, Crikelair GF, Corliss S: Creation of a burn center. Plast Reconstr Surg 43:260–265, 1969.
33. Shirani KZ, McManus AT, Vaughan GM, et al: Effects of environment on infection in burn patients. Arch Surg 121:31–36, 1986.
34. Wiklund PE: Intensive care units: Design, location, staffing ancillary areas, equipment. Anesthesiology 31:122–136, 1969.

35. Burn JMB: Design and staffing of an intensive care unit. Lancet 1:1040–1043, 1970.
36. Favero MS, Carson LA, Bond WW, Peterson NJ: Factors that influence microbiologic contaminations of fluids associated with hemodialysis machines. Appl Microbiol 28:822–823, 1974.
37. du Moulin GC, Stottmeier KD: The ecology and health effects of waterborne mycobacteria. ASM News 52:525–529, 1986.
38. Bancroft ML, du Moulin GC: Re-evaluating the role of respiratory care equipment and practices in the prevention of nosocomial pneumonia. Respir Care 28:165–168, 1983.
39. Teres D, Schweers P, Bushnell LS, et al: Sources of Pseudomonas aeruginosa infection in a respiratory/surgical intensive care unit. Lancet 1:415–417, 1973.
40. Arnow PM, Allyn PA, Nichols EM, et al: Control of methicillin-resistant Staphylococcus aureus in a burn unit: Role of nurse staffing. J Trauma 22:954–959, 1982.
41. Mayhall CG, Lamb VA, Gayle WE Jr, Haynes BW Jr: Enterobacter cloacae septicemia in a burn center: Epidemiology and control of an outbreak. J Infect Dis 139:166–171, 1979.
42. Pierson CL: Infection control in burn care facilities. In Roderick MA (ed): Infection Control in Critical Care. Rockville, MD, Aspen Systems Corporation, 1983, pp 143–154.
43. Fujita K, Lilly HA, Ayliffe GAJ: Spread of resistant Gram-negative bacilli in a burns unit. J Hosp Infect 3:29–37, 1982.
44. Espersen F, Bo Nielsen P, Lund K, et al: Hospital-acquired infections in a burns unit caused by an imported strain of Staphylococcus aureus with unusual multi-resistance. J Hyg Camb 88:535–541, 1982.
45. Lowbury EJL: Control of infection in the hospital: Problems in surgery and the management of burns. Rev Infect Dis 3:728–733, 1981.
46. Larson E, McGinley KJ, Grove GL, et al: Physiologic, microbiologic, and seasonal effects of handwashing on the skin of health care personnel. Am J Infect Contr 14:51–59, 1986.
47. Holzman BH, Scott GB: Control of infection and techniques of isolation in the pediatric intensive care unit. Pediatr Clin North Am 28:703–721, 1981.
48. Hambraeus A, Ransjö U: Attempts to control clothes-borne infection in a burn unit. I. Experimental investigations of some clothes for barrier nursing. J Hyg Camb 79:193–202, 1977.
49. Thomsen M, Sorensen B: A modern burns unit. Ann Chir Gynaecol 69:173–177, 1980.
50. du Moulin GC, Dasse P, Miller MG, et al: Staphylococcal outbreak in an intensive care unit—a narrative account of its management. Heart Lung 8:94–99, 1979.
51. Scheidt A, Drusin LM: Bacteriologic contamination in an air-fluidized bed. J Trauma 23:241–242, 1983.
52. Robinson DW: KUMC Burn Center. First six months. J Kansas Med Soc July 1974, pp 233–237.
53. du Moulin GC, Paterson DG, Hedley-Whyte J, Lisbon A: Aspiration of gastric bacteria in antacid-treated patients: A frequent cause of postoperative colonization of the airway. Lancet 1:242–245, 1982.
54. Ruddell WSJ, Axon ATR, Findlay JM, et al: Effect of cimetidine on the gastric bacterial flora. Lancet 1:672–674, 1980.
55. Tryba M, Zevounou F, Torok M, Zenz M: Prevention of acute stress bleeding with sucralfate, antacids, or cimetidine. Am J Med 79(Suppl 2C):55–61, 1985.
56. Morris DL, Youngs D, Burdon DW, Keighley MRB: The influence of sucralfate or cimetidine on gastric juice pH, bacterial flora and mutagenicity. Dig Surg 1(1):6–9, 1984.
57. Wexler H, van Deventer G, Olson C, et al: Effects of acute ulcer healing therapy on gastric microbiology and nitrite presence in gastric aspirates [abstract]. Dig Dis Week 86(5, pt 2):1297, 1984.
58. Kahn RJ, Serruys-Schoutens E, Brimioulle S, Vincent J-L: Influence of antacid treatment on the tracheal flora in mechanically ventilated patients [abstr]. Crit Care Med 10(3):229, 1982.
59. Hedley-Whyte J, du Moulin GC: The environment of endotracheal tubes: Role of tracheal tubes in the colonization of the upper airway and development of pneumonia. King of Prussia, PA, Tracheal Tube Workshop, Annual Meeting of the Pennsylvania Society of Anesthesiology, 1981, pp 91–99.
60. Johanson WG, Pierce AK, Sanford JP, Thomas GD: Nosocomial respiratory infection with gram-negative bacilli. The significance of colonization of the respiratory tract. Ann Intern Med 77:701–706, 1972.
61. Stevens RM, Teres D, Skillman JJ, Feingold DS: Pneumonia in an intensive care unit: A 30 month experience. Arch Intern Med 143:106–111, 1974.

62. Brook I: Bacterial colonization, tracheobronchitis, and pneumonia following tracheostomy and long term intubation in pediatric patients. Chest 76:420–424, 1979.
63. Bryant LR, Trinkle JK, Mobin-Uddin K, et al: Bacterial colonization profile with tracheal intubation and mechanical ventilation. Arch Surg 104:647–651, 1972.
64. Redman LR: Colonization of the upper respiratory tract with gram-negative bacilli after operation, endotracheal intubation and prophylactic antibiotic therapy. Anaesthesia 22:220–227, 1967.
65. Dominquez de Villota E, Arello F, Granados MA, et al: Early post-surgical bacterial contamination of the airways: A study of 28 open heart patients. Acta Anaesth Scand 22:227–233, 1978.
66. Reinarz JA: Nosocomial infections. Clin Symp 30:2–32, 1979.
67. Greenfield S, Teres D, Bushnell LS, et al: Prevention of gram-negative bacillary pneumonia using aerosol polymyxin as prophylaxis. I. Effect on the colonization pattern of the upper respiratory tract of seriously ill patients. J Clin Invest 52:2935–2940, 1973.
68. Schwartz SN, Dowling JN, Benkovic C, et al: Sources of gram-negative bacilli colonizing the tracheae of intubated patients. J Infect Dis 138:227–231, 1978.
69. Ramphal R, Small PM, Shands JW, et al: Adherence of *Pseudomonas aeruginosa* to tracheal cells injured by influenza infection or by endotracheal intubation. Infect Immun 27:614–619, 1980.
70. Feeley TW, du Moulin GC, Hedley-Whyte J, et al: Aerosol polymyxin and pneumonia in seriously ill patients. N Engl J Med 293:471–475, 1975.
71. Klick JM, du Moulin GC, Hedley-Whyte J, et al: Prevention of gram-negative bacillary pneumonia using polymyxin aerosol as prophylaxis. II. Effect on the incidence of pneumonia in seriously ill patients. J Clin Invest 55:514–519, 1975.
72. Eckhauser FE, Billote J, Burke JF, et al: Tracheostomy complicating massive burn injury: A plea for conservatism. Am J Surg 127:418–422, 1974.

# 19

# Burn Wound Infections

MARISSA SELIGMAN and J. A. JEEVENDRA MARTYN

Despite the significant advances made in the last 40 years in the treatment of burn patients, infections continue to represent a serious complication of burn injury. Up to 75 per cent of critically burned patients who survive the initial resuscitation period but develop a burn wound infection subsequently die from sepsis despite intensive local and systemic antibiotic therapy.[1] Accordingly, the primary role of drugs in the management of severe burn wound is to prevent the development of wound infections and to effectively treat those that develop.

## ETIOLOGY, RISK FACTORS, AND MICROBIOLOGY

Following a critical burn injury, the wound surface is sterile and sparsely populated by surface microorganisms. During the next 48 to 72 hours, however, bacteria from the environment, from adjacent undamaged epithelium, and from deeper surviving hair follicles and sweat glands seed onto the wound eschar.[1] These bacteria rapidly reproduce and colonize the area of damage. In fact, the organisms so proliferate that by the second post-burn day, they usually number in the millions per gram of wound tissue.[2] Until the 1960s, the prevailing colonizing organisms were gram-positive ones, primarily *Staphylococcus aureus* and streptococci.[2, 3] At present, however, these microbes can be isolated from the wound only during the first one to three post-burn days. On or about the third post-wound day, and almost universally by the seventh, the microorganisms that colonize the burn wound are gram-negative, primarily *Pseudomonas aeruginosa* but also *Klebsiella pneumoniae* and *Escherichia coli*.[2, 3]

Bacterial colonization of burn wounds occurs for a number of reasons. First, there is the loss of epithelium and mucous membranes, which are integral physical barriers to the proliferation and systemic invasion by microorganisms. Second, burn wound eschar is dead tissue, an ideal medium for microbe growth. Finally, burn wounds are often covered by dressings and kept warm, moist, and dark, thereby providing optimal conditions for bacterial proliferation. The combination of these factors supports rapid microorganism replication within the burn wound. It should be noted that superficial eschar colonization occurs after any burn injury and does not necessarily result in burn wound infection. Rather, there are specific patient- and microbe-related factors that increase the likelihood of a burn wound infection materializing.[2] The most important of these factors are those relating to the vascular and immunological abnormalities that develop following a burn injury.[4]

Partial- and full-thickness burns cause varying degrees of blood vessel damage; the degree of vascular abnormality within a burn wound appears to be in proportion to the extent of the injury.[5] After a burn injury, the center of the wound is coagulated,[6] and the resultant eschar tissue is totally devoid of blood flow, i.e., avascular. This zone of blood flow stasis results from the formation of platelet microthrombi and red cell packing within the burn wound.[7] In a full-thickness wound, this area is fully occluded until approximately three weeks after the injury.[5] In partial-thickness burns, the circulation in the center of the wound is occluded only in the first 24 to 48 hours.[5, 7] Infection can convert a partial-thickness burn wound to a full-thickness wound.[8] Regardless of the thickness of a burn wound, the surrounding tissue peripheral to the area of avascularity may have markedly variable blood flow. All of these vascular abnormalities can lead to the development of infection of the burn wound because they impair the delivery of host defense mediators to the burn area.[5]

Critically ill burned patients are also at high risk for developing infection owing to marked functional abnormalities in the mechanisms of cellular and humoral immunity.[2, 4] Defects that have been identified include decreased neutrophil phagocytosis and killing ability,[9–11] decreased neutrophil chemotaxis,[12–14] decreased macrophage activity,[4, 15] decreased lymphocyte response,[13] decreased number and function of helper T cells,[15, 16] decreased gamma globulin,[17, 18] decreased lymphocyte stimulator interleukin-2,[19–21] decreased fibronectin,[17] and increased circulating immunosuppressors[22] and suppressor T cells.[13, 23] Of these, the depression of neutrophil activity has been proposed as the major factor that predisposes burn patients to infection.[6] Other patient and microbe-related factors that influence the development of burn wound infections are listed in Table 19–1.

Given the marked derangement of burn patients' host defenses and the usual occurrence of microbial growth and proliferation within a burn wound, it

**TABLE 19–1. Risk Factors Leading to Development of Burn Wound Infection**

1. Greater than 30% TBSA burn
2. Full-thickness burn
3. Very young, elderly
4. Pre-existing disease(s)
5. Wound dryness
6. Wound temperature
7. Impaired blood flow
8. Acidosis
9. Greater than $10^5$ microorganisms per gram of tissue
10. Motility of colonizing/infecting microorganisms
11. Metabolic products of colonizing/infecting microorganisms
    a. Endotoxin
    b. Exotoxin
    c. Permeability factors
12. Antimicrobial resistance

is not surprising that these patients commonly develop wound infections. Because burn wound infections often progress to septicemia, much attention should be given to preventing the progression of injury, to controlling bacterial colonization of the wound, and to averting the development of infection. The primary goals of burn therapy immediately after a burn injury include stabilization of the patient to ensure sufficient delivery of oxygen, nutrients, and mediators of cell and humoral immunity to the wound.[4] Surgical excision of necrotic tissue and wound closure are of utmost importance, as they remove dead necrotic tissue and its inherent bacterial contaminants, thereby lessening the risk of burn wound infection.[23]

The primary pharmacological method of reducing the incidence of burn wound infection is by the use of topical antimicrobial agents. Systemic antibiotics are not used for prophylaxis in burned patients because the avascularity of eschar tissue limits the ability of antibiotics to diffuse from the blood stream and penetrate the burn wound.[8] In addition, the unrestricted use of parenteral antibiotics tends to induce the development of resistance by the colonizing microorganisms.[1, 8, 20] Therefore, systemic antibiotic therapy should be reserved for the treatment of suspected or documented burn wound infection or sepsis.

## BACTERIAL INFECTIONS

As previously discussed, bacterial infections of burn wounds arise from opportunistic microorganisms that colonize the wounds. The species of colonizing microorganisms vary from institution to institution and, in many hospitals, from month to month. The organisms most commonly isolated from burn wounds are *Staphylococcus pyogenes*, *S. aureus*, *S. epidermidis*, and alpha- and beta-hemolytic and enterococcal streptococci.[1, 2] Gram-negative organisms frequently isolated from burn wounds include *Pseudomonas aeruginosa*, *Escherichia coli*, and species of *Klebsiella*, *Enterobacter*, *Citrobacter*, *Proteus*, and *Bacteroides*.[1, 2]

Overall, *Staphylococcus aureus*, *Klebsiella pneumoniae*, and *Pseudomonas aeruginosa* are the microorganisms that most commonly cause burn wound infections.[2]

## Common Sites of Infections

### Wound Infections

Burn wound infections can be clinically characterized by their causative microorganisms. They usually become infected by a single strain of a pathogen. Gram-positive microbes such as staphylococci and streptococci tend not to be invasive.[1, 2] Therefore, they usually do not penetrate the fascial layers of the wound but remain within the skin and subcutaneous tissue. Accordingly, these organisms cause such local complications of a burn wound as cellulitis of the surrounding skin.[8] Rarely, a gram-positive organism disseminates and precipitates a systemic infection.[1]

In contrast to gram-positive organisms, gram-negative microorganisms, most commonly *Pseudomonas aeruginosa*, tend to rapidly proliferate in necrotic tissue and invade underlying and adjacent healthy tissue, including blood vessels.[2, 24] It is not uncommon, therefore, for gram-negative organisms to cause burn wound infections of healthy, viable tissue adjacent to and beneath a burn wound (subeschar tissue). In clinical practice, uncontrolled proliferation of gram-negative organisms can induce wound ischemia and hemorrhage. These changes commonly result in the conversion of a partial-thickness burn wound to a full-thickness one.[6] The development of a full-thickness wound can, in turn, lead to bacteremia and the hematogenous spread of these pathogens, whereby distant healthy tissue is seeded with a gram-negative pathogen and becomes infected. Dissemination of gram-negative pathogens almost universally leads to the development of septicemia.[1, 2, 5]

Burn wound infection occurs if there are more than $10^5$ bacteria per gram of tissue.[8, 25] Although surface cultures of wounds are useful in determining which microorganisms are colonizing the burn wound and which potential pathogens exist within the hospital burn unit environment, they do not provide direct information about the bacterial content of the burn wound itself. This can be detected only by biopsy of the wound.[25] Several studies have demonstrated that systematic evaluation of burn injuries by biopsying all areas of the wound allows for early detection of invasive wound infections.[25-27] Therefore, it appears that the combined use of biopsy and culture techniques can provide early diagnosis of the development of burn wound infection as well as the identity and antimicrobial sensitivity of the causative organism.[2]

The bacterial concentration per gram of tissue is the most sensitive indicator of the development of a burn wound infection. The conversion of a burn wound to a progressive and invasive burn wound infection may also be presumed if there is a change in the appearance or character of the wound.[23] Hemorrhage, conversion of a partial- to a full-thickness wound with rapid eschar separation and advancing wound margin, and black or greenish discoloration of the eschar or subeschar fat imply bacterial invasion of the wound.[2, 5, 8, 23]

The development of bacteremia or septicemia from a burn wound infection should be suspected if the clinical signs of sepsis develop, e.g., hypo- or hyperthermia, hypotension, ileus, thrombocytopenia, neutropenia, hyperglycemia, and decreased urine output. Often bacteremia cannot be documented.[23]

## Pulmonary Infections

Serious pulmonary infections may develop in the burned patient, particularly in those individuals who have lung damage secondary to a thermal or chemical inhalation injury.[4] Because of the resultant destruction of respiratory epithelium, loss of mucociliary function, and loss of the protective barrier formed by tracheobronchial secretions, bacteria from the environment readily colonize the respiratory tree.[21] Bacteria may also seed the lung from a burn wound or from invasive equipment such as feeding tubes and ventilators.[2] Use of central venous, pulmonary artery, or cardiac catheters can result in endothelial damage with overlying thrombus in the pulmonary artery.[28, 29] Subsequent embolism and infarction can induce pulmonary ischemia and can also result in pulmonary infection if bacteria from a burn wound disseminate to the lung. Cellular debris within the respiratory tree and decreases in postinjury ventilatory function may result in atelectasis and possibly pneumonia.[4]

Prior to the advent of topical antimicrobial therapy and effective wound management, pulmonary infections most commonly resulted from hematogenous seeding of the lungs from a burn wound; other common sources of bacterial contamination of the lung include suppurative thrombophlebitis, soft tissue abscesses, and intraperitoneal infection.[2, 4, 30] Although hematogenous pneumonia is now less common, it remains a serious complication.[4, 31] Treatment should be directed at removing the source by wound debridement, for example.[21] Systemic antibiotics should be used only in patients with documented bronchopneumonia. Choice of agent should be based on endobronchial culture and sensitivity tests. There is no value in using either prophylactic antibiotics or aerosolized antibiotics in burned patients with pulmonary infections.[32] They are of no clinical value and may actually induce the emergence of multiple drug-resistant microorganisms.

### Miscellaneous Sites

Suppurative thrombophlebitis occurs in at least 5 per cent of burn patients.[21] Mortality, even in treated patients, is very high—almost 60 per cent.[33, 34] Suppurative thrombophlebitis is commonly associated with the use of peripheral intravenous catheters. Persistent fevers and persistently positive blood cultures in the burned patient, in the absence of an obvious source, should be diagnosed as septic thrombophlebitis until proven otherwise.[1, 21] Changing infusion catheters and rotating the site of insertion have minimized the incidence of suppurative thrombophlebitis.[4]

The use of central venous, pulmonary, and cardiac catheters also represents a potential infectious source in burn patients.[35–38] An increased incidence of bacterial endocarditis in burned patients is related to the use of central catheters. The intracardiac placement of catheters may injure the myocardium, particularly of the right heart, and result in the formation of nonbacterial thrombi or vegetations and aseptic thrombotic endocarditis.[38] Bacteremia emanating from burn wounds or infections such as pneumonia or suppurative thrombophlebitis can seed these endocardial thrombi and result in septic endocarditis. The incidence of endocarditis has been estimated to be as high as 9.4 per cent in patients with a central catheter.[39] The incidence of catheter-induced heart injury can be reduced if central catheters are inserted only in patients who will derive the maximum benefit, such as those exhibiting marked hemodynamic instability, if the catheters are inserted under aseptic conditions, and if the catheters are changed frequently, at least once every 72 hours. If a burn patient with a central catheter manifests fever and persistent bacteremia in the absence of an obvious source of infection, echocardiographic and angiographic studies may be necessary to rule out injury to the heart and heart valves from infecting organisms.[40]

Like other hospitalized patients, burn patients with indwelling Foley catheters in place for prolonged periods are at high risk for developing urinary tract infections.[4] These infections include pyelonephritis and prostatic abscess.

Burn patients may develop intra-abdominal infections, the diagnosis of which is often complicated by difficulties in physically examining the burn patient for peritoneal signs of abdominal infection.[4] The burn patient is at high risk for developing intra-abdominal infections secondary to paralytic ileus, gastrointestinal hemorrhage, or perforation due to stress ulcers.[4, 5] Other infrequent causes of intra-abdominal sepsis include cholecystitis, appendicitis, and pancreatitis.[1]

Burn patients may develop sinusitis and middle ear infections as a result of prolonged nasotracheal intubation or the use of nasogastric or feeding tubes.[1, 4] These infections arise from irritation and the resultant swelling of the mucosa or nasopharynx.

Following a burn injury or aggressive patient care, the eyes may be susceptible to corneal damage by ulceration or perforation and subsequent infection.[4] The incidence of these complications may be reduced by careful taping and padding to keep the eyes closed and by intensive use of methylcellulose drops and topical antibiotic ointments.

## Fungal Infections

Over the past 20 years, fungal infections have emerged as an important cause of morbidity and mortality in the burned patient.[41] The most commonly isolated fungi are species of *Candida*, but aggressive pathogens such as *Phycomycetes* have also been isolated.

*Candida* organisms commonly colonize burn wounds, especially in those areas treated with wide-spectrum topical antimicrobials. Significant growths of the organisms are very uncommon and *Candida* have a low potential of invading into the burn wound.[2, 42] However, candidal wound infections have been reported most commonly in patients with extensive burn injuries (greater than 40 per cent total body surface area [TBSA]).[41] Clinically, burn wound infections due to *Candida* are similar to those caused by staphylococci in that the organisms tend to remain localized, but systemic candidiasis has been seen, especially in the presence of major burns.[1]

*Phycomycetes* is isolated from burn wounds less frequently than *Candida* species.[43] When phycomycotic infections do occur, they tend to disseminate. Once *Phycomycetes* wound sepsis occurs, the overall mortality is 50 per cent.[1] Accordingly, the wounds of burn patients must be carefully monitored for the presence of *Phycomycetes* and other aggressive fungi.

Fungal infections limited to the subcutaneous tissue are best treated by local excision of the wound. Systemic antifungal therapy with amphotericin B, 5-

fluorocytosine, or fluconazole (investigational) should be reserved for patients with suspected or documented disseminated infection.[2]

## Viral Infections

Viral infection of burn wounds is rare. Although viral organisms can be isolated from biopsy specimens, their clinical importance is usually minimal. Viral pathogens reported to have caused infections in burned patients include herpesvirus, cytomegalovirus, varicella, and vacinia.[1, 44] Herpes viral infections are the most common.[45] In addition to infecting the wound, viral infections may disseminate to infect distant tissues such as the lungs and gastrointestinal tract.[4]

## USE OF TOPICAL ANTIMICROBIAL THERAPY

Topical antimicrobial therapy is an important aspect of the management of burn injuries. The goal of this therapy is the prevention of wound infection by controlling the extent of microbial colonization of the wound, thereby decreasing the risk of bacterial wound invasion.[8] Although the use of topical antimicrobials decreases the risk of conversion of partial-thickness to full-thickness wounds by preventing local infection and prolongs the sterility of full-thickness wounds, the need for aggressive surgical treatment of burn wounds cannot be overemphasized. In addition, it should be noted that topical antibiotic therapy has not decreased the mortality of patients with significant burns, especially those patients with greater than 70 per cent TBSA burns.[46]

For a drug to be topically effective in the treatment of burn wounds, it must possess certain characteristics.[47] It must act against the major pathogens responsible for burn wound infection and burn wound sepsis; it must concentrate within the burn wound at levels effective against these pathogens; it must be both locally and systemically nontoxic; if it is absorbed systemically, it should be rapidly excreted or metabolized; and it should be easy to use and inexpensive.

The use of topical drugs in the treatment of burn injury was first investigated more than 60 years ago. Drugs that were tested clinically but found to be minimally effective include tannic acid, various dyes, sulfa compounds, and penicillin.[47] Despite the fact that topically applied penicillin products were of limited benefit, their use remained popular until the 1960s. The first drug to be developed which possessed many of these characteristics was $p$-aminomethylbenzene, or mafenide.

## Mafenide Acetate

Mafenide is commercially available as the acetate salt (Sulfamylon). It is a synthetic antibiotic closely related chemically, but not pharmacologically, to the sulfonamides.[48] The mechanism of its action remains to be defined, although the drug appears to interfere with bacterial cellular metabolism.[48] Mafenide is a bacteriostatic agent active against many gram-positive and gram-negative organisms, including *Staphylococcus aureus* and *epidermidis*, hemolytic streptococci, *Pseudomonas aeruginosa*, and some strains of anaerobes including *Clostridium*.[1] Microbial resistance to mafenide has not been reported.

For topical administration, mafenide acetate is used as an 8.5 per cent cream in a water-miscible base. Following application, the drug promptly diffuses through burn eschar and is absorbed systemically.[47, 48] Mafenide is rapidly metabolized in the blood stream to a metabolite devoid of antimicrobial effects, *p*-carboxybenzenesulfonamide,[48] and therefore cannot be administered systemically.

A complication of mafenide therapy arises from the fact that *p*-carboxybenzenesulfonamide is a weak carbonic anydrase inhibitor[47, 48] that is responsible for impairment of the renal mechanisms involved in buffering the blood.[47] This causes increased bicarbonate and decreased ammonia and chloride excretion in the urine. The outcome of carbonic anhydrase inhibition is increased pulmonary ventilation to maintain normal acid-base equilibrium. For this reason hyperventilation is characteristic of extensively burned patients treated with mafenide acetate.[1, 49] If the compensatory hyperventilation is not sufficient, systemic acidosis results. In patients with renal failure, mafenide and its metabolite accumulate because of their decreased urinary excretion (mafenide and *p*-carboxybenzenesulfonamide are eliminated only by the kidneys). Therefore, the drug should be used cautiously in burn patients with acute renal failure and/or pulmonary dysfunction.[48]

Pain or burning sensations are commonly experienced by patients after the application of mafenide.[1, 47] The pain is of varying intensity and duration for the first 7 to 10 post-burn days, and its intensity is roughly inversely proportional to the burn depth.[47]

Approximately 3 to 5 per cent of patients develop sensitivity to mafenide in the form of a maculopapular rash in unburned areas.[48, 50] Allergic reactions, manifested by dermal reactions including pruritus, facial edema, swelling, urticaria, blisters, and eosinophilia, have been reported. When allergic reactions occur, mafenide therapy should be discontinued and antihistamines administered. Other side effects of mafenide rarely reported are hemolytic anemia with disseminated intravascular coagulation and methemoglobinemia.[51]

Superinfection with nonsusceptible organisms, including fungi, may occur within the burn eschar, in the subeschar tissue, or in viable tissue adjacent to the burn wound.[1]

Mafenide acetate cream should be applied to clean, debrided burn wounds once or twice a day up to a maximum thickness of 16 mm. It is not necessary to use dressings with mafenide as long as the wounds are covered with cream at all times.[48] Mafenide therapy should be continued until healing is apparent or the site is grafted.

## Silver Nitrate

Silver nitrate is used as a 0.5 per cent solution in distilled water and is applied to bulky gauze dressings every two hours. Unfortunately, these bulky dressings restrict patient mobility, an important factor in rehabilitation.[8] This complication is somewhat overcome by the fact that because the dressings must be changed every 12 hours, debridement of the wound is promoted.

Silver nitrate is a bacteriostatic drug that inhibits a wide variety of gram-positive and gram-negative organisms, including *Pseudomonas*.[8, 47, 49, 52] The antimicrobial effects of the drug are due to the actions of the silver ion component, which acts on the surface of bacteria causing marked alterations in the cell wall and membrane.[52] In addition, the silver ion interacts and denatures bacterial proteins, leading to their inactivation and precipitation.

The major disadvantage of silver nitrate therapy is that the silver ion interacts nonspecifically with protein. Its tissue diffusion is therefore limited, and it cannot penetrate burn wounds effectively.[47] Thus, the interaction of silver ion with microorganisms may be minimal if the organisms are located deep within the wound. There are also a number of local and systemic complications of silver nitrate use. When applied to tissues, the silver ions immediately interacts with chloride ions to form a black silver chloride precipitate that discolors both the burn wound and the adjacent tissues.[1] This hampers the visual inspection of wounds essential to surveillance of the injury. When a low concentration of silver is applied, deep tissue penetration is impossible. When a high concentration is applied, cellular toxicity, including intracellular damage to healthy tissue, may occur. In addition, the nitrate ion may be systemically absorbed and converted to nitrite, which has been reported to cause significant methemoglobinemia.[52]

Silver nitrate must be applied as a 0.5 per cent aqueous solution. Accordingly, large amounts of water may be absorbed from the dressing site, and this may result in electrolyte abnormalities. These electrolyte disorders may be worsened by the hypochloremia that may result when silver ion binds chloride ion and precipitates as silver chloride within tissues.[1] Thus, burn patients treated with silver nitrate commonly manifest hyponatremia and hypochloremic alkalosis.

Silver nitrate is used prophylactically to prevent surface colonization of burn wounds with microorganisms. Because of its inability to penetrate tissue, silver nitrate is ineffective if applied more than 72 hours following a burn injury.[52]

## Silver Sulfadiazine

Silver sulfadiazine 1 per cent cream is the most commonly used topical antimicrobial drug. The drug acts on the cell membrane and the cell wall of susceptible bacteria and binds to cellular DNA.[1] Interestingly, neither the silver ion nor the sulfadiazine individually appears to be responsible for the antimicrobial effects of the silver sulfadiazine.[53]

Silver sulfadiazine is bactericidal and is effective against a wide variety of microbes. Susceptible gram-positive organisms include *Staphylococcus* and *Streptococcus*, and gram-negative organisms include *Escherichia coli* and species of *Klebsiella, Pseudomonas, Proteus, Corynebacterium, Citrobacter, Providencia, Serratia,* and *Enterobacter*.[53] *Clostrium* is inhibited at high concentrations of silver sulfadiazine.[8] Microbial resistance to the drug has been rarely reported.

Following topical application, silver sulfadiazine reacts with sodium chloride and protein and releases the sulfadiazine component. Sulfadiazine is systemically absorbed, particularly from second- and third-degree burns.[53, 54] Because it is a sulfonamide, it may induce adverse effects common to sulfonamides. Hemolytic anemia may occur in patients with glucose-6-phosphate dehydrogenase deficiency. Hematologic effects including leukopenia have also been reported.[55]

Silver sulfadiazine is formulated in a propylene glycol base. Propylene glycol absorption has been documented in a number of patients and has been implicated as a cause of hyperosmolality and elevated osmolol gap.[56, 57] It has been recommended that osmolol gap be monitored in patients treated with silver sulfadiazine who are at risk for increased absorption or decreased elimination of propylene glycol. This includes patients with large burns, infants and young children, patients with hepatic or renal dysfunction, and patients with large areas of abnormal epidermis such as toxic epidermal necrolysis.[56, 57]

Pain and burning have been reported infrequently after the topical application of silver sulfadiazine. Sensitization and rashes also may occur.[47] Because the drug is a sulfonamide, it should be used with caution in patients with known allergy to sulfonamides.

Silver sulfadiazine should be applied to clean, debrided burn wounds once or twice a day; the burned area should be covered with cream at all times.

## WHICH TOPICAL ANTIMICROBIAL: MAFENIDE, SILVER NITRATE, OR SILVER SULFADIAZINE?

Although no topical antimicrobial sterilizes burn wounds, the drugs do suppress microbial proliferation. Average microbial counts of $10^3$ to $10^4$ are typical during mafenide therapy and silver sulfadiazine therapy.[1, 2, 8] Silver sulfadiazine is probably as effective as mafenide in suppressing microbial colonization of burn wounds and burn wound sepsis. While mafenide may penetrate eschar better than sulfadiazine, eshar separation and removal appear to be easier following sulfadiazine therapy. In contrast to mafenide, silver sulfadiazine has no effect on carbonic anhydrase, and metabolic acidosis has not been associated with its use. Unlike silver nitrate, neither silver sulfadiazine nor mafenide acetate stains and discolors the burn wound or adjacent viable tissue. In addition, silver sulfadiazine has not been reported to alter electrolyte homeostasis, although silver nitrate can. Both mafenide acetate and silver sulfadiazine are probably more effective than silver nitrate in preventing burn wound sepsis. Because silver sulfadiazine has the lowest incidence and severity of local and systemic toxicity, it is the preferred topical antimicrobial drug in many burn units.[58] Mafenide is often reserved for those patients who are intolerant of or fail silver sulfadiazine therapy. Comparative studies on the use of mafenide acetate, silver sulfadiazine, and silver nitrate are lacking.

Any topical antimicrobial may inhibit the regeneration of new epithelium. Because the drugs are discontinued when the wound is clean and healing starts, this is of minor clinical importance. Mafenide acetate and silver sulfadiazine have also been reported to induce hypertrophic scarring, which is the direct result of inhibited bacterial growth and, in turn, leads to spontaneous healing of deep dermal burns. Burn wounds characteristically heal with hypertrophic scarring, however, regardless of the topical therapy applied. Another consequence of inhibited bacterial growth common to all topical antimicrobials is a profound delay in eschar separation of full-thickness burn wounds.

## Other Topical Antibiotics

A variety of agents has been investigated for use in the treatment of burn injuries; most are of little clinical benefit in suppressing burn wound colonization. Gentamicin and tobramycin creams have been used for their known efficacy against gram-negative bacteria, especially the *Pseudomonas*. Microbial resistance may develop from their use, however. In addition, the drugs are readily absorbed and may cause ototoxicity and/or nephrotoxicity.[8] Therefore, the prophylactic use of gentamicin and tobramycin topical preparations should be discouraged.[1, 4, 8] Another topical antimicrobial cream, nitrofurazone, also possesses gram-negative activity. Like gentamicin cream, nitrofurazone may produce microbial resistance and systemic toxicity.[1] In addition, because nitrofurazone is formulated using polyethylene glycol, hyperosmolality may occur with its use.[1, 56]

Povidone-iodine has been used in the treatment of burn wounds. The drug does not penetrate eschar tissue, however, and is only moderately effective in controlling infection.[1, 8] In addition, its iodine component may give rise to problems in thyroid function. The use of povidone-iodine often results in excessive wound drying.[8]

Recent investigations have centered on the use of cerium nitrate and cerium sulfadiazine. In vitro studies have documented the antimicrobial activity of these drugs; they appear to be more effective against gram-negative organisms, including *Pseudomonas*, than against gram-positive ones.[59–62] Most clinical studies have used a combination of cerium nitrate with silver sulfadiazine and/or cerium sulfadiazine. It is interesting to note that cerium may interfere with the action of silver sulfadiazine and reduce its efficacy.[58] Studies evaluating cerium and silver mixtures are continuing.

## SUBESCHAR ANTIBIOTIC THERAPY

As previously discussed, topical antimicrobial agents do not sterilize a burn wound. Rather, they suppress bacterial colonization, thereby reducing the risk of bacterial invasion and septicemia. Despite the extensive use of topical antimicrobials, patients continue to develop burn wound infection and subsequent wound sepsis. Accordingly, research continues into techniques and therapies to further decrease the incidence of burn wound infection. One such method is the subeschar administration of antibiotics.

A number of studies have demonstrated the benefit of subeschar treatment of burn wound infection.[63-65] Subeschar administration of antibiotics offers a theoretical advantage over systemic and topically administered antibiotics in that the drug is applied directly into the infected burn wound, an area that is often inaccessible to intravenous and topical anti-infectives.

Baxter et al administer subeschar antibiotics by the following technique[65]: Once the diagnosis of burn wound infection has been established and the decision made to administer antibiotics, the daily systemic dose of the appropriate antibiotic(s) is delivered into the subeschar space at 7.5-cm intervals with 22-gauge needles. Twenty-five milliliters of normal or half-normal saline containing the antibiotic are delivered by pediatric drip-set into each needle site once a day. The choice of antibiotic(s) is based on the sensitivity of the specific organisms colonizing the individual burn wounds. The effectiveness of this therapy is monitored by serial full-thickness wound biopsies taken at two-day intervals.

Subeschar administration of antibiotics, including semisynthetic penicillins and aminoglycosides, appears to be a promising and effective adjunct in the care of the patient with burn wound infections.[65] Confirmatory evidence of its efficacy is lacking.

## SYSTEMIC ANTIBIOTICS

Because of the anatomical and vascular abnormalities that develop in the area of burn wounds, the efficacy of systemically administered antibiotics in treating burn wound infection is markedly decreased. This is especially true of full-thickness wounds and burn wound infection, which may be associated with occlusive vasculitis and tissue avascularity.[1, 2]

The use of parenteral antibiotics in the burn patient should be reserved for the treatment of any and all uncontrolled septic events. In the burn patient, sepsis commonly occurs in the absence of positive blood cultures. A positive blood culture, however, should be treated immediately by the administration of parenteral antibiotics to temporarily prevent bacterial dissemination from the burn wound. Unfortunately, the penetration of systemic antibiotics into burn wounds is not predictable. Thus, systemic antibiotics should not and do not negate the need for surgical excision and debridement of the burn wound, which is the definitive method for treating burn wound infection.

Irrespective of the etiology of burn wound sepsis, the choice of systemic antibiotic agent should be based on culture of infected material such as blood, urine, and the wound tissue; the species of infecting organism; the pattern of sensitivity; the status of the patient; and the impact of the drug on the flora endogenous to the unit. It should be noted that no single agent or combination of agents is effective against all pathogens to which burn patients are exposed. Moreover, combinations of antibiotics are not necessarily synergistic or even additive in antimicrobial effect, whereas multiple-drug therapy may precipitate superinfection by resistant bacteria, yeast, fungi, or viruses. Antibiotic drug therapy for treatment of burn wound infection must be individualized; burn patients usually require higher doses of drugs to achieve sufficient clinical effect, particularly drugs that are cleared primarily by glomerular filtration.

During the time when culture results are unavailable or are being processed, choice of antibiotic should be made empirically based on the flora known to be colonizing the patient's wound, as detected by surface cultures and wound biopsy cultures, if available, or on organisms known to inhabit the particular burn unit where the patient is located.[1, 2, 4] There is a wide variety of parenteral antibiotics available for the treatment of infection. This chapter reviews only the general characteristics of the drugs most commonly used in the treatment of burn wound infections.

## Penicillins

Against susceptible organisms, penicillins are bactericidal, extraordinarily effective, and of relatively low toxicity.[66] Penicillin G has a broad spectrum of activity, including streptococci, staphylococci, *Corynebacterium*, and *Neisseria*. However, it is not commonly used to treat burns in hospitalized patients, because most gram-positive organisms that colonize burn wounds are resistant to penicillin G; most of these organisms, especially staphylococci, produce beta-lactamases that rapidly hydrolyze the beta-lactam ring of all natural and semisynthetic penicillins such as ampicillin.[1, 2] In contrast, the most commonly used penicillins in burn patients are those with activity against penicillinase-producing *Staphylococcus aureus* and *S. epidermidis*, primarily nafcillin and oxacillin.[67] Although these drugs have some in vitro activity against other gram-positive bacteria such as streptococci and enterococci and some gram-negative bacteria such as *Haemophilus influenzae*, they are generally less effective than other penicillins.[67] Accordingly, the use of nafcillin and oxacillin is generally limited to the treatment of infections caused by sensitive penicillinase-producing staphylococci.

Extended-spectrum penicillins, which encompass the ureidopenicillins azlocillin, mezlocillin, and piperacillin and the carboxypenicillins ticarcillin and carbenicillin, are frequently used in the treatment of burn wound sepsis. These drugs, especially the ureidopenicillins, have high intrinsic activity against the gram-negative organisms most often responsible for burn wound sepsis: *Pseudomonas aeruginosa* and *Escherichia coli*.[66, 67] In addition, azlocillin, mezlocillin, and piperacillin are active against some strains of *Klebsiella*, *Serratia*, and *Enterobacter*.[66, 67] Although extended-spectrum penicillins may be used alone in the treatment of gram-negative infections, they are almost universally used in conjunction with another antibiotic to reduce the likelihood of superinfection or emergence of resistant organisms. This is particularly important in the burn patient who may manifest marked derangements in cellular and humoral defense mechanisms.[67]

## Cephalosporins

Cephalosporins are currently divided into three groups based on their spectrum of activity. The first-generation cephalosporins are usually active against gram-positive cocci, including penicillinase-producing strains of *Staphylococcus aureus* and *S. epidermidis* and *Streptococcus*, including *pyogenes* and *pneumoniae* strains.[67] Their gram-negative spectrum is limited, but some strains of *Klebsiella* and *Proteus* and *Escherichia coli* may be inhibited by these drugs.[67] All cephalosporins are inactive against the enterococci. The first-generation cephalosporins most frequently used in the burn patient are cefazolin, cephapirin, and cephalothin, and they are used less often than penicillinase-resistant penicillins.

The parenteral second-generation cephalosporins are cefoxitin, cefuroxime, cefamandole, cefonicid, and cefotetan. They possess in vitro activity similar to that of first-generation cephalosporins.[68] In addition, the second-generation drugs, particularly cefuroxime, are active against most strains of *Haemophilus influenzae* and also have activity against some strains of *Klebsiella, Neisseria, Proteus,* and *Enterobacter* and *Escherichia coli*.[68] Cefoxitin and cefotetan have activity against *Bacteroides fragilis*.

The third-generation cephalosporins include ceftazidime, cefotaxime, cefoperazone, ceftriaxone, ceftizoxime, and moxalactam. They are generally less active than first-generation agents against staphylococci.[68] These agents have significant activity against a number of gram-negative bacteria, especially *Escherichia coli* and species of *Klebsiella, Proteus,* and *Enterobacter*.[67] In addition, ceftazidime has marked activity against *Pseudomonas aeruginosa*.[68]

## Vancomycin

Vancomycin is the drug of choice for the treatment of infections due to methicillin-resistant staphylococci and enterococci.[69] Although the drug is reported to be both ototoxic and nephrotoxic, the incidence of both side effects has decreased tremendously as the purity of the drug has increased.[69]

## Aminoglycosides

The aminoglycosides—gentamicin, tobramycin, amikacin, and netilmicin—are highly effective against a number of gram-negative organisms, including *Escherichia coli, Serratia, Shigella, Salmonella, Proteus,* and, most importantly, *Pseudomonas*.[70] They are also active against most strains of staphylococci but are minimally active against streptococci; many strains of enterococci are resistant.

The aminoglycosides are nephrotoxic and ototoxic, particularly when used with loop diuretics and cephalosporin antibiotics. In addition, burn patients require high dosages of aminoglycosides because their elevated glomerular filtration rate results in rapid aminoglycoside clearance.[71–75]

## Other Antibiotics

Other antibiotics used in the treatment of burn wound sepsis are clindamycin and metronidazole. These drugs are used for treatment of anaerobic infections, primarily *Bacteroides*.

A new class of antimicrobials has recently been introduced into clinical use: the fluoroquinolones ciprofloxacin and norfloxacin. The fluoroquinolones are chemically related to nalidixic acid and act by inhibiting the bacterial DNA gyrase, an intracellular enzyme essential to the reproduction of all bacteria.[75] Fluroquinolones have in vitro activity against a wide variety of gram-positive and gram-negative enteric organisms, including *Pseudomonas aeruginosa, Haemophilus influenzae,* and *Neisseria gonorrhoeae.*[76] Ciprofloxacin also has activity against *Staphylococcus,* including methicillin-resistant strains. Norfloxacin is less potent than ciprofloxacin against *Pseudomonas aeruginosa*[75, 77] and is indicated only for the treatment of urinary tract infections. Ciprofloxacin is indicated for the treatment of lower respiratory tract infections, bone and joint infections, skin and soft tissue infections, and urinary tract infections. The use of the fluoroquinolones in burn patients and other seriously ill patients appears promising.[75, 76]

## REFERENCES

1. Goodwin CW Jr, Pruitt BA Jr: Burns. *In* Kagan M (ed): Antimicrobial Therapy. Philadelphia WB Saunders Co, 1980, pp 397–409.
2. Pruitt BA Jr: The diagnosis and treatment of infections in the burn patient. Burns 11:79–91, 1984.
3. Pruitt BA Jr, Lindberg RP: *Pseudomonas aeruginosa* infections in burn patients. *In* RG Doggett (ed): Pseudomonas Aeruginosa. New York, Academic Press, 1979, pp 339–351.
4. Luterman A, Dasco CC, Curreri PW: Infections in burn patients. Am J Med 81(S1A):45–51, 1986.
5. Moncrief JA: Burns. N Engl J Med 288:444–454, 1973.
6. Arturson NG: The pathophysiology of severe thermal injury. J Burn Care Rehabil 6:129–146, 1985.
7. Boykin JV, Eridsson E, Pittman RN: Microcirculation of the scald burn: An in vivo experimental study of the hairless mouse ear. Burns 7:335–337, 1980.
8. Pegg SP: The role of drugs in the management of burns. Drugs 24:256–260, 1982.
9. Alexander JW, Ogle CK, Stinnett SD, et al: A sequential prospective analysis of immunologic abnormalities and infection following severe thermal injury. Ann Surg 188:809–816, 1978.
10. Grogran JB, Hered A: Neutrophil function in burn patients. J Trauma 16:734–737, 1976.
11. Balch HH, Watters BS, Kelly D: Resistance to infections in burned patients. Ann Surg 188:809–816, 1978.
12. Davis JM, Dineen P, Gallin JI: Neutrophil degranulation and abnormal chemotaxis after thermal injury. J Immunol 124:1467–1471, 1980.
13. Fibrig SM, Karl SC, Suntharaling AMK: Neutrophil chemotaxis in patients with burns. Ann Surg 186:746–749, 1977.

14. McCabe WB, Rebuck JW, Kelly AP, et al: Leukocyte response as a monitor of immunologic depression in burn patients. Arch Surg 106:155–159, 1973.

15. Miller CL, Baker CC: Changes in lymphocyte activity after thermal injury: The role of suppressor cells. J Clin Invest 63:202–210, 1979.

16. Antonacci AC, Good RA, Gupta S: T-cell subpopulations following thermal injury. Surg Gynecol Obstet 155:1–6, 1982.

17. Lanser ME, Saba TM, Scovil WA: Opsonic glycoprotein (plasma fibronectin) levels after burn injury: Relationship to the extent of burn and development of sepsis. Ann Surg 192:776–782, 1980.

18. Munster AM, Hadland HC, Pruitt BA Jr: The effect of thermal injury on serum immunoglobulins. Ann Surg 172:965–969, 1970.

19. Antonacci AC, Calvanto SE, Reaves LE, et al: Restoration of autologous mixed lymphocyte responses in burn patients following in vitro addition of interleukin-2; analysis of responder cell populations with monoclonal antibodies. Surg Form 34:108–110, 1983.

20. Ninnemann SL, Stockland AE, Condre JT: Induction of prostaglandin synthesis–dependent suppressor cells with endotoxin: Occurrence in patients with thermal injuries. J Clin Immunol 3:142–150, 1983.

21. Woods SS, O'Mahoney JB, Rodrick ML, et al: Abnormalities of antibody production after thermal injury: An association with reduced interleukin-2 production. Arch Surg 121:108–115, 1986.

22. Wolfe JM, Wu AVO, O'Connor Ne, et al: Anergy, immunosuppressive serum and impaired lymphocyte blastogenes in burn patient. Arch Surg 117:1266–1271, 1982.

23. Ninnemann SL: Suppression of lymphocyte response following thermal injury. In Ninnemann SL (ed): The Immune Consequences of Thermal Injury. Baltimore, William & Wilkins, 1981, pp 66–79.

24. Pruitt BA Jr, Lindberg RB, McManus WF: Current approaches to prevention and treatment of *Pseudomonas aeruginosa* infections in burn patients. Rev Infect Dis 5(S5):889–898, 1983.

25. Pruitt BA Jr, Foley FD: The use of biopsies in burn patient care. Surgery 73:887–891, 1973.

26. Bretano L, Gravens AC: A method for the quantification of bacteria in burn wounds. Appl Microbiol 15:670, 1967.

27. Lawrence JL, Lilly HA: A quantification method for investigating the bacteriology of skin: Its applicability to burns. Br J Exp Pathol 53:550–553, 1972.

28. Foote GA, Schnabel SI, Hodges M: Pulmonary complications of the flow-directed balloon-type catheter. N Engl J Med 290:927–931, 1974.

29. Chan GMH, Ellestad MH: Perforation of the pulmonary artery with a Swan-Ganz catheter. N Engl J Med 284:1041–1042, 1971.

30. Pruitt BA Jr, DiVincenti FC, Mason ADP, et al: The occurrence and significance of pneumonia and other pulmonary complications in burned patients: Comparison of conventional and typical treatments. J Trauma 10:519–531, 1970.

31. Pruitt BA Jr, Flenna CJ, DiVincenti FC, et al: Pulmonary complications in burn patients: A comparative study of 697 patients. J Thoracic Cardiovasc Surg 59:7, 1970.

32. Levine BA, Petroff PA, Stade CL, et al: Prospective trials of dexamethasone and aerosolized gentamicin in the treatment of initial injury in the burned patient. J Trauma 18:188–192, 1978.

33. Pruitt BA Jr, McManus WF, Kin SH, et al: Diagnosis and treatment of cannulae-related intravenous sepsis in burn patients. Ann Surg 191:546, 1980.

34. Stein JM, Pruitt BA Jr: Suppurative thrombophlebitis: A lethal iatrogenic disease. N Engl J Med 282:1452, 1970.

35. Sasaki TM, Panke TW, Dorethy JF, et al: The relationship of central venous and pulmonary artery catheter position to acute right-sided endocarditis in severe thermal injury. J Trauma 19:140–143, 1979.

36. Srivastava RF, MacMilliam BG: Cardiac infection in acute burn patients. Burns 6:48–54, 1979.

37. Hyams KC, Mador JT, Pollard RB: Serratia endocarditis in a pediatric burn patient. JAMA 246:983–984, 1981.

38. Ehrie M, Morgan AP, Moore FD, et al: Endocarditis and the indwelling balloon-tipped pulmonary artery catheters in burn patients. J Trauma 18:664–667, 1978.

39. Greene JF, Fitzwater JE, Clenmer TP: Septic endocarditis and indwelling pulmonary artery catheters. JAMA 233:891–897, 1975.

40. Powell DC, Bivins BA, Bell RM, et al: Bacterial endocarditis in the critically-ill surgical patient. Arch Surg 116:311–314, 1981.
41. Nash G, Foley FD, Pruitt BA Jr: Candida burn-wound invasion. Arch Pathol 90:75–81, 1970.
42. Bruck HM, Nash G, Stein JM, et al: Studies on the occurrence and significance of yeast and fungi in the burn wound. Ann Surg 176:108–111, 1972.
43. Bruck HM, Nash G, Foley FD, et al: Opportunistic fungal infections of the burn wound with Phycomycetes and Aspergillus. Arch Surg 102:470–473, 1971.
44. Matthews SCW, Levick PL, Coombs EJ, et al: Viral infections in a group of burned patients. Burns 6:55–58, 1980.
45. Foley FD, Greenwald KA, Nash G, et al: Herpes infections in burn patients. N Engl J Med 282:652–654, 1970.
46. Burke JF, Quinby WC Jr, Bondoc CC: Primary excision and prompt grafting as routine therapy for the treatment of thermal burns in children. Surg Clin North Am 56:477–494, 1976.
47. Moncrief JA: Topical therapy of the burn wound: Present status. Clin Pharm Ther 10:439–448, 1969.
48. Anonymous: Mafenide acetate. In McEvoy GK, 1989 (ed): AHFS Drug Information 1989. Bethesda, MD, American Society Hospital Pharmacists, 1989, pp 1964–1965.
49. Albert LT, Lewis NS, Warpeha RL: Late pulmonary complications with use of mafenide acetate. J Burn Care Rehabil 3:375–377, 1982.
50. Richards RME, Mahlangu GM: Therapy for burn wound infections. J Clin Hosp Pharm 6:233–243, 1981.
51. Monies-Chass I, Simon K, Sternman P: Methaemoglobinemia resulting from the absorption of 4% sulfamylon acetate gel. Burns 4:143–144, 1976.
52. Anonymous: Silver nitrate. In McEvoy GK (ed) 1989: AHFS Drug Information 1989. Bethesda, MD, American Society of Hospital Pharmacists, 1989, p 1487.
53. Anonymous: Silver sulfadiazine. In McEvoy GK (ed): AHFS Drug Information '89. Bethesda, MD, American Society of Hospital Pharmacists, 1989, pp 1968–1969.
54. Lockhart SP, Rushworth AA, Azmy AAF: Topical silver sulfadiazine. Burns 10:9–12, 1983.
55. Caffee HH, Bingham HG: Leukopenia and silver sulfadiazine. J Trauma 22:586–587, 1982.
56. Anonymous: Burns and PEG. FDA Drug Bull 12:25–26, 1982.
57. Flinger CL, Jack R, Twiggs GA, et al: Hyperosmolality induced by propylene glycol. JAMA 253:1606–1609, 1985.
58. Hartford CE: Topical therapy for infection control. J Burn Care Rehabil 8:49–53, 1987.
59. Bridges K, Cason JS, Jackson DM, et al: Topical chemoprophylaxis with cerium (cerous) nitrate cream. Burns 6:231–234, 1979.
60. Hermans RP: Topical treatment of serious infections with special reference to the use of a mixture of silver sulphathiazine and cerium nitrate: Two clinical studies. Burns 11:59–62, 1984.
61. Fox Cl, Monafo WW, Ayvazian VH, et al: Topical chemotherapy for burns using cerium salts and silver sulfadiazine. Surg Gynecol Obstet 144:668–672, 1971.
62. Monafo WW, Tandon SN, Ayvazian V, et al: Cerium nitrate: A new topical antiseptic for extensive burns. Surgery 80:465–476, 1976.
63. MacManus WF, Manson AD, Pruitt BA Jr: Subeschar antibiotic infusion in the treatment of burn wound infection. J Trauma 20:1021–1023, 1980.
64. MacManus WF, Goodwin CW Jr, Pruitt BA Jr: Subeschar treatment of burn-wound infection. Arch Surg 118:291–294, 1983.
65. Baxter CR, Currerri PW, Marvin JA: The control of burn wound sepsis by the use of quantitative bacteriologic studies and subeschar clysis with antibiotics. Surg Clin North Am 53:1509–1513, 1973.
66. Anonymous: Penicillins. In McEvoy GK (ed): AHFS Drug Information '89. Bethesda, MD, American Society of Hospital Pharmacists, 1989, pp 191–299.
67. Weinstein L: Penicillins and cephalosporins. In Goodman LS, Gilman A, Gilman AG, Koelle GB (eds): The Pharmacological Basis of Therapeutics, 6th ed. New York, MacMillan, 1985, pp 1130–1166.
68. Anonymous: Cephalosporins. In McEvoy GK (ed): AHFS Drug Information '89. Bethesda, MD, American Society of Hospital Pharmacists, 1989, pp 82–142.
69. Cooper GL, Given DB: Clinical use of vancomycin. In Cooper GL, Given DB (eds): Vancomycin: A comprehensive review of 30 years of clinical experience. Indianapolis, Park Row, 1986, pp 39–69.

70. Weinstein L: Streptomycin, gentamicin, and other aminoglycosides. *In* Gilman AG, Koelle GB (eds): The Pharmacological Basis of Therapeutics, 7th ed. New York, Macmillan, 1985, pp 167–182.
71. Glew RH, Moehlering RC, Burke JF: Gentamicin dosage in children with extensive burns. J Trauma 16:819–823, 1976.
72. Zaske DE, Cipolle RJ, Strate RJ: Gentamicin dosage requirements: Wide interpatient variations in 242 surgery patients with normal renal function. Surgery 84:164–169, 1980.
73. Loirat P, Rohan J, Baillet A, et al: Increased glomerular filtration rate in patients with major burns and its effect on the pharmacokinetics of tobramycin. N Engl J Med 299:915–919, 1979.
74. Zaske DE, Cipolle RJ, Solem LD, et al: Rapid individualization of gentamicin dosage regimens in 66 burn patients. Burns 7:215–220, 1980.
75. Nix DE, DeVito JM: Ciprofloxacin and norfloxacin, two fluoroquinone antimicrobials. Clin Pharm 6:105–117, 1987.
76. Wolfson JS, Hooper DC: The fluoroquinones: structures, mechanisms of action and resistance, and spectra of activity in vitro. Antimicrob Agents Chemother 28:581–586, 1985.
77. Anonymous: Quinolones. *In* McEvoy GK (ed): AHFS Drug Information '89. Bethesda, MD, American Society of Hospital Pharmacists, 1989, pp 391–407.

# 20

# The Social Worker and the Family:

## A Long-Term Relationship in Burn Care

SUE S. CAHNERS and PATRICIA P. KARTIGANER

Only a generation ago, people who suffered major burns seldom survived, and when they did, they often became housebound because of their profound disfigurement and depression. When they were able to leave home, it was often to work at such jobs as night watchman or projectionist in a theater.[1]

Life-saving expertise and techniques in plastic surgery have advanced burn care to the point where immediate survival is less uncertain, and, as a result, the long-term functional and cosmetic consequences have become as important as survival. Rehabilitation is an integral part of burn care; surgeons recognize that there is much treatment needed beyond the operating room to ensure a successful outcome and a return to productive normal living; and the nursing staff, providing daily care, need to know that the patient will not go on to suffer "social death."[1]

Because of the myriad social and psychological needs of burn patients and their families, social workers are involved in their care from admission to discharge and throughout all subsequent reconstructive admissions. The Shriners Burns Institute is a pediatric burn facility unique in that it provides treatment for the acute as well as the reconstructive patient. The authors, therefore, have the opportunity to work with patients from infancy to young adulthood and with their families and to observe and treat their psychological responses to burn injuries over the entire course.

Early intervention with the patient and his family ensures the social, emotional, and psychological support essential to a positive outcome. The family is the primary resource for the patient because the patient does better when the family adapts better to the injury. At the same time, the injury presents a formidable challenge to family adaptation. One major role of the social worker is the psychosocial evaluation and treatment of the family and patient in order to enhance their strengths. Another, which is part of continuing care, is outreach education to ensure acceptance of the severely disfigured person back into the community. In conjunction with these, ongoing psychosocial research to validate the effectiveness of the total burn effort continues.

Acute burn care is a three-phase process, with some overlap from one phase to the other.

306

## ADMISSION

The social worker endeavors to meet the family at the earliest possible moment. While the patient is being examined by the medical staff, families have their first quiet moments, and the impact of the accident and its attendant panic are experienced. This is the optimal time for a social worker to intervene because people are most open to help and most responsive to helpers when beset by crisis.[2] Emotional support is offered as well as concrete services such as financial and housing assistance, orientation to the hospital, and education about what the family can expect. The first meeting also provides an opportunity for initial assessment of the special needs of each family and their distinctive styles of coping. This assessment is recorded in the chart for the information of all the staff. This is only one of several ways in which the social worker acts as a liaison between family and staff.

At the time of admission, families are bombarded with information such as the status of the patient, details of burn treatment, issues of infection, and the complications of an inhalation injury, among others, all couched in unfamiliar terminology and presented by innumerable staff people. The social worker is present as often as possible during these sessions so that she can later repeat, explain, and reinforce all the data, which are difficult for the family to absorb and integrate at first hearing. Meeting with an empathic person whose job is directed at family needs cushions the traumatic impact of the crisis and marks the beginning of an enduring relationship.

## THE FIRST PHASE: THE IMPACT

The impact of a burn injury on families is enormous. In a moment their lives change dramatically, and the suddenness of the crisis leaves them in a shocked state of disbelief. At the same time, they are anxious about the adjustments they must make in their everyday lives in response to the accident. During the first phase the family and patient experience parallel processes: What the patient undergoes physically, the family suffers emotionally. If the injury is relatively small, the family must accept the need for hospitalization and possible surgery. Few people are acquainted with serious burn injuries; relatives often remark that it is almost unbelievable that brief contact with a source of heat such as hot water can have serious consequences. When the injury is more profound, families are overwhelmed by the horror of the accident. The patient's life may be at risk and may remain so for an extended period. Families face the possibility of the patient's death while they must encourage him to fight for his life, and they are torn between grief and hope. They usually resolve this conflict by relying on optimism, and they are sustained by confidence in the medical team and by their own particular religious faith. Their display of optimism often leads staff to wonder whether they are keeping in mind the reality of the consequences of the burn injury. Social workers assess this issue while assuring staff that some degree of denial helps families cope, particularly during the "impact" phase.

The hospitalization itself causes a major disruption of family life. Job commitments and other responsibilities continue, while families have all they can do to focus on what has happened to the patient. Moreover, since burn units do not exist in all localities, hospitalization frequently represents a geographical dislocation for family members who must travel to be with the patient. This uprooting and separation from support systems when they are most needed are other reasons why families require much help during this phase. The presence of social workers who empathize with these burdens and who can help them prepare for the ordeal ahead sustains families until they are able to cope more independently.

Other families at the hospital are an additional source of support. Meeting people with similar experiences can ease the sense of isolation. Sharing their experiences has proven very beneficial; the social worker therefore encourages family members to attend group therapy sessions, which provide access to this avenue of mutual support.

Families, overwhelmed with feelings of helplessness and dealing with partial separation from the patient, struggle with their role in his recovery. Although doctors and nurses have become primary caregivers, the family still provides a special form of care. They represent security to the patient, and they are a link to his pre-burn world. The presence of a parent at the bedside can be extremely reassuring to a child thrust into the strange and frightening world of intensive care. This role demands new strengths from families. Shock, pain, and the effects of medication often render the patient unresponsive to the family's customary methods of comfort. If a bacteria-controlled nursing unit is required, its plastic barrier represents additional separation. The patient's lack of response causes family members to wonder whether their presence actually does make a difference, and they need help recognizing the importance of their relationship to the patient. The social worker reinforces the fact that while the professional staff can do many things for their loved one, they cannot replace the family. Moreover, the family knows the patient best and is an invaluable source of the medical and psychological history essential to comprehensive treatment.

Families attempt to present a smiling face to the patient and to utter reassuring words, frequently in direct opposition to what they feel. They are fearful of displaying their real feelings, yet they need a place where they may express sadness, fear, anger, guilt, and helplessness. The social worker can provide time for individual therapy to help them express these painful emotions.

Chief among these emotions is guilt. Whether it is valid or not, parental guilt is universal, particularly during the first phase, when parents are trying to understand what has befallen the child. Self-blame is a common response to an accident to one's child. Parents often blame themselves rather than attributing an occurrence to fate or the improbable. This creates a diminished sense of worth as a parent and many self-doubts as a person. Guilt impedes coping mechanisms and emotional recovery. Families are reluctant to take part in pleasurable experiences while a loved one is suffering the rigors of burn treatment; this occasionally extends even to their willingness to eat and to rest. While grief, shock, and depression can contribute to a loss of appetite and disturbed sleep, guilt compounds the problem if the family performs a self-imposed penance. Family members frequently refuse to leave the hospital or even the bedside, thereby denying themselves opportunities to replenish their strength. The social worker is able to give them permission to leave, thereby relieving some of their guilt.

Child protection agencies are occasionally notified when a burned child arrives in the emergency room. The law requires that the slightest suspicion of abuse or neglect must be reported, and investigation proceeds immediately. Just when their vulnerability as parents is most profound, they are required to answer questions as to the circumstances of the accident. This increases their already mounting self-doubts as parents. The social worker recognizes this threat to their self-esteem and is able to describe the investigation in less threatening terms and to present it as an opportunity for getting help, thus reinforcing their importance as a family. The natural alliance of the staff with the patient makes it difficult for them to allow the parents a supportive role in such circumstances. The social worker meets with staff continually to help them understand that the patient must rely on his family regardless of the deficits that seem to be present.

Families also need to share their parenting functions with staff and to eventually become comfortable with their altered role. The patient must learn to trust the professionals who care for him and to be able to seek comfort from his nurse, particularly when a family member is not available. This is a challenge to families, who may feel disenfranchised by the patient's necessary dependence on staff. It takes great strength for them to relinquish their role of caring for the patient in order to enhance his adjustment to hospitalization.

Balancing their former role with the demands imposed by burn treatment extends throughout the inpatient stay. That balance shifts as the three phases of acute care are negotiated, and each shift presents new challenges to families. Ongoing communication between social worker and staff helps to successfully accomplish this balance.

## THE MIDDLE PHASE: SETTLING IN

The middle phase is usually the longest, and it is characterized by uncertainty, which represents another obstacle to family coping. Complex multiple surgical procedures are performed during this period, and they result in complications and sudden changes. Family members have often remarked of this phase that they are never sure what they will be facing from day to day. They describe themselves as being on an emotional roller-coaster. Just as they manage to cope with one crisis, they are confronted by another. They begin to understand that the body's response to burn injury is somewhat unpredictable and that treatment may consequently be altered. Despite the uncertainty, some expectation of the length of stay is now established, and families can set up a schedule that conforms to their understanding of the patient's needs. Even while the patient's life may hang in the balance, an adjustment to the hospital routine occurs. They may now be able to consider some of their responsibilities for other family members and jobs.

During the middle phase the patient usually experiences more pain. Individual treatment continues with the social worker. Family members feel helpless when their efforts to comfort do not alleviate suffering. They feel that the patient looks to them to intercede for relief, and this presents a further challenge. Information provided by the medical staff has given them some understanding of burn and pain treatment, and they wonder about their degree of involvement in pain control and direct care. Family approaches to these problems range from one of questioning every detail of treatment to one of appearing completely disinterested. The social worker acts as a liaison, helping families maintain an appropriate role and encouraging staff to value their contributions. This issue is complicated by the patient's attitude. If the requisite trust in staff discussed previously is not established, the patient may split the staff and the family. Children know very well how to manipulate parents and/or nurses when roles are not clear. For example, they may beg the family to extend visiting time in order to delay painful procedures. Parents, especially, fall prey to such manipulation because the patient's pain renders them helpless and their own guilt feelings interfere with their ability to say no.

It is also during the middle phase that the reality of scarring is confronted. During the impact phase, families tend to focus on immediate survival issues, and scarring is a secondary concern. The miracles of plastic surgery presented in the media lead them to assume that all scars can eventually be removed. By the middle phase families have been exposed to the disfigurement of other patients, and they realize that their loved one may never look the same again. Assistance in accepting this reality is part of the ongoing social work intervention. Families defend themselves against such unwelcome truths in a variety of ways, usually by complete denial or by anger that gets displaced onto staff. Parents begin to grieve the loss of their "perfect child." They learn what can be done to minimize scars and how to help the patient adjust to a new body image. Social workers help with this process through individual and group therapy. The appropriate involvement of the family in patient care can mediate family adjustment to the patient's scars. Families often cope better when they can do something to help the patient; prolonged feelings of uselessness only add to their feelings of helplessness.

Family disorganization is noted in approximately 70 per cent of pediatric burns.[3] Hospitalization for burn treatment stretches all family resources, and the outcome is dependent on the experience they bring with them. Disorganized families can often pull together in the initial phase, but they need extra help in maintaining support for the extended duration of burn hospitalization. Families with pre-existing psychopathology require even more intervention and certainly more understanding from the entire team. The increase of divorce in society is evident in families of burn patients. The previously cited stresses are magnified when parents are divorced. Competition between the parents complicates all areas of family involvement, and the children are often caught in the middle, particularly during this middle phase. Such triangulation is detrimental to the patient's medical progress. It is essential that social workers continually assess and document the family dynamics in the record so that special considerations can be given by all disciplines on the team.

## THE FINAL PHASE: PREPARING FOR DISCHARGE

Preparation for discharge is a time of transition. Families have become less needy and they have adjusted to most aspects of acute care. Emphasis is now on re-empowering the entire family.[4]

Discharge planning is the traditional domain of the social worker. It begins with the initial family assessment on admission and is a goal throughout the three phases of acute care. Emerging psychosocial data form an expanded view of family dynamics, which is incorporated into the discharge plan. The social worker helps the family and the patient make use of their former supports and of additional resources in their community.

This third phase, although brief, is an important testing ground as roles begin to revert to patient-family autonomy. Families are usually reluctant to relinquish the significant act of feeding the patient; when arms and fingers are contracted and stiff, self-feeding can be slow and painful. Families excuse their unwillingness to stop assisting the patient by rationalizing that it takes too much time for him to feed himself and to maintain his therapeutic calorie level. The patient, in frustration with the same problem and sometimes enjoying the special attention, often allows relatives to continue to help, despite the admonitions of occupational therapists. Once again, as the patient progresses, so too must the family.

Families begin to feel more competent, but staff are still relied on for primary care. This is a safe time for family members to test resumption of their former roles while remaining in a supportive setting. Hands-on care is strongly encouraged for families. Adult patients are expected to do more for themselves. Family members are instructed in skin care, the application of support garments, and the performance of physical therapy exercises with the patient.

For families not previously involved in direct care, this can be a difficult transition. Skin care is uncomfortable for the patient, and the necessary exercises frequently cause pain. Responsibility for a loved one's pain is not one that families assume willingly. Although they may accept that these treatments are for the ultimate well-being of the patient, some families find it difficult to urge the patient to do something that will be painful. Early and ongoing involvement in care tends to fortify families to persist in spite of complaints of pain. Persistence is required for all aspects of restored autonomy. If scars are to be flattened, support garments must be worn, regardless of how uncomfortable or unsightly they may be. Opportunities to observe professionals dealing with the patient's resistance may encourage families to do the same at home. Families need time during this predischarge phase to test the methodologies of persistence demonstrated by the staff. When parents are more involved before discharge, they will be more comfortable when the entire responsibility is theirs and the patient's. The patient is regaining his autonomy, but he may test his family to determine whether he can use his injury to gain special favors. If parents participate in care and apply some discipline during hospitalization, it is easier for them to resume normal parent-child relationships at home. All of these should be accomplished before the discharge plan can be considered complete.

The social worker aggressively encourages attendance at group sessions at this time because it is in these groups that transition issues are discussed.[5] Group exposure enables families to learn that what the patient needs most is a sense of normalcy. Although he may look different, it is understood that if he is treated as he has always been, his changed body will not result in a changed sense of self. While families agree with this concept, it is a difficult one to act on; it conflicts with their desire to compensate for all the patient has suffered and to protect him from future injury. Social workers look for signs of this conflict, most evident in this predischarge phase.

The emphasis on regaining control and independence applies to all areas of patient-family functioning. Friends and neighbors need to be rallied for support at home, and the social worker encourages families to accept all offers of assistance, recognizing that the first few weeks at home, no matter how eagerly awaited, are particularly exhausting. These renewed connections also facilitate a smoother re-entry.

Hospitalization often brings into focus problems which had troubled the family before the injury but which had not been identified and for which no help had been sought or offered. Needs peculiar to the injury as well as pre-existing ones are addressed. The burn crisis has brought the family into contact with professionals who pay attention to the whole problem. Services of a hospital social worker often represent a family's first mental health intervention.[6] Having accepted this kind of help in connection with the burn, families tend to be less threatened by the idea of psychotherapy in the future. Referrals to community mental health agencies for individual and family therapy are frequently made as part of the discharge plan, and these are more successful because of the family's psychotherapeutic experience in the hospital.

As the family and the patient begin the termination phase of treatment, they rely less on staff and more on themselves and have increased contact with pre-burn associations. Separating from the security of the hospital and the supportive relationships formed there is difficult, but the desire to return home is stronger. The patient and his family are both fearful of the unknown future.

A key element of the third phase is exposure to the outside world. Particularly in the case of burn disfigurement, it is essential that patients have the opportunity to leave the hospital on an interim outing. If a family member accompanies the patient, they can experience together how it feels when people respond to the patient's appearance. The hospital staff can help them integrate their reactions to "going public" and how it feels when people stare or point, and they also help each other cope. The outing symbolizes the tasks of the final phase of acute care during which the patient and family resume their interdependent relationship and reconnect with the world outside the hospital.

## GROUPS

Group therapy, under the direction of the social worker, addresses family needs during all phases of acute and follow-up care. For those participants who have uprooted themselves to be near the hospitalized patient, groups provide much needed friendships and the nucleus of a support system to see them through the separation from home. Those in the predischarge phase find themselves reaching out to help families still in the earlier stages of acute care. In so doing they realize how far they have come, and they are fortified by this recognition of their own ability to cope. The challenges of discharge seem less frightening when they are approached with this new sense of mastery.

Participation in a group session during follow-up clinic visits affords an opportunity for returning families to interact with those who are still experiencing the acute phase. The veterans can report on the problems encountered and how they have coped since discharge. They are a fine resource for inpatient families preparing for the future. In addition, as returning group members, they can measure their own progress since the acute care phase.

Regardless of the length of time since acute care, experienced participants still value the group sessions. They refer to a sense of isolation in the community because others do not understand what they have experienced and what they feel. While acknowledging that it is important to talk about feelings, most participants know that it is only in the group that they are able to do so with ease. They consider the family support group a vital part of the clinic appointment because it enhances their ability to cope. Veteran group members welcome the opportunity to share what they have learned since the patient's acute care. At the other end of the spectrum, families new to the experience are eager to learn about the effects of a burn injury on other patients. The more experienced participants reinforce the need for normalcy for burned people, and they are in a position to advise others that guilt and overprotection produce poor results.

Even those unable to act on their own advice tend to verbalize (perhaps still trying to teach themselves) that what these patients need most is families who love them enough to treat them in the same way as before the injury, to let them learn to be independent, and to accept them as whole.

It is frequently during group sessions that the reality of burn scars or the chronic nature of aftercare is first recognized by families of acute care patients. Other participants are usually sensitive to this and offer support to help them accept what is to follow. In the group setting families share their various responses to the burn experience. They express their feelings about scarring and the pain of acknowledging that the patient's body will never look the same. They discuss the difficulties that burn scars present and the impact of parental guilt on discipline, sibling rivalry, and general family functioning. They talk about how they deal with the public's response to scars. Group participants hear a broad range of approaches from which to draw, and they feel a renewed sense of self-esteem when offering their own opinions for others to consider.

Participants in these groups share many common feelings, the strongest of which is guilt. Sharing this feeling enables families to see that although their self-blame is profound, it is not necessarily valid. They realize this when they hear another participant blame himself for a patient's injury and find themselves saying, "You shouldn't feel responsible." This advice is more meaningful when it comes from someone with the same experience. Shared experience gives permission to verbalize within the group what is difficult to say elsewhere. A parent will sometimes disclose some thought considered taboo such as his own initial revulsion at the child's disfigurement or the wish to escape the burden of a child with chronic needs. This frees other group members to acknowledge the same thoughts, to recognize that they are not alone, and to safely admit negative feelings. This is a liberating and a positive experience. Regardless of the various stages of burn involvement of the participants, the universality of the burn experience engenders mutual support in each group. What group members offer to each other is distinct from professional input: They *know* how it feels to have a loved one who has been burned.

Providing the setting for this mutual support and facilitating the group process are important aspects of the social worker's intervention. Social workers also lead groups for teenage patients. These groups focus mainly on the patient's anxiety about re-entry and on social concerns. The same process of mutual help seen in parent groups is also evident in teen groups as they draw on each other's experience and feelings. They derive much support from others who do not see them as different.

Leading each kind of group gives the social worker an opportunity to assess patient and family coping skills.[7] Previously unknown strengths and hidden anxieties frequently emerge in this supportive atmosphere. Specific intervention can then be productively directed to further enhance patient and family rehabilitation.

## HOUSING

In addition to the extremely high cost of medical/surgical burn care, which is disruptive and threatening to most families, the financial and emotional stress of living near the burn center for weeks or months takes its toll. Burn units are usually in large cities where the cost of living is high and the pace of life is strange. Since it is important for the family to be present as much as possible, it is essential that every effort be made to assist them in this adaptation. While a mother or spouse may at times want to sleep at bedside, either before surgery or during a life-threatening crisis, a good night's sleep away from the hospital in comfortable surroundings is important.

Social workers at the Shriners Burns Institute have for many years referred families to nearby private homes that offer rooms with or without kitchen privileges; a neighboring convent welcomes parents for a minimal fee, and the Y.W.C.A. offers a safe night for travelers. Rooming houses are usually managed by older women who take pleasure in mothering their guests who have loved ones in the hospital. Shriners Burns Institute in Boston has more recently become affiliated with a group of parents who have organized for the purpose of providing a comfortable, inexpensive, and supportive place where parents can stay together. This ensures that family visitors are not alone, that they can eat and share with others, and that they are within easy reach of the hospital. This facility also relieves the social worker of competing for available rooms when the city is crowded.

## RE-ENTRY

Families with a severely burned relative often have feelings of helplessness which pervade the entire experience and which are not limited to the acute stage. While returning home to family, neighbors, and the community at large should bring relief from the arduous hospital stay, it more often brings renewed feelings of isolation and helplessness. Families and patients longing for their lost autonomy must at the same time confront the reality of the burn and all its implications. First meetings face to face with strangers elicit a desire to flee and to seek the comfort of those who understand. When people in the community ask, "What happened to your child?" parents hear it as, "What did you do to your child?" and there is a resurgence of all the guilt and anger that had been eased during the hospital stay.

Returning home after a physically disfiguring burn injury is a major step for both family and patient. The ease or difficulty with which this crucial adjustment is made depends on a variety of factors, not the least of which is the attitudes of neighbors, teachers, and employers and their biases and needs for information. Social re-entry is as critical for life survival as was stabilization and wound healing for physical survival. For the school-age child, re-entry means a return to school.[8]

Planning for the return to school occurs simultaneously with planning for discharge. It is the role of the social worker to assess the attitudes and informational needs of school personnel and other community agencies.[9] Burns and scars evoke fears in those who are not familiar with that type of injury, and can result in a tendency to withdraw or reject. Thus, although the child is ready to return to school, the school may not be ready for the child's return.

The social worker's visit to the school is very helpful in easing the anxiety of school staff, classmates, and the patient. It also relieves parents of having to explain once again what has happened. The re-entry team of the Shriners Burns Institute is composed of a social worker, a hospital school teacher, and often the nurse or physical therapist who was close to the patient. A typical visit consists of a meeting with the school staff to answer questions about the special needs of the child and anticipated emotional responses. The team then makes a classroom presentation tailored to the appropriate age level. This may include a film strip about how burns occur followed by open discussion. When practical, a film and discussion session is also presented to the entire school to encourage the students to talk openly about burns and their feelings about scars and to be comfortable asking questions. It is most advantageous for teachers to observe how easily young people talk about these issues that adults feel uncomfortable addressing. Rejection usually occurs when fear of confronting the issues and lack of knowledge exist; acceptance results when information is shared and fears are dispelled.

The patient is given the choice of being present at these sessions, and he is asked if he would be willing to answer questions himself. The opportunity to observe the hospital team talk with his friends reassures him that his friends will understand what he has experienced and that they will treat him like a normal person again.

The major obstacle for all age groups returning home and one that must be addressed by the social worker is the tendency of families, teachers, or psychotherapists to overprotect and pamper the patient. Too often poor behavior is forgiven and deeper emotional problems are not addressed; instead, blame for all problems is placed on the burn injury. For this reason the social worker should continue to be available after discharge to the patient and his community to help them focus their efforts productively.

## ADULT CARE

The social worker helping an adult burn patient and his family deals with many of the same issues seen in helping children, as well as some additional ones. The ability of the family to rally and to persevere through the trauma is, again, key. Marriages without strong bases may not survive the demands placed on them. The depth of trust and commitment is tested; adults who had arrived at a point of self-knowledge are more keenly aware of their losses. While maturity and self-esteem can carry patients to a productive re-entry, any gaps in one's level of maturity become evident and may result in regression and depression. Young adults previously on their way to full independence may feel conflict as they find they need parental care once again.

The social worker can help by making a careful assessment of the support available from family, friends, co-workers, and community agencies. This is often more difficult with adult patients than with children, who are always in someone's care and who may also be more socially appealing. If the patient is not married or has no available and concerned close family members, or if his job is not secure, rehabilitation can be more arduous and more lonely. The social worker can locate a community agency or rehabilitation center that may be needed and prepare them to ensure a successful transfer and to prevent the patient from feeling fearful and distrustful.

The patient with few social or personal supports may do everything possible to deter his discharge. Adult patients are even more fearful than children of facing the public and of having to be independent again. Brief visits outside the hospital are therefore important. The patient needs the opportunity to discover whether he is able to resume his everyday activities at home and to be responsible for himself in public. Chronic depression, which may have been present before the burn injury and indeed may have been a factor in the accident, needs to be treated in therapy before the consequences of the injury become the major focus. Loss of income and the possibility of not returning to familiar work can exacerbate the depression. Vocational rehabilitation, along with psychological and physical rehabilitation, can bring about a positive social re-entry.

Returning to work is similar in many ways to the child's return to school. Fellow workers may not understand the disfigurement and may be fearful of close contact; they may avoid the person instead of communicating naturally. The social worker should approach an employer in the same way she would approach a school in order to provide the necessary educational information and psychological expertise.

A referral to a community social worker should always be considered for adult patients, especially where family support systems are weak. Long-term reconstructive burn care is often not provided because patients become "lost" in the community. Hospital systems that try to provide good follow-up care and referral to plastic surgeons are unsuccessful when the patient remains depressed or when he is not readily available. A community-based social worker who has been prepared by the hospital social worker can follow up and carry out the work initiated by the hospital and can help with vocational and rehabilitative counseling.

Alcoholism and homelessness are known factors in the adult burn population. Derelicts have been known to manipulate a readmission to the hospital because they have no other home. Their vast social problems cannot be easily corrected, but the burn unit staff needs to be aware of them and work with advocacy groups to alleviate problems and to deal with the immediate issues of burn rehabilitation.

## RECONSTRUCTIVE SURGERY

Many patients require years of reconstructive surgery. Frequent hospitalization may become a part of their lives. Reconstructive surgery is performed to improve function and appearance; it is a long, slow process and it cannot completely restore the skin to normal. The social worker who is able to maintain an ongoing relationship with the family and the patient can help them accept these limitations and the need for patience to achieve the best possible result. Parents are called on to help children live with the pain and disruption of many readmissions for plastic surgery, while they are also continually reminded of the traumatic injury.

The emotional responses noted earlier—denial, grief, helplessness, and guilt—may resurface repeatedly during the reconstructive process, and they need to be addressed so that they do not hamper rehabilitation. Some families struggle for control by seeking miracles from plastic surgery, whereas others resist the surgeries that are offered. By being present during the family's visits with the surgical team, the social worker has the opportunity to support the doctors' goals while allowing the family to work through their conflicting emotions.

## BURN PREVENTION

Teaching burn prevention is always an integral part of good burn treatment. Outreach on behalf of patients at the time of discharge most naturally includes teaching prevention. Since the subject is considered less surgical and more educational, it is welcomed by schools, employers, and community groups. Films depicting the many sources of heat which can cause burns and those illustrating human negligence that results in burns are acceptable. Scenes of operating rooms where wounds are being debrided are not. Some studies have shown that education does not have a strong impact on the incidence of burn injuries.[10] Patients often report, however, that repetitive television spots may have been responsible for their response to "stop, drop, and roll" when their clothes ignited, and this speaks strongly for such educational techniques.

The social worker often receives requests from the community for prevention information. Callers most frequently ask for help with children who play with matches and do not seem to respond to discipline. This is very frightening to parents and teachers, and it affords an excellent opportunity for prevention work. A brief telephone interview usually reveals a source of depression or conflict in the child's life, such as loss of a parent by death or divorce, parental depression resulting in lack of consistency and structure, and a learning disability leading to frustration, anger, and jealousy. The social worker can urge that the child be taken to a community mental health facility for evaluation. In the case of a chronic fire setter, family therapy may be necessary to achieve the structure that is lacking. When straightforward preventive education seems appropriate, the school can be contacted and encouraged to provide it. State agencies such as SCIPP (Statewide Childhood Injury Prevention Program) and local fire departments are excellent resources for educational programs in the community.

## SUMMARY

A productive treatment plan for burn injuries includes all members of the burn team in order to heal the patient and his family. The social worker is responsible for co-ordinating all members of the team, including the family, to facilitate a cohesive plan of discharge and continuing care. Families cannot be disenfranchised; patients do not place emotional needs on hold while being physically healed. Emotional energy is extended to its limit when one is trying to restore balance and stability. While the medical staff works to heal the patient, the social worker is the advocate and family therapist whose goal it is to dissolve psychological scars and create a therapeutic milieu for the patient and his family as they work through the painful maze of a burn injury.

## REFERENCES

1. Bernstein NR: Emotional Care of the Facially Burned and Disfigured. Boston, Little, Brown, 1976, pp 78, 93, 94, 105.
2. Golan N: Treatment in Crisis Situations. New York, The Free Press, 1978, p 16.
3. Cope O, Long RT: Emotional problems of burned children. New Engl J Med 264:1121–1127, 1961.
4. Cahners SS, Bernstein NR: Rehabilitating families with burned children. Scand J Reconstr Surg 13(1):173–175, 1979.
5. Cahners SS: Group meetings benefit families of burned children. Scand J Reconstr Surg 13:169–171, 1979.
6. Cahners SS: Social Services. *In* Bernstein NR, Robson M (eds): Comprehensive Approaches to the Burned Person. New Hyde Park, NY, Medical Examination Publishing, 1983, pp 235–244.
7. Cahners SS: Coping strategies of children and their families. *In* Milunsky A (ed): Coping with Crisis and Handicap. New York, Plenum Press, 1981, pp 289–293.
8. Cahners SS, Dumont J, McLaughlin E, O'Connor M: The Burned Child Returns to School. Shriners Burns Institute, 1975.
9. Cahners SS: A strong hospital-school liaison: A necessity for good rehabilitation planning for disfigured children. Scand J Reconstr Surg 13(1):167–168, 1979.
10. McLaughlin E, Vince C, Lee AM, Crawford JD: Project burn prevention: Outcome and implications. M J Public Health 72:241–247, 1982.

# 21

# Rehabilitation of the Burn Patient

AMY E. FLYNN and LAURIE L. GUNTER

Advances in medical care have made it possible for more patients suffering major thermal injuries to survive and to re-enter society. For this reason one major focus of treatment must be rehabilitation. To ensure maximum cosmetic outcome and functional independence, occupational and physical therapy must begin on the day of admission and continue throughout the hospital course and after discharge. This chapter offers information that will help therapists deliver optimal rehabilitation care to the burn patient.

## POSITIONING AND SPLINTING

Positioning and splinting are amoung the most effective methods by which occupational and physical therapists can help the acute burn patient achieve mobility and independence. When a patient is admitted, the therapist evaluates the extent of the injury in terms of the total percentage of body involvement. He notes the joint surfaces involved. He evaluates the depth of the burn wounds and checks for the presence of edema in both involved and uninvolved extremities. Following this evaluation, with consideration of the patient's age and mental status, a determination is made regarding necessary splints and proper extremity position.

### Positioning

The burn wound begins to contract immediately after trauma. Several researchers have identified the presence of myofibroblasts, which contain bundles of contractile elements similar to those in smooth muscle, as being responsible for the wound contraction. These cells increase in number during the inflammatory reaction phase and at 120 days post burn comprise up to 75 per cent of the total fibroblasts present in the healing wound. The "pull theory," described by Baur, states that the tight matrix of collagen fibers and the myofibroblasts pull on the margins of the wound, resulting in wound closure.[1]

Wound contraction, however, continues after wound closure is complete. If this continued contraction occurs across a flexed joint, the outcome is a debilitating flexion contracture. It is well known that patients sustaining a burn injury assume the flexed position, which is the position of comfort. For this reason, immediately upon admission, the patient is positioned in the antideformity, extension position with elevation for control of edema.

## Splinting

Three types of splinting for burn patients exist: static splints, dynamic splints, and conformers.[2]

### Static Splinting

Static splinting is done immediately on admission to maintain the antideformity position mentioned above. It is also done immediately after grafting to immobilize the part and facilitate graft take. Most splints are custom-fabricated and must be assessed daily for fit, skin tolerance, and potential complications such as pressure sores, skin breakdown or maceration, and graft shearing.

Splinting the burned hand is critical to maintain function when deep dorsal hand burns leave delicate tendons and joints exposed. These hands must be positioned in the lumbrical plus position or the position of protection, with the wrist in 20 to 30 degrees of dorsiflexion, the metacarpophalangeal (MCP) joints in 75 to 80 degrees of flexion, the interphalangeal (IP) joints fully extended, and the thumb opposed.[3, 4] In the first 24 to 48 hours, it is often difficult to achieve full MCP joint flexion because of pain and swelling. At this time, 45 degrees of MCP joint flexion with full IP flexion are adequate. As edema resolves, MCP joint flexion is gradually increased until full flexion is reached.

Maintenance of the lumbrical plus position through splinting protects against the development of two common hand deformities: the clawed hand and the boutonniere deformity. The clawed hand deformity can be observed within the first 24 hours after trauma when capillary permeability in the tissues increases in response to trauma and results in excessive intercellular fluid or severe edema.[5] As the hand swells, the increased tension causes the MCP joints to hyperextend and the IP joints to flex. With time, collagen is laid down in the protein-rich fluid, resulting in fibrosis and contractures in these joints. Left untreated, these contractures become fixed.

The intricate balance between the intrinsic and extrinsic musculature of the hand must also be maintained to prevent deformity. Disruption of the central slip of the extensor mechanism by tearing of the transverse fibers of the dorsal hood over the proximal interphalangeal joint (PIP) causes the lateral bands to fall volarly. This results in flexion rather than extension of the PIP joints and hyperextension of the distal interphalangeal joints (DIP). This is known as the boutonniere deformity.[2] If the extensor mechanism is involved but the PIP joints remain in extension, it is possible for scar to form and tether down the lateral bands, maintaining proper alignment and function. Passive flexion of the PIPs and full fisting are, therefore, contraindicated. Only supervised, active flexion of the PIP joints while viewing the wounds is allowed. The hand is securely wrapped into the splint at all times, except during exercise and functional activities, and elevated until wounds are closed and range of motion is regained. Proper positioning in very young children with small hands is difficult. However, by using ⅟₁₆-inch thermoplastic material and supporting the wrist with a T strut, the thumb web space, MCP flexion, and IP extension can be maintained.

Full-thickness burns of the thick fibrous pads of the palmar surface of the hand are less common but no less difficult to treat. The hand is naturally held in slight flexion, and the position of comfort further encourages this flexion. Hands with this type of burn must be splinted with all joints in full extension and the thumb radially abducted and extended.

Static splints are also used for immobilization in order to facilitate graft take. Immobilizing joints over or near where grafts have been placed reduces the possibility of graft movement and formation of hematomas and blisters and creates a more favorable condition for healing. The burn pan splint can be adapted to allow open treatment of grafts so that the nursing staff can expel fluid that collects under the graft and inhibits graft take. Traction by means of rubber bands and hooks applied to the intact finger nails is used to immobilize the digits.[3]

A great deal of splinting for patients undergoing reconstructive surgery can be done in the operating room. This is especially beneficial for very young and fearful patients.

### Dynamic Splinting

Dynamic splinting is usually initiated in the rehabilitation phase of treatment to increase range of motion (ROM), strength, and mobility. This form of splinting enhances recovery because it combines the dynamic stretching of opposing contractile forces with the strengthening of weakened muscles. It is most commonly used and effective on metacarpal and interphalangeal joints in the hand; however, recent advances in commercially available equipment such as continuous passive motion machines and Dynasplints have proven beneficial for other joints involved in the burn injury.

Application of dynamic forces begins gently and progresses slowly. The involved areas are closely monitored for complications including skin breakdown, extremity edema, and increased joint pain. Evidence of any of these complications necessitates postponing or discontinuing the splint or decreasing wearing time. If the splint is well tolerated, dynamic forces and wearing schedule are increased.

To prevent skin breakdown and damage to the small joints of the hand, dynamic hand splints are most often used in conjunction with static splints. The dynamic splint is worn during the day when it can be monitored and the static splint is worn at night. Continuous passive motion devices and Dynasplints usually can be worn both during the day and at night without resulting complications. All types of dynamic splints are maintained until active motion is sufficient to overcome contractile forces.

### Conformers

Occupational and Physical Therapists can assist burn patients in their overall recovery and acceptance of scars by maximizing the cosmetic appearance of the healing skin. Conformers—garments or devices fabricated from various materials and used for the purpose of additional pressure on skin grafts—function to accomplish this by remodeling scar tissue. The work of Malick and Carr[6] with Elastomer molds and inserts has enabled therapists to better control scar formation on concave surfaces of the body where, previously, other types of pressure garments had been unsuccessful. Several other devices have been conceived and researched, including the transparent face mask and the Elastomer face mask, which most recently has been used as an integral part of the postoperative primary dressing following autografting procedures to the face.

A discussion follows of the different types of conformers and materials, their applications, and advantages and disadvantages. Vital to this discussion is the understanding that the final outcome is directly influenced by patient compliance.

**SOFT FOAM CONFORMERS.** After a reconstructive procedure involving the release of tight scar tissue and placement of a split-thickness skin graft and following the removal of the primary dressing, raised edges of old scar tissue remain. In addition, the new graft tends to wrinkle under the forces of gravity and to contract as it heals. Foam conformers fabricated from a closed-cell, nonabsorbent foam and a pressure-sensitive foam are fit into the newly grafted areas and help to keep the graft flat and to reduce its edges as healing proceeds. Graft take must be 80 per cent or greater for this pressure to be well tolerated.

To make the conformer, the new graft is traced and a template is made. The foams are adhered to each other by their sticky-back surfaces. Using the template, the conformer, precisely matching the shape of the graft, is cut from the foam and applied to the graft with the closed-cell, nonabsorbent foam facing toward the skin. A thin layer of gauze is placed between the foam and the graft to absorb any drainage. The foam edges are beveled to overlap the graft edges to provide continuous pressure as the skin heals and the edges recede. The conformers are wrapped securely in place with gauze and elastic wraps and used for approximately three to seven days before pressure garments are applied.

The patient or primary caregiver is instructed to remove the conformer twice each day for skin care and massage. Massage of the healed areas, in conjunction with an exercise program, begins immediately. Massage along the suture line begins at approximately three to five days. An alternate set of conformers is fabricated to facilitate a 23-hour-per-day wearing schedule and conformer care.

**ELASTOMER AND PROSTHETIC FOAM T-SHIRTS.** The use of Elastomer inserts to aid in controlling scar formation has been well documented.[6] These Silastic inserts have greatly enhanced the cosmetic results of burn scars in hard-to-control areas such as the axilla and the supraclavicular notch. Keeping these inserts in place without constant repositioning, however, poses a problem. As a workable solution, Elastomer and prosthetic foam are impregnated into a T-shirt, which enables the patient to simply don the T-shirt under the pressure garment, with little or no repositioning needed.

Elastomer insert fabrication begins by mixing together elastomer, prosthetic foam, and catalyst. When this mixture begins to froth, it is poured over the area requiring additional pressure. The T-shirt is then pulled down over the body and, just prior to completely setting of the mixture, the shirt is pressed lightly against the foam to secure adherence. The mixture is allowed to set for approximately 5 minutes. Care must be taken to stay away from hair lines or skin surface hairs, as hairs will be extracted when the set mold is removed. Two garments are made for continuous wear under pressure garments until the scars have reached maturity.

BURN-QUALITY AQUAPLAST FACE MASKS. Burn-quality Aquaplast has been used for three years at the Shriners Burns Institute in Boston to fabricate total and partial face masks. The properties of the material make it desirable to use for this purpose for several reasons. First, it can be molded directly on the patient. Second, because of its temporary transparency when heated, the effects of pressure can be observed during the fabrication process. Third, patients can see and breathe during the fabrication process, enhancing cooperation. Finally, the cost and fabrication time are minimal compared with those of high-temperature materials requiring fabrication of positive and negative molds.

With the patient in a supine position, a paper tracing of the face is made. The eyes, nose, mouth, and edges of the desired mask are marked. The pattern is traced onto the Burn-quality Aquaplast and cut out and the material is heated until transparent; it is often necessary to rub lotion over the Aquaplast to prevent it from sticking to itself and to other surfaces. The mask is then allowed to cool until the patient can wear it comfortably, but the material remains malleable. At this time the mask is placed over the face, and the eyes, nose, and mouth are properly positioned, with the nares opened for easy breathing. While maintaining the primary anchor at the bridge of the nose, the mask is smoothed into place. Usually the material cools before the mask is complete, necessitating spot heating in stages to complete fabrication—first each eye independently, then the nose including nasolabial folds, the upper lip, the mouth, and finally the chin. Care is taken not to overheat the material, as the heat dissipates to already completed areas and shape is lost. Fingertip massage and molding with lotion-soaked cotton swabs facilitate precise fit and pressure to facial contours.

Like other conformers and pressure garments, the mask is worn most of the time during the day and at night. It can be removed for bathing and eating and vigorous physical activity. It should also be removed periodically for skin checks, cleaning, and skin massage.

BREAST CONFORMERS. Sustained prior to development, burns of the chest in female patients resulting in the formation of thick or hypertropic scar tissue can inhibit formation of breast tissue or cause misshapen development. Surgical procedures have been developed to release scar tissue, allowing reshaping of the breast, proper growth of the breast, and insertion of breast implants. The release procedure involves excision of all or a portion of the inhibiting scar, placement of autografted skin, and follow-up care by physical or occupational therapy.

One aspect of the postoperative follow-up care includes wearing both soft and hard conformers to prevent skin contracture and graft wrinkling. Conformer application is contingent on graft take and occurs for most patients usually no later than one week after the removal of the primary dressing. Soft foam conformers are worn until the graft is sufficiently healed and tough enough to accept increased pressure; conformers fabricated from low-temperature thermoplastic material are then applied.

The procedure for fabricating the hard conformer begins by tracing the graft with clean or sterile paper. Patterns for conformers fabricated for day wear are taken while the patient is in a relaxed sitting position with arms resting at her side. Night wear patterns are taken with the patient lying supine, also with arms resting at her sides. The pattern parallels the grafted area and extends one inch beyond the suture lines to assure adequate pressure along the margins of the graft. The pattern is then traced onto the thermoplastic material. The material most suited for use in the breast conformer is a medium-thickness, low-temperature plastic with elastic memory because it permits greatest support, conformity, and frequent remolding. The material is cut and heated and then molded to the grafted area with the breasts slightly elevated to prevent creasing in the natural fold below the breast tissue. When molding is complete, final adjustments are made to maximize fit.[9]

The conformer is held in place with Velcro and Betapile straps or a brassiere or long-line brassiere, depending upon the size and location of the release and the size of the breasts. For best results, the conformer is worn at all times for six months to one year, or until the grafts are mature. After several months, however, if the conformer can be removed without the graft becoming raised and rigid and without a change in breast shape, a 12-hour-per-day schedule may be instituted.

Patients are seen in therapy once a week for two to three weeks, then every two to three weeks for several months. The purpose of these visits is to check skin condition, noting areas of wrinkling, raised edges, or scar thickening. These signs usually indicate insufficient pressure, while red or blistered pressure areas indicate too much pressure. In such cases, conformers are remolded or refabricated for proper fit and conformity.

The nature of the procedure and the age of the patient dictate that psychosocial issues be carefully considered. A concerted effort must be made to keep the conformer as inconspicuous as possible. Preoperative instruction, including a detailed description of follow-up treatment, helps prepare the patient for the procedure and enhances compliance with essential rehabilitation treatment procedures.

## EXERCISE

Therapeutic exercise is used in addition to positioning and splinting to maintain joint mobility and extremity function. In the acute stage of treatment, the goals of exercise include maintaining or increasing ROM of involved and uninvolved joints, preventing skin contractures, preventing muscle weakness resulting from disuse and a loss of protein structures in the presence of a high metabolic state, reducing edema, and preventing venous stasis and possible subsequent thrombus formation. These goals are best met through immediate implementation of a treatment program including active, active-assisted, passive, and occasionally resistive exercises.[10-15]

Active exercises most effectively maintain ROM and prevent weakening of muscles. They most greatly benefit patients with significant pain or fear, since this type of exercise allows some control over the treatment program. Active-assisted exercises are used most with patients incapable of independently completing full ROM, whereas a passive exercise program is designed for patients incapable of active participation because of altered mental status or neurological impairment. Passive exercises are also indicated for uncooperative patients, young children, patients with large injuries and a debilitated medical status, and, as will be discussed in more detail later, patients under anesthesia in the operating room. Although resistive exercises are most frequently initiated in the rehabilitation stage, in some instances they can be initiated in the acute stage. For example, patients whose burn involves a small percentage of total body surface area and who tolerate activity well can participate in a resistive program as soon as they are stable medically.

Some suggestions for exercise during the rehabilitation stage include proprioceptive neuromuscular facilitation (PNF) rhythmic rotation of the extremities for relaxation; PNF rhythmic initiation and slow reversals in diagonal movement patterns for strengthening and increasing ROM; and gentle contract-relax and hold-relax of indicated muscles to facilitate relaxation and increase ROM.[16] All exercises are done to prepare for functional mobility and must be translated into meaningful daily living activities such as ambulation. All exercises are performed at least once each day but preferably two or three times per day, in short treatment sessions that do not overstress the patient. Respiration, temperature, heart rate, and blood pressure are monitored at regular intervals as determinants of the patient's response to activity.

The goals of exercise in the acute stage continue into the rehabilitation stage, with the additional goal of cardiovascular system conditioning. Aerobic and endurance training activities such as the treadmill, ergometry, progressive ambulation, and jogging reverse the deconditioning effects of prolonged immobilization and prepare the patient for the increased demands of normal daily activities and independent functional mobility.

Joint mobilization to increase ROM is an appropriate treatment modality in both the acute and rehabilitation stages. It functions to increase ROM by causing relaxation of reflexively contracted muscles through reciprocal inhibition, inhibition of the muscles through facilitation of the Golgi tendon organ, mechanical stretching of tight tissues, and breaking of intra-articular adhesions.

Again, exercises in the rehabilitation stage are done at least once a day, but preferably two or three times per day in short sessions. Exercises continue until the threat of the development of contractures no longer exists and until muscle strength is regained and the patient is functioning well in daily activities.

## TREATMENT IN THE OPERATING ROOM

Exercises done while the patient is anesthetized in the operating room allow the therapist to better perform ROM and result in improved functioning. They enable the therapist to view the wounds during exercise and allow him to accurately assess muscle length and joint status with the patient's pain and apprehension eliminated.[10, 15, 17, 18] Because normal protective mechanisms are not functioning when the patient is under anesthesia, exercises must be done slowly and gently to allow sufficient time for the tissues to stretch. Fast, vigorous movements can lead to tears and bleeding in the tissues, fibrosis, and formation of adhesions. ROM exercises preceded or accompanied by massage with a moisturizing cream or lotion facilitate stretching and movement.

Some splint fabrication is also done in the operating room. This is especially beneficial for pediatric patients when the neck and face are the areas to be splinted, as well as for patients who have had surgical releases of joint contractures with skin graft placement requiring splints for postoperative immobilization and positioning. Under anesthesia the part to be splinted is more easily placed and maintained in the desired position while the splint is molded. All preliminary splint work, such as measuring the part and cutting the material, is done before entering the operating room so that anesthesia time is not unnecessarily prolonged.

## ACTIVITIES OF DAILY LIVING

Activities of daily living (ADLs) are self-help tasks that individuals perform daily and include things such as feeding, personal hygiene, grooming, dressing, and school and vocational activities. Performance of these tasks in terms of appropriateness and timing depends on age, cultural or ethnic background, role within the family or social structure, and physical abilities, but in most cases independent performance is essential for a sense of autonomy and self-worth.

ADL activities are initiated as soon as the patient is medically stable enough to participate. Most often, feeding is the point at which treatment begins. Independence then follows a sequential developmental pattern to include continence, transfers, toileting, dressing, and bathing. A program that facilitates this pattern and adapts to meet the individual needs of each patient assists in the physical and psychological recovery.

Built-up handles, Dycem mats, extended straws, and other types of adaptive equipment produce successful performance of ADL. The ultimate challenge for therapists working with burn patients is the fabrication of this adaptive equipment. Some are commercially available but often do not meet the needs of the patient, especially if the patient has lost digits or joint motion. This is frequently the case with patients who have sustained a burn injury. Possibilities for adaptive techniques are limited only by the patient's and therapist's imagination.

## AMBULATION

The debilitating effects of immobilization, even for very short periods of time, can be manifested in all body systems. Some changes that occur in the major body systems include the following: in the cardiovascular system, orthostatic hypotension, increased cardiac workload, and thrombus formation; in the respiratory system, decreased respiratory movement, decreased movement of secretions, and decreased oxygen-carbon dioxide balance; in the musculoskeletal system, osteoporosis, contracture, and loss of muscle strength; and in the integumentary system, decubitus ulcer formation. Urinary function, gastrointestinal function, and psychosocial development may also be adversely affected.[20]

Ambulation can prevent or reverse these debilitating changes and maintain optimal functional mobility. The decision to begin ambulation is based on a careful evaluation of the patient's wound and overall medical status. Approximately two to three days post burn, stabilization of cardiac and respiratory function is achieved and fluid resuscitation is complete.[18] Ambulation activity should begin at this time, even when support or monitoring equipment is in use. However, it is contraindicated in patients with exposed joint structures, exposed tendons, or severe edema in the lower extremities.[18] Postoperative ambulation should begin as soon as healing progresses to a point where the dependent position of the lower extremities does not jeopardize graft take[10, 18, 21, 22] and should continue regularly throughout the hospital course. Timing varies among patients and facilities, usually ranging from one to ten days.

Before upright activity is begun, the lower extremities must first be prepared with appropriate burn dressings and elastic pressure bandages. Elastic bandages help prevent venous stasis and edema as well as provide comfort and support to the new grafts when the patient is upright. Meticulous attention is paid to the method of applying these bandages in order to prevent excessive pressure and consequent breakdown of tissue. Bandages are applied with the legs elevated using a figure-8 technique. Wraps begin distally just proximal to the toes and move proximally to the groin. Folds in the bandage material are avoided.[23]

Gait training in the acute stage begins in the parallel bars with frequent short walks and rest periods and progresses to increased distances, fewer rest periods, and more difficult ground surfaces. The use of parallel bars provides maximal support to weak or deconditioned patients and helps alleviate fear. Patients demonstrating orthostatic hypotension require a closely monitored tilt table program or a program of activities progressing from sitting to standing.

During rest periods the lower extremities are elevated to assist venous return. When the upright position is well tolerated, ambulation begins and progresses as described above. Heart rate, blood pressure, respiration, and pain are carefully monitored, as these parameters help determine activity tolerance; progression of ambulation is dependent on that tolerance.

Gait training in the rehabilitation stage helps to improve general body condition and to increase endurance, muscle strength, and functional mobility. Therefore, ambulation is done in conjunction with a program of stretching and strengthening exercises as well as postural and balance activities. Ambulation should expand to include greater distances, faster speeds, and more challenging ground surfaces.

## PRESSURE THERAPY

The principle of pressure therapy in the treatment of burn scars was first applied in 1881 by Unna.[1] Today we continue to use pressure therapy as a treatment for scars and over the years have gained a better understanding of the physiological changes caused by this pressure.

Histologically, hypertrophic scar contains an increased number of fibroblasts compared to normal skin. Its collagen fibers are arranged in a nodular as opposed to parallel fashion. The interstitial space is decreased. The vascular supply is increased, resulting in increased production of collagen. Finally the concentration of chondroitin sulfate A is increased and the concentration of hyaluronic acid decreased. The increased numbers of myofibroblasts produce a rigid link between collagen fibers and may play a role in the contractile forces of hypertrophic scar.[1, 24] Application of pressure garments causes vascular shutdown, tissue hypoxia, degeneration of fibroblasts, and reduced production of collagen. The collagen fibers become organized in a more parallel manner. Interstitial space is increased, the concentration of chondroitin sulfate A is decreased, and the concentration of hyaluronic acid is increased.

Patients who develop hypertrophic scars are frequently those whose deep, partial-thickness burn wounds heal without grafting but whose healing process requires longer than two weeks; patients who undergo excision and grafting of deep, partial-thickness or full-thickness burn wounds; and patients who frequently develop infections in burn wounds, grafts, or donor sites. For this reason pressure garments should be provided prophylactically for all patients except those whose wounds involve only the superficial, epidermal layer. Most hypertrophic scar responds to pressure as long as it remains immature and in the healing phase, indicated by redness, thickening, and rigidity.

Clinically, the effects of pressure on hypertrophic scar are seen immediately as blanching, mild flattening, and formation of a softer, more pliable scar tissue texture. The amount of tension required to produce these changes is controversial; values range from 4 to 55 mm Hg.[26, 27, 28] However, in order to achieve vascular shutdown with subsequent tissue hypoxia, degeneration of fibroblasts, and decreased collagen production, pressure must exceed the intercapillary pressure, or 20 mm Hg.[25]

During the active scar-healing phase, these clinical changes can be maintained only through constant and prolonged daily use of the prescribed garments. If the garments are removed before full maturity, the scar reverts back to its red, raised, and rigid state. A suggested wearing schedule is 24 hours a day, with removal only for bathing, skin care, and vigorous exercise. Their use is continued for a period of time ranging from six months to two years.

Pressure therapy is contraindicated when there are large remaining open areas in the burn wound and when open areas greater than 2 cm are located directly over joint surfaces. Because prolonged use of high-pressure garments can cause structural changes in immature bone, very young children must be closely monitored, and parents or guardians must be apprised of the possible complications. Children under the age of one should be limited to wearing pressure garments for three- to four-hour intervals, with one- to two-hour rest periods.

A variety of prefabricated and custom-made garments is available in today's market, each with its own advantages and disadvantages. Prefabricated garments such as Tubigrip, Ace wraps, and Coban, are readily available and can be applied early in the healing process. Variations in tension in these garments are difficult. Custom-made garments, such as Jobst, deliver more consistent tension and are fabricated to fit the individual needs of the patient, but because the high pressure provided can cause some delay in healing, wounds must be well healed prior to their application.

## DISCHARGE PLANNING AND TEACHING

The rehabilitation team should provide information at discharge on skin care, exercise, and splints.

### Skin Care

To care for skin properly, the patient must have a basic understanding of burn wound healing and scar formation. He should be taught to clean and dress any remaining open wounds or donor sites, to clean newly grafted areas with soap and water, and to moisturize these areas twice daily with a lanolin-based, low-alcohol cream or lotion. Deep friction or deep pressure massage is taught as a means of effectively minimizing scar and skin contracture formation and controlling edema. The patient is cautioned against exposure to direct sunlight and instructed to use SPF-15 sunblock to prevent further burning of fragile, healing skin.

## Exercise

The contractile forces of scar continue as long as scar is immature. Patients and family members are often under the misconception that scar formation ends when wounds area healed; they must understand that contractile forces can continue for up to two years and that exercise is an excellent method to counteract these forces. Individualized exercise programs are designed for each patient and taught in advance of discharge.

## Splints

To enhance compliance, the patient must be made fully aware of the purpose of splinting and of the functional limits and deformities that can occur when prescribed treatment is not followed. Indications for splinting include active scarring around a joint surface, disuse of an involved extremity, and poor cosmesis. Splints are continued until optimal functional and cosmetic results are achieved; then they are often worn during sleep to maintain position and removed during the day to allow participation in normal daily activities.

### REFERENCES

1. Baur PS, Parks DH, Larson DL: The healing of burn wounds. Clin Plast Surg 4:389–407, 1977.
2. Malick MH, Carr JA: Manual on Management of the Burn Patient. Pittsburgh, PA, Harmarville Rehabilitation Center, 1982.
3. Malick MH: Management of the severely burned patient. Br J Occup Ther 38:76–80, 1975.
4. Covey MH: Occupational Therapy. In Boseick JA (ed): The Art and Science of Burn Care. Rockville, MD, Aspen Publishers, 1987, pp 285–298.
5. Vasudevan SV, Melvin JL: Upper extremity edema control: Rationale for the techniques. Am J Occup Ther 33:520–523, 1979.
6. Malick MH, Carr JA: Flexible elastomer molds in burn scar control. Am J Occup Ther 34:603–608, 1980.
7. Rivers EA, Strate RG, Solem LD: The transparent face mask. Am J Occup Ther 33:108–113, 1979.
8. Engrav LH, MacDonald LB, Covey MH, et al: Do splinting and pressure devices damage new grafts? Journal of Burn Care and Rehabilitation 4:107–108, 1983.
9. Mullison, Alison: In press.
10. DiGregoria VR: Rehabilitation of the burn patient. New York, Churchill Livingstone, 1984.
11. Bartlett RH, Wengerson E, Simonton S, et al: Rehabilitation following burn injury. Surg Clin North Am 58:1249–1262, 1978.
12. Helm PA, Head MD, Pullium G, et al: Burn rehabilitation: A team approach. Surg Clin North Am 58:1236–1277, 1987.
13. Parks DH, Evans EB, Larson DL: Prevention and correction of deformity after severe burns. Surg Clin North Am 58:1279–1289, 1978.
14. Dobbs ER, Curreri PW: Burns: Analysis of results of physical therapy in 681 patients. J Trauma 12:242–248, 1972.
15. Givliani CA, Perry GA: Factors to consider in the rehabilitation aspect of burn care. Phys Ther 65:619–623, 1985.
16. Knott M, Voss D: Proprioceptive Neuromuscular Facilitation Patterns and Techniques. New York, Harper and Row, 1969.
17. Nicosia J, Stien ED, Stein JM: The advantages of physiotherapy for burn patients under anaesthesia. Burns 6:202–204, 1980.

18. Helm PA, Kevorkian GC, Lushbaugh M, et al: Burn injury: Rehabilitation management in 1982. Arch Phys Med Rehabil 63:6–16, 1982.
19. Trombly CA, Scott AD: Occupational Therapy for Physical Dysfunction. Baltimore, Williams & Wilkins, 1977.
20. Effects on cardiovascular function. Am J Nurs 67:781–797, 1967.
21. Golden GT, Power CG, Skinner JR, et al: A technique of lower extremity mesh grafting with early ambulation. Am J Surg 133:646–647, 1977.
22. Badenham DC, Watson R: The early ambulation of patients with lower extremity burn grafts. Br J Plast Surg 24:20, 1971.
23. Whitmore JJ, Burt MM, Fowler RS, et al: Bandaging the lower extremity to control swelling: Figure 8 versus spiral technique. Arch Phys Med 53:487–490, 1972.
24. Garcia-Velasco M, Ley R, Mutch D, et al: Compression treatment of hypertrophic scars in burned children. Can J Surg 21:450–452, 1978.
25. Kischer WC, Shetlar MR, Shetlar CL: Alteration of hypertrophic scars induced by mechanical pressure. Arch Dermatol 111:60–64, 1975.
26. Rose MD, Deitch EA: The clinical use of a tubular compression bandage. Tubigrip for burn scar therapy: A critical analysis. Burns 12:58–64, 1985.
27. Judge JC, May RS, DeClement FA: Control of hypertrophic scarring in burn patients using tubular support bandages. J Burn Care Rehabil 5:221–224, 1984.
28. Leung KS, Cheng JCY, Ma GFY, Leung PC: Complications of pressure therapy for post-burn hypertrophic scars. Burns Inc Therm Inj 10:434–438, 1984.

# Index

Note: Page numbers in *italics* refer to illustrations.

Abdomen, infections of, bacterial, 293
Abortion, spontaneous, from electrical injuries, 73
Abuse, child, burns and, 107
  social worker and, 309
Acalculous cholecystitis, post-burn, 171–172
Acetaminophen, renal function and, 249
Acidosis, metabolic, in major burn, 18
Acrolein, as toxin in smoke, 27–31
Activities of daily living (ADLs), in rehabilitation, 327–328
Adrenal insufficiency, post-burn, 175
Adrenergic agonists, studies of, in burned patients, 191–193
Adult care, social worker in, 316–317
Adult respiratory distress syndrome (ARDS), scald burns and, 32–34
  smoke inhalation and, 32, 89
Airway(s). *See also* Upper airway.
  damage to, 110
  management of, in major burns, 5, 38
  post-burn, anesthetic management and, 217–218
Alveolar damage, 110
Ambulation, in rehabilitation, 328–329
Aminoglycosides, renal function and, 248–248
  systemic, for burn wounds, 301–302
Amphotericin, renal function and, 249
Amputations, in electrical injuries, 80–81
Analgesics, for débridement and dressing changes, deficiencies of, 201
  for intubation, 52
  in psychiatric management, 264–265
Anemia, post-burn, 172–173
Anesthesia, for intubation, 52
Anesthetic agents, in pain management, 205–206
  studies of, in burned patients, 189–191
Anesthetic management, 217–229
  calcium homeostasis and, 227
  induction in, 224
  intravenous lines and, 222–224
  maintenance of anesthesia in, 224–225
  monitoring lines and, 222–224
  of upper airway injury, 61–62
  pathophysiological considerations for, 217–220
    for airways, 217–218

Anesthetic management (*Continued*)
  for central nervous system, 220
  for circulatory system, 218
  for electrical injuries, 219–220
  for renal function, 219
  patient preparation in, 221
  postanesthetic management and, 228
  preoperative evaluation in, 220–221
  preoperative medication in, 222
  temperature regulation and, 226–227
Antacids, for stress ulcer prevention, 280–281
Anthropometric measurements, in nutritional assessment, 154
Anti-anxiety agents, in psychiatric management, 265
Antibiotics, for toxic epidermal necrolysis, 133–134
  in major burn management, 8
  prophylactic, 283–284
  renal function and, 248–249
  studies of, in burned patients, 183–184
  subeschar, for burn wounds, 298–299
  systemic, for burn wounds, 299–302
  topical, for burn wounds, 294–298
Antidepressants, in psychiatric management, 265
Antimicrobial therapy, topical, for burn wounds, 294–298
Antipsychotic agents, in psychiatric management, 265
Aquaplast face masks, burn-quality, in rehabilitation, 324
Arrhythmia, cardiac, post-burn, 161
Arterial blood gas determination, serial, in patient assessment, 39
Arterial oxygen tension, in inhalation injury, 48
  maintenance of, in post-burn pulmonary dysfunction, 89
Artery, innominate, perforation of, complicating prolonged intubation, 58
Atelectasis, complicating major burn, 35
  in inhalation injury, 28–29
Ativan, in psychiatric management, 265
  studies of, in burned patients, 187, *188*
Atracurium, studies of, in burned patients, 195
Auditory tube, blocking of, complicating prolonged intubation, 57
Autonomic nervous system, effects of electrical injuries on, 72

Bacterial flora, of patient, in infection prevention, 280–281
Bacterial infection(s), burn wound and, 290–291
   endocarditis as, 292–293
   intra-abdominal, 293
   middle ear, 293
   ocular, 293
   pulmonary, 291–292
   sinusitis as, 293
   suppurative thrombophlebitis as, 292
   urinary tract, 293
Bedding, in infection prevention, 279
Benzodiazepines, in psychiatric management, 265
   studies of, in burned patients, 186–187
Biochemical indices, in nutritional assessment, 154–156
Blood, flow of, renal, in acute phase, 242
   loss of, excisional, decreasing, 236–237
      perioperative fluid requirements and, 233–235
   volume of, restoration of, post-burn, 91
Blood vessels, complications involving, 176–177
   effects of electrical injuries on, 73
Bones, complications involving, 176–177
Brain, effects of electrical injuries on, 71
Breast conformers, in rehabilitation, 324–325
Bronchodilators, indications for, 40–41
Bronchoscopy, fiberoptic, in inhalation injury diagnosis, 48–49
   in patient assessment, 37–38
Burn(s), acute phase of, treatment in, 19–22
   burn source removal as, 19
   hematological change management as, 23
   initial fluid resuscitation as, 19–21
   metabolic change management as, 23
   pulmonary support as, 21
   wound management as, 22
   classification of, 4–5, 12–14, 102–104
   prevention of, social worker and, 318–319
   size of, calculation of, 6–8
Burn injury, complication(s) of, 159–177
   acalculous cholecystitis as, 171–172
   adrenal insufficiency as, 175
   anemia as, 172–173
   cardiac, 159–162
   electrolyte imbalances as, 175–176
   gastrointestinal, 166–170
   hemoglobinuria as, 162–163
   hepatic, 163–166
   hyperosmolar hyperglycemic nonketotic coma as, 176
   hypertension in children as, 174
   leukopenia as, 173
   multiple organ failure as, 166
   muscle, 176–177
   pancreatitis as, 172
   skeletal, 176–177

Burn injury *(Continued)*
   superior mesenteric artery syndrome as, 170–171
   vascular, 176–177
   depth of, 12–14
   severity of, 14–15
Burning process, cessation of, 1, 19
Burnout, staff, preventing, 267–268

Calcium, homeostasis of, post-burn, anesthetic management and, 227
   imbalance of, post-burn, 175–176
Caloric goals, compliance with, in nutritional assessment, 154
*Candida* infections, burn wound and, 293
Carbamazepine, in psychiatric management, 265
Carbohydrates, requirements in nutritional support for, 144, 146
Carbon monoxide poisoning, 110
   in patient evaluation, 47
   in smoke inhalation, 5, 26, 27
   signs of, 36
Carboxyhemoglobin levels, measurement of, in patient assessment, 36–37
Cardiac output, in major burn, 16
   post-burn, 159–160
      pharmacologic effects of, 180–181
Cardiopulmonary changes, acute, 15–16
   fluid shifts and, 15–16
   hematological response and, 18–19
   hemodynamic instability and, 15–16
   metabolic changes and, 18
   pulmonary changes and, 17–18
   temperature change and, 16–17
Cardiovascular assessment, of burn patient, 101–102
Cardiovascular stabilization, for intubation, 52
Cardiovascular system, changes in, pharmacologic effects of, 180–181
Catheterization, bladder, 106
   Swan-Ganz, 39
Causalgia, from electrical injuries, 72
Central nervous system, effects of electrical injuries on, 71–72
   post-burn, anesthetic management and, 220
Cephalosporins, renal function and, 249
   systemic, for burn wounds, 301
Cerium, topical, for burn wounds, 298
Chemical burns, emergency treatment of, 1, 19
Chest radiographs, in patient assessment, 37
Child abuse, burns and, 107
   social worker and, 309
Chlordiazepoxide, studies of, in burned patients, 187
Chlorpromazine, in psychiatric management, 265
Cholecystitis, acalculous, post-burn, 171–172

Cimetidine, for stress ulcer prevention, 280–281
  studies of, in burned patients, 184–186
Circulatory system, post-burn management and, 218
Clindamycin, for burn wounds, 302
Clonazepam, in psychiatric management, 265
Colloids, nonprotein, for fluid resuscitation, 20
Coma, hyperosmolar hyperglycemic nonketotic, post-burn, 176
Complement activation, in major burns, lung injury and, 32, 33
Conduction, in heat exchange, burn injury and, 17
Conformers, in rehabilitation, 322–325
Congestive heart failure, post-burn, 160
Continuous arteriovenous hemofiltration (CAVH), for renal failure, 252
Convection, in heat exchange, burn injury and, 17
Cooling, of thermal burns, 3
Cricothyroidotomy, emergency, for endotracheal intubation, 56
Crystalloid solutions, for fluid resuscitation, 20
Curling's ulcer, post-burn, 166–170

Débridement, analgesia for, deficiencies of, 201
  of electrical injuries, 77–79
Delirium, burn, 260–261
Dermal burn, deep, 13–14
Dextran, for fluid resuscitation, 20, 21
Dialysis, for renal failure, 252–253
Diazepam, in psychiatric management, 265
  studies of, in burned patients, 187
Discharge, planning and teaching for, 330–331
  preparing for, social worker and, 311–313
Disinfection, in infection prevention, 280
Diuretics, renal function and, 249
Dopamine, studies of, in burned patients, 191–192
Dressing changes, analgesia for, deficiencies of, 201
Dynamic splinting, in rehabilitation, 322

Edema, glottic, in inhalation injury, 28
  in major burn, 15
  upper airway, 46–47
Elastomer, and prosthetic foam T-shirts in rehabilitation, 323–324
Electrical injury(ies), acute, 66–84
  amputations in, 80–81
  clinical management of, 73–76
  gastrointestinal, 72
  neurological, 71–72
  ophthalmological, 73
  pulmonary, 73

Electrical injury(ies) (Continued)
  reconstructive surgery in, 81–83, 84
  types of damage from, 74
  vascular, 73
  wound care in, 76–80
  anesthetic management of, 219–220
  cardiac, 71
  emergency treatment of, 2–3
  pathophysiology of, 67–70
  renal, 71
  tissue effects of, 70–73
Electricity, physics of, 67–68
Electrolyte imbalances, post-burn, 175–176
Emergency treatment, of burns, 1–4
  chemical, 1, 19
  electrical, 2–3
  flame, 1–2, 19
Emotional care, 114–115
Endocarditis, bacterial, 292–293
  post-burn, 161, 163
Endogenous modulation, of pain, 203–204
Endogenous toxins, post-burn, renal function and, 250–251
Endotracheal intubation, 49–58
  difficult, 55–56
  emergency cricothyroidotomy for, 56
  equipment for, 50–52
  extubation in, 59–60
  fiberoptic, 55
  guidelines for, 52–53
  oral versus nasal, 54–55
  prolonged, complications of, 56–58
  with retrograde translaryngeal guide wire, 55–56
Endotracheal tube, securing, 53, 54
Energy, requirements in nutritional support for, 142–143
Enflurane, studies of, in burned patients, 190
Enteral nutrition, 153–154
  post-burn, 94
Epinephrine, topical, studies of, in burned patients, 192–193
Erythrocytes, perioperative fluid requirements and, 232–233
Eschar, daily removal of, 92–93
  respiratory movement restriction by, 47
Escharotomy, determining need for, 8
  in electrical injuries, 77
Excision, fascial, techniques for, 124–125
  surgical, of burn wound, 92–93
  tangential, techniques for, 122–124
  techniques for, 122–125
Exercise, in discharge planning and teaching, 331
  in rehabilitation, 325–327
Extubation, 59–60
Eye(s), effects of electrical injuries on, 73
  infections of, 293
  toxic epidermal necrolysis involving, 132

Face masks, of burn-quality Aquaplast in rehabilitation, 324
Family, emotional care of, 114–115
  psychiatric management of, 263–264
  social worker and, 306–319. *See also* Social worker.
Fascial excision, techniques for, 124–125
Fasciotomy, determining need for, 8
  in electrical injuries, 77
Fat, requirements in nutritional support for, 149–150
Fetal death, from electrical injuries, 73
Fiberoptic bronchoscopy, in inhalation injury diagnosis, 48–49
Fiberoptic endotracheal intubation, 55
First aid, for burns, 1–4
  chemical, 1
  electrical, 2–3
  flame, 1–2
First-degree burn, characteristics of, 103
  definition of, 4, 12–13
Fistula, tracheoesophageal, complicating prolonged intubation, 57
Flame burns, emergency treatment of, 1–2, 19
Flaps, in electrical injury closure, 79–80
Fluid(s), perioperative administration of, 235–236
  complications of, 237
  perioperative requirements for, 231–238
    blood loss and, 233–235
    decreasing, 236–237
    fluid administration and, 235–236
    fluid therapy complications and, 237
    for red blood cells, 232–233
    hyperalimentation and, 233
    insensible water loss and, 232
    postoperative considerations and, 237–238
Fluid and electrolyte balance, 111–113
  in toxic epidermal necrolysis, 132–133
  maintenance of, post-burn, 91–92
Fluid resuscitation, calculating requirements for, 6–8
  in electrical injuries, 75
  initiation of, 7–8, 19–20
  nursing interventions for, 101–102
Fluoroquinolones, for burn wounds, 302
Food, in infection prevention, 279–280
Full-thickness burn, characteristics of, 103–104
  definition of, 4–5, 14
Fungal infections, burn wound, 293–294

Gait training, in rehabilitation, 328–329
Gastric decompression, in major burn management, 8
Gastrointestinal tract, complications involving, 166–170
  effects of electrical injuries on, 72

Gastrointestinal tract (*Continued*)
  in assessment of burn patient, 106
Genitourinary tract, in assessment of burn patient, 106
Gentamicin, renal function and, 248–249
  topical, for burn wounds, 298
Glomerulus, function of, between four and seven days, 245
  in acute phase, 242
Glottic edema, in inhalation injury, 28
Gluconeogenesis, post-burn, 93
Grafts, skin, choice of, 125–127
  in electrical injury closure, 79–80
Granulocytopenia, post-burn, 173
Grieving patient, managing, 262–263
Group therapy, for family, 313–314
Guilt, in response to pediatric burn, 308–309

$H_2$–receptor antagonists, studies of, in burned patients, 184–186
Haloperidol, in psychiatric management, 265
  studies of, in burned patients, 187–189
Halothane, studies of, in burned patients, 190, 225
Hand washing, in infection prevention, 278–279
Head burn management, in reconstructive stages, 60–61
Heart, complications involving, 159–162
  effects of electrical injuries on, 71
  monitoring of, in electrical injuries, 75–76
Hematological changes, in major burn, management of, 22
Hematological response, in major burn, 18–19
Hemochromogens, urinary, in electrical injuries, 75
Hemodialysis, for renal failure, 252
Hemodynamic changes, post-burn, 90–92
Hemofiltration, continuous arteriovenous, for renal failure, 252
Hemoglobinuria, post-burn, 162–163
  renal function and, 250
Hetastarch, for fluid resuscitation, 20, 21
High-efficiency particle arresting (HEPA) filters, in infection prevention, 274
Hormones, counterregulatory, release of, post-burn, 139–140
Housing, near burn center, 315
Humidity, room, in infection prevention, 275–276
Hydrotherapy, infection potential and, 277–278
Hyperalimentation, perioperative fluid requirements and, 233
Hyperbilirubinemia, post-burn, 165
Hypercoagulable state, in major burn, 19
Hyperglycemia, post-burn, 93
Hyperkalemia, post-burn, 175
Hypermetabolism, post-burn, 93, 140
  pharmacologic effects of, 181

Hyperosmolar hyperglycemic nonketotic coma (HHNKC), post-burn, 176
Hypertension, in children, post-burn, 174
Hyperthermia, in major burn, 17
Hypertonic salt solutions, for fluid resuscitation, 20
Hypertrophic scar, pressure therapy for, 329–330
Hypnosis, in pain management, 205, 261–262
Hypocalcemia, post-burn, 175–176
    anesthetic management and, 227
Hyponatremia, post-burn, 175
Hypophosphatemia, post-burn, 176
Hypoproteinemia, in major burns, lung injury and, 32–33
Hypothermia, in major burn, 17
Hypovolemia, in fluid resuscitation, signs of, 102
  in major burn, 15
  post-burn, 159
    anesthetic management and, 218
    pharmacologic effects of, 180–181
Hypoxia, management of, for intubation, 52

Ileus, paralytic, post-burn, 170
Infection(s), burn wound, 288–302
    bacterial, 290–293
    etiology of, 288–290
    fungal, 293–294
    microbiology of, 288–290
    organ dysfunction and, 87–88
    prevention of, 273–284
        antibiotic prophylaxis in, 283–284
        bedding in, 279
        disinfection in, 280
        food in, 279–280
        humidity in, 275–276
        lighting in, 276
        nursing in, 278–279
        temperature of room in, 275–276
        treatment space in, 276
        ventilation systems in, 273–275
        wet and moist environment of burn unit and, 276–278
    risk factors for, 288–289
    subeschar antibiotic therapy for, 298–299
    systemic antibiotics for, 299–302
    topical antimicrobial therapy for, 294–298
    viral, 294
  in nursing care plan, 108–109
Inflammation, of burn tissue, organ dysfunction and, 87–88
Inhalation anesthetics, studies of, in burned patients, 190–191
Inhalation injury, acute, 31–32
  assessment of, 5–6
  delayed, 32–34

Inhalation injury (Continued)
  early, 6–31
  late complications of, 34–35
  pathophysiology of, 88–89
Injury, burn. See Burn injury.
Innominate artery, perforation of, complicating prolonged intubation, 58
Integumentary assessment, of burn patient, 102–104
Intensive care nursing, of burned patient, 97–117
  approach to, 107
  initial assessment in, 97–107
    cardiovascular, 101–102
    gastrointestinal, 106
    genitourinary, 106
    integumentary, 102–104
    respiratory, 100–101
    thermostability in, 104–106
  operative nursing concerns and interventions in, 115–117
  planning in, 107–115
Intensive care unit, major burn management in, 87–95
Intravenous anesthetics, studies of, in burned patients, 189–190
Intubation, endotracheal. See Endotracheal intubation.
  indications for, 38–39, 101
  pneumonia potential from, 281–283
Isotonic salt solutions, for fluid resuscitation, 20

Ketamine, in pain management, 205–206
  studies of, in burned patients, 189–190
Kidney(s), changes in, pharmacologic effects of, 183
  effects of electrical injuries on, 71
  failure of, acute, 246–248
    caloric and L-amino acid supplementation for, 252
    dialysis for, 252–253
    prophylaxis for, 251–252
    sepsis and, 251
    treatment of, 251–253
  function of, 239–253
    after seven days, 246
    between four and seven days, 245–246
    effects of endogenous therapy on, 250–251
    effects of therapy on, 248–250
    hypovolemia and, 239
    in acute phase, 241–245
  post-burn management and, 219
  ultrafiltration for, 252–253
Klonopin, in psychiatric management, 265

Lactated Ringer's solution, for fluid resuscitation, 20

Laminar air flow, in infection prevention, 274
Laryngoscopy, for intubation, 53
Larynx, structures of, erosion of, complicating prolonged intubation, 57
Leukocytosis, in major burn, 19
Leukopenia, post-burn, 173
Librium, studies of, in burned patients, 187
Lighting, in infection prevention, 276
Lithium carbonate, in psychiatric management, 265
Liver, changes in, pharmacologic effects of, 182–183
   complications involving, 163–166
Lorazepam, in psychiatric management, 265
   studies of, in burned patients, 187, *188*
Lung(s). *See also* Pulmonary *entries.*
   changes in, pharmacologic effects of, 183
   disorders of, 25–42
      acute, 31–32
      clinical examination for, 35–36
      delayed, 32–34
      early, 26–31
      laboratory tests for, 36–38
      late, 34–35
      patient assessment in, 35–38
      prognosis for, 41
      treatment of, 38–41
   dysfunction of, post-burn, 88–90
   effects of electrical injuries on, 73
   infections of, bacterial, 291–292
   major burn and, 17–18
   supporting, in acute phase, 21
   toxic epidermal necrolysis involving, 132

Mafenide acetate, for burn wounds, 294–295, 297–298
Major burn(s), immediate care of, 5–8
   airway management in, 5
   burn size calculation in, 6–8
   escharotomy need determination in, 8
   fasciotomy need determination in, 8
   fluid resuscitation in, 6–8
   inhalation injury assessment in, 5–6
   secondary priorities in, 8
   management of, in intensive care unit, 87–95
      burn tissue changes and, 87–88
      hypermetabolism in, 93
      nutrition in, 94
      pulmonary dysfunction and, 88–90
      systemic hemodynamic changes and, 90–92
      wound management in, 92–93
Mechanical ventilation, for post-burn pulmonary dysfunction, 90
   in acute phase, 21
   pain management and, 209–213
   with PEEP, 39
Meperidine, in pain management, 207–208

Meperidine *(Continued)*
   in psychiatric management, 264–265
Metabolic acidosis, in major burn, 18
Metabolic changes, in major burn, 18
   management of, 22
Metabolic rate, altered, nutritional support and, 143–144
Metabolic response, to injury, 138–141
   ebb phase in, 138–140
   flow phase in, 140–141
Methoxyflurane, in pain management, 205–206
Metocurine, studies of, in burned patients, 195
Metronidazole, for burn wounds, 302
Micronutrients, requirements in nutritional support for, 150, *151*
Middle ear, infections of, bacterial, 293
Minor burns, immediate care of, 9–11
Minute ventilation, maintenance of, in post-burn pulmonary dysfunction, 89–90
Morphine, in pain management, 207–208
   for mechanically ventilated patients, 209–213
   in psychiatric management, 264–265
   studies of, in burned patients, 189, 190–191
Multiple organ failure (MOF), post-burn, 166
Muscle(s), complications involving, 176–177
   relaxation of, for intubation, 52–53
Myocardial depressant factor (MDF) activity, post-burn, 160
Myoglobinuria, post-burn, renal function and, 250

Naloxone, for respiratory depression from narcotics, 208
Narcotics, in pain management, 206–214
   for mechanically ventilated patients, 209–213
   side effects of, 208–209
   studies in burned patients on, 189
Nasal arches, erosion of, complicating prolonged intubation, 56–57
Nasal endotracheal intubation, versus oral endotracheal intubation, 54–55
Nasal septum, erosion of, complicating prolonged intubation, 56–57
Nasogastric suction, for intubation, 53
Nasotracheal intubation, bacterial infections and, 293
   prolonged, versus tracheotomy, 58–59
Neck burn management, in reconstructive stages, 60–61
Necrolysis, toxic epidermal, 128–137. *See also* Toxic epidermal necrolysis (TEN).
Nephropathy, pigment, 250–251
Nerves, peripheral, effects of electrical injuries on, 72
Nervous system, effects of electrical injuries on, 71–72

Neuromuscular relaxants, studies of, in burned patients, 193–196, 225
Nitrofurazone, topical, for burn wounds, 298
Nitrogen balance, in nutritional assessment, 154–156
Nitrous oxide, in pain management, 205–206
Nonprotein colloids, for fluid resuscitation, 20
Nonsteroidal anti-inflammatory drugs, renal function and, 249
Norfloxacin, for burn wounds, 302
Nursing practices, in infection prevention, 278–279
Nutrition, enteral, 153–154
    in nursing care plan, 113–114
    parenteral, 152–153
    post-burn, 94
Nutritional support, 138–156
    assessment for, 154–156
    enteral nutrition for, 153–154
    future directions in, 156
    metabolic response to injury and, 138–141
    parenteral nutrition for, 152–153
    requirements for, 141–151
        altered metabolic rate and, 143–144
        for carbohydrates, 144, 146
        for energy, 142–143
        for fat, 149–150
        for micronutrients, 150, 151
        for protein, 146–149

Operating room, treatment in, rehabilitative, 327
Operative nursing concerns and interventions, 115–117
Ophthalmological damage, from electrical injuries, 73
Oral endotracheal intubation, versus nasal endotracheal intubation, 54–55
Oral mucosa, toxic epidermal necrolysis involving, 132
Oxygen therapy, 38, 100

Pain, 201–214
    endogenous modulation of, 203–204
    management of, 204–214
        anesthetic agents in, 205–206
        hypnosis in, 205, 261–262
        narcotic agents in, 206–214
    problems associated with, 201–203
Pancreatitis, post-burn, 172
Pancuronium, studies of, in burned patients, 195
Panse's syndrome, from electrical injuries, 71–72
Paralysis, spinal atrophic, from electrical injuries, 71–72

Paralytic ileus, post-burn, 170
Parenteral nutrition, 152–153
Partial-thickness burns, characteristics of, 103
Penicillins, renal function and, 249
    systemic, for burn therapy, 300–301
Percocet, in pain management, 206–207
Peripheral nerves, effects of electrical injuries on, 72
Peritoneal dialysis, for renal failure, 252
Pharmacology, 180–197. *See also specific drug.*
    cardiovascular changes affecting, 180–181
    hepatic changes affecting, 182–183
    pathophysiological changes affecting, 180–183
    protein-binding changes affecting, 181–182
    pulmonary changes affecting, 183
    renal changes affecting, 183
    studies in burned patients and, 183–196
Pharynx, structures of, erosion of, complicating prolonged intubation, 57
Phosphorus imbalance, post-burn, 176
*Phycomycetes* infections, burn wound, 293
Pigment nephropathy, 250–251
Plasma loss, in major burn, 16
Pneumonia, complicating major burn, 34–35, 89
    intubation and, 281–283
Positioning, in rehabilitation, 320–321
Positive end-expiratory pressure (PEEP), mechanical ventilation with, 39
Postoperative considerations, in fluid therapy, 237–238
Post-traumatic stress disorders (PTSD), 259–260
Potassium imbalance, post-burn, 175
Povidone-iodine, topical, for burn wounds, 298
Preoperative medications, 222
Pressure therapy, in rehabilitation, 329–330
Promethazine, in psychiatric management, 265
Protein(s), excretion of, tubular function and, in acute phase, 242–243
    requirements in nutritional support for, 146–149
Protein solutions, for fluid resuscitation, 20
Protein-binding, pharmacologic effects of, 181–182
Proteinuria, between four and seven days, 245–246
Psychiatric management, 256–269
    coping strength assessment in, 256–257
    for dying patient and family, 257–258
    of family, 263–264
    of staff stress/burnout, 267–268
    outcome studies on, 266–267
    psychobiological responses to acute burns in, 258–263. *See also* Psychobiological responses to acute burns.
    psychopharmacological, 264–266
    risk factor assessment in, 256–257

Psychobiological responses to acute burns, 258–263
  burn delirium as, 260–261
  grief as, 262–263
  pain management and, 261–262
  post-traumatic stress disorders as, 259–260
Psychopharmacological agents, studies of, in burned patients, 187–189
Psychopharmacological management, 264–266
Pulmonary. *See also* Lung(s).
Pulmonary edema, smoke-induced, 32
  experimental data on, 29–31
Pulmonary embolism, complicating major burn, 35
Pulmonary function tests, in patient assessment, 37
Pulmonary toilet, for post-burn pulmonary dysfunction, 90

Radiation, in heat exchange, burn injury and, 17
Radiographs, chest, in patient assessment, 37
Ranitidine, studies of, in burned patients, 186
Reconstructive surgery, in electrical injuries, 81–83, *84*
  social worker and, 318
Red blood cells, perioperative fluid requirements and, 232–233
Re-entry after burn, 315–316
Reflex sympathetic dystrophy, from electrical injuries, 72
Rehabilitation of burn patient, 320–331
  activities of daily living in, 327–328
  ambulation in, 328–329
  discharge planning and teaching in, 330–331
  exercise in, 325–327
  positioning in, 320–321
  pressure therapy in, 329–330
  splinting in, 321–325
  treatment in operating room in, 327
Renal tubules, function of, between four and seven days, 245–246
  in acute phase, 242–245
Respiratory assessment, of burn patient, 100–101
Respiratory injury, 109–111
Respiratory therapy, for intubated patient, 53
Ringer's solution, lactated, for fluid resuscitation, 20
Rule of nines, 7, 14–15

Salt solutions, isotonic and hypertonic, for fluid resuscitation, 20
Scar, hypertrophic, pressure therapy for, 329–330
Second-degree burn, characteristics of, 103

Second-degree burn *(Continued)*
  deep dermal, 13–14
  definition of, 4, 13–14
  superficial, 13
Sedation, for intubation, 52
Sedatives, studies of, in burned patients, 186–189
Sepsis, invasive, in electrical injuries, 76
  renal failure and, 251
Shock, burn, 101
Silver nitrate, for burn wounds, 296, 297, 298
  renal function and, 249–250
Silver sulfadiazine, for burn wounds, 296–298
Sinusitis, complicating prolonged intubation, 57
  nasotracheal intubation and, 293
Skeletal complications, 176–177
Skin, anatomy of, 12, *13*
  care for, in discharge planning and teaching, 330
  function of, 12
  in assessment of burn patient, 102–104
Skin grafts, choice of, 125–127
  in electrical injury closure, 79–80
Smoke toxicity, 5, 27–29
Social worker, and family, 306–319
  burn prevention and, 318–319
  group therapy and, 313–314
  housing and, 315
  in adult care, 316–317
  in final phase, 311–313
  in first phase, 307–309
  in middle phase, 309–311
  on admission, 307
  reconstructive surgery and, 318
  re-entry and, 315–316
Sodium, excretion of, post-burn, between four and seven days, 246
  fractional, 239, *241*
  imbalance of, post-burn, 175
  tubular handling of, in acute phase, 243
Soft foam conformers, in rehabilitation, 323
Spinal atrophic paralysis, from electrical injuries, 71–72
Spinal cord, effects of electrical injuries on, 71–72
Spirometry, in upper airway injury assessment, 48
Splinting, in rehabilitation, 321–325
Splints, in discharge planning and teaching, 331
Staff, stress and burnout of, 267–268
Static splinting, in rehabilitation, 321–322
Steroids, controversy over, 40
  for toxic epidermal necrolysis, 133
Stress, staff, managing, 267–268
Stress response, in major burn, 18
Stress ulcer, post-burn, 166–170
  prevention of, antacids and cimetidine in, 280–281

Subeschar antibiotic therapy, for burn wounds, 298–299
Substrate metabolism, post-burn, 140–141
Succinylcholine, studies of, in burned patients, 193–195
Sufentanil, studies of, in burned patients, 189
Sulfamylon, for burn wounds, 294–295
  renal function and, 249
Superior mesenteric artery syndrome (SMAS), post-burn, 170–171
Suppurative thrombophlebitis, 292
Surgical approach, acute, excision and grafting techniques in, 122–125
  patient selection for, 118–121
  rationale for, 118–127
  skin graft selection for, 125–127
Surgical excision, of burn wound, 92–93
Swan-Ganz catheterization, 39
Systemic antibiotics, for burn therapy, 299–302

Tangential excision, techniques for, 122–124
Tegretol, in psychiatric management, 265
Temperature, change in, major burn and, 16–17
  regulation of, post-burn, anesthetic management and, 226–227
  room, in infection prevention, 275–276
Thermostability, in assessment of burn patient, 104–106
Third-degree burn, characteristics of, 103–104
  definition of, 4–5, 14
Thrombophlebitis, suppurative, 292
Tobramycin, topical, for burn wounds, 298
Tolerance, to narcotics, 208–209
Toxic epidermal necrolysis (TEN), 128–137
  etiology of, 129–131
  management of, 133–136
    approach to, 134–136
    controversy in, 133–134
  pathophysiology of, 131–133
Toxins, endogenous, post-burn, renal function and, 250–251
Tracheoesophageal fistula, complicating prolonged intubation, 57
Tracheostomy, emergency, for endotracheal intubation, 56
Tracheotomy, prolonged, nasotracheal intubation versus, 58–59
Transcutaneous electrical nerve stimulation (TENS), in pain management, 213
Transfusion, blood, for excisional blood loss, 234–235
Translaryngeal guide wire, retrograde, endotracheal intubation with, 55–56

Treatment space design, in infection prevention, 276
Tricyclic antidepressants, in psychiatric management, 265–266
Tube feeding, 153–154
d-Tubocurarine, studies of, in burned patients, 195–196

Ulcer, Curling's, post-burn, 166–170
  stress, prevention of, antacids and cimetidine in, 280–281
Upper airway, injury to, clinical assessment of, 47–49
  management of, 46–62
    anesthetic, 61–62
    endotracheal intubation in, 49–58. See also Endotracheal intubation.
  pathophysiology of, 46–47
  obstruction of, in inhalation injury, 28
Urinary tract infections, bacterial, 293

Valium, studies of, in burned patients, 187
Vancomycin, systemic, for burn wounds, 301
Vascular complications, 176–177
Vascular damage, from electrical injuries, 73
Vascular structures, erosion of, complicating prolonged intubation, 57–58
Vecuronium, studies of, in burned patients, 195
Ventilation, burn unit, in infection prevention, 273–275
  for intubation, 52
  mechanical, for post-burn pulmonary dysfunction, 90
    in acute phase, 21
    pain management and, 209–213
    with PEEP, 39
Viral infections, burn wound, 294

Water, excretion of, between four and seven days, 246
  in burn unit, in infection prevention, 277
  loss of, insensible, perioperative fluid requirement and, 232
  tubular handling of, in acute phase, 243–245
Wound, from electrical injuries, care of, 76–80
  major burn, management of, 92–93
  management of, in acute phase, 22
  skin, treatment of, for toxic epidermal necrolysis, 134

Xenon-133 lung scanning, in patient assessment, 37–38